How COVID-19 Took Over the World

How COVID-19 Took Over the World

Lessons for the Future

Edited by Christine Loh

Hong Kong University Press
The University of Hong Kong
Pok Fu Lam Road
Hong Kong
https://hkupress.hku.hk

© 2023 Hong Kong University Press

ISBN 978-988-8805-65-5 (*Paperback*)

British Library Cataloguing-in-Publication Data
A catalogue record for this book is available from the British Library.

Digitally printed

Contents

Illustrations

Tables

Preface

COVID-19's place in history is assured as the first pandemic to emerge in the twenty-first century. There were earlier threats. In 2003, soon after the start of the twenty-first century, a new infectious disease, a coronavirus known as SARS, was identified in South China and spread to Hong Kong and elsewhere. A decade later, another coronavirus, named MERS, was identified in the Middle East and South Asia. These two epidemics were quite lethal although they were not highly transmissible. A third coronavirus, COVID-19, was first identified in the city of Wuhan and Hubei Province at the end of 2019. COVID-19 turned out to be extremely nimble in human-to-human transmission although much less virulent than SARS and MERS. Its ability to spread, with the help of global air travel, led to the COVID-19 pandemic.

In 2003, I was the chief executive officer of the non-profit think tank, Civic Exchange. SARS created a major scare in Hong Kong, as the city's activities ground to a frightening halt after the World Health Organization recommended that people postpone non-essential trips to Hong Kong and Guangdong on 2 April. Our city was portrayed as a 'ghost town' via the international media. Many people from all walks of life wanted to help to lessen local concerns because we all knew we needed to unite to fight SARS and to look to the future. At that time, Civic Exchange helped create Fearbusters, a community campaign to develop short- and longer-term projects related to disease prevention and public hygiene improvement. At Civic Exchange, we followed events closely and, as a think tank, we thought we were best suited to record what was happening and provide analysis. This led to Hong Kong University Press inviting us to put our observations and insights together into a book. I was privileged then to work with a group of authors to produce *At the Epicentre: Hong Kong and the SARS Outbreak*, published by Hong Kong University Press in 2004. The then-publisher, Colin Day, gave us enormous encouragement to put the book together.

As COVID-19 spread around the world in 2020, Hong Kong University Press suggested that I put a book together again. In mid-2020, we did not know how COVID-19 would evolve and how long the pandemic would last. The writing team started to write in the latter part of 2021, as we had a general sense about COVID-19's possible trajectory, and that the pandemic might ease by the end of 2022. Most importantly, we could see which were the issues we could usefully address. I am privileged to act as editor and co-author of this book, working with a diverse and collegial group of scholars and experts. As a team, we decided to use governance, social contract, and trust as a framework to address our various issues—these are explained in Chapter 1, the introduction.

I hope this book adds to the large and growing literature on COVID-19 and that it adds insights and perspectives on a complex subject.

Christine Loh
Hong Kong
December 2022

Acknowledgements

I am grateful to Hong Kong University Press for the opportunity to put this book together. I need to thank the staff at the Press for their guidance and assistance to get the manuscript in order. Most of all, I am grateful to the authors. I owe each one of them an enormous debt of gratitude for their willingness to write and for their conviviality—I know the effort it took. They were also willing to read each other's draft chapters and gave helpful comments. They made my task as editor considerably easier, and they were forgiving of my disorderliness.

I also need to thank three institutions for their support. I am grateful to the Hong Kong University of Science and Technology for giving me the time and flexibility to take on this writing project. Many thanks to colleagues Michael Edesess at the Division of Environment and Sustainability for his contribution, and to Renu Singh, when she was still at the Division of Public Policy for her participation. Over the years, I have worked with many distinguished scholars from the University of Hong Kong. On this project, I am grateful to Ben Cowling at the School of Public Health and Richard Cullen and Hualing Fu at the Faculty of Law for their chapters. I must also thank Christopher Tang, the faculty director of the Center for Global Management in the Anderson School of Management at the University of California at Los Angeles, for his support in contributing a chapter together with ManMohan Sodhi, who is at City University of London. I am grateful to have spent time at the Center for Global Management to teach and learn over the past five years, and to have participated at the events there about COVID-19. This book would not be complete without the contribution of Judith Mackay, a world-renowned expert on public health, who has done so much and for so long to promote public health in Hong Kong and globally. It has been my honour and privilege to work with this writing team.

There are two more people I should mention—Gabriela Gutierrez and Isabel Andreatta—student interns who helped me initially to gather information in 2020. I am grateful for their assistance.

Christine Loh
Hong Kong
December 2022

Abbreviations

CARES	Coronavirus Aid, Relief, and Economic Security Act (USA)
CDC	Centre for Disease Control and Prevention (mainland China)
CDH	commercial determinant of health
CDNDRS	Contagious Disease National Direct Reporting System (mainland China)
CEPI	Coalition for Epidemic Preparedness Innovation
COVAX	COVID-19 Vaccines Global Access
CSR	corporate social responsibility
DHHS	Department of Health and Human Services (USA)
FDA	Food and Drug Administration (USA)
FENSA	WHO Framework of Engagement with Non-State Actors
GAVI	Vaccine Alliance
GDP	Gross Domestic Product
GHSI	Global Health Security Index
HA	Hospital Authority (Hong Kong)
HAEA	Hospital Authority Employees Alliance (Hong Kong)
HKSAR	Hong Kong Special Administrative Region
HoA	homeowners' association (mainland China)
ICU	intensive care units
IFC	International Financial Centre
IHR	International Health Regulations
IMF	International Monetary Fund
IP	Intellectual Property
mRNA	Messenger RNA (ribonucleic acid)
NCD	non-communicable diseases
NGO	non-government organisations

NHC	National Health Commission (mainland China)
OECD	Organisation for Economic Cooperation and Development
PCS	neighbourhood police station (mainland China)
PHEIC	Public Health Emergency of International Concern
PMC	property management company (mainland China)
PPE	personal protective equipment
ProMED	Program for Monitoring Emerging Diseases
RC	Residential Committee (mainland China)
SaH	Stay-at-Home Order
SARS	severe acute respiratory syndrome
SDMs	social distancing measures
SIR	Susceptible-Infected-Removed (SIR) model
SNS	Strategic National Stockpile (USA)
SO	Street Office (mainland China)
SPRP	UN's Strategic Preparedness and Response Plan
STEM	science, technology, engineering, and mathematics
TRIPS	Trade-Related Aspects of Intellectual Property Rights
UNCMT	UN Crisis Management Team
UNDP	United Nations Environment Programme
UNICEF	United Nations International Children's Emergency Fund
UNSDGs	United Nations Sustainable Development Goals 2030
USCDC	United States Center for Disease Control
WHO	World Health Organization
WHO FCTC	WHO Framework Convention on Tobacco Control
WTO	World Trade Organization

Contributors

Benjamin J. Cowling

Benjamin Cowling is currently chair professor of epidemiology and head of the Division of Epidemiology and Biostatistics in the School of Public Health at the University of Hong Kong, and co-director of the WHO Collaborating Centre for Infectious Disease Epidemiology and Control. Originally from the United Kingdom, he moved to Hong Kong in 2004 after the SARS epidemic, to build capacity in Hong Kong for a better response to a future SARS epidemic. He has been conducting scientific research on the epidemiology of respiratory virus infections, with a focus on transmission dynamics and the effectiveness of control measures including vaccination. Since early 2020, he has conducted research on the epidemiology and control of SARS-CoV-2 including highly cited publications in *NEJM*, *Science*, and *Nature Medicine*. He has authored more than 500 peer-reviewed journal publications to date.

Richard Cullen

Richard Cullen is a visiting professor in the Faculty of Law at the University of Hong Kong. He has spent over 25 years based in Hong Kong since he first arrived to teach in the new Law School at the then City Polytechnic of Hong Kong in late 1991. He was a professor at Monash University in Melbourne, Australia until 2006. He has written and co-written over 200 books, articles, notes, and commentaries and he has been a recurrent visiting scholar in Austria, Canada, China, Japan, South Korea, and Switzerland. His 2014 essay, 'Land Revenue and the Chinese Dream', was recognised by the *China Policy Review* as one of the Top 20 Economic Essays of 2014 on China. It was subsequently published in the 2014 *Almanac of China's Economy*, an important annual publication that has been recording the changes in China's national economy since 1981. Richard Cullen co-wrote with Christine Loh *No Third Person: Rewriting the Hong Kong Story* (Abbreviated Press, 2018), which examines the rewriting of the Hong Kong story. He recently wrote *Hong Kong Constitutionalism: The British Legacy and the Chinese Future* (Routledge, 2020).

Michael Edesess

Michael Edesess, PhD, is a mathematician and economist with expertise in the finance, energy, and sustainable development fields. He is an adjunct associate professor in the Division of Environment and Sustainability at the Hong Kong University of Science and Technology and a research associate of the EDHEC-Risk Institute. He is the author or co-author of two books and numerous articles and was a co-founder and chief economist of a financial company that was eventually sold to BNY Mellon. He also chaired the boards of three major non-profit organisations in the fields of energy, environment, and international development.

Hualing Fu

Hualing Fu is the Warren Chan Professor of Human Rights and Responsibilities and dean of the Faculty of Law at the University of Hong Kong. He holds an LLB from the Southwestern University of Politics and Law in China, an MA from the University of Toronto, and a doctor of jurisprudence from Osgoode Hall Law School. His research is in the areas of human rights, public law, and comparative Chinese law. He is a China law editor of the *Hong Kong Law Journal*, an editorial board member of *The China Quarterly*, and co-editor of the Routledge Rule of Law in China and Comparative Perspectives series. He has widely published in local and international journals, including *The China Quarterly*, *The China Journal*, and the *Journal of Contemporary China*.

Christine Loh

Christine Loh, OBE, SBS, JP, is the chief development strategist in the Institute for the Environment at the Hong Kong University of Science and Technology (HKUST), where she also has various research and teaching assignments, and she taught a course on non-market risks for five years in the UCLA Anderson School of Management. She was a former undersecretary for the environment at the HKSAR government and a legislator for nearly a decade. She has edited and co-authored many academic and popular publications, including *At the Epicentre: Hong Kong and the SARS Outbreak* (Hong Kong University Press) in 2004. Apart from her university-related work, she serves on the boards of a number of listed and non-listed organisations in Hong Kong and overseas. She received her LLB from the University of Hull in England and LLM in Chinese and comparative law from the City University of Hong Kong. She was a commodities trader for a US multinational firm and was its regional managing director before embarking on a career in politics. Her wide experience in law, business, politics, and policy makes her a sought-after speaker and presenter on many topics including geopolitics and environmental issues.

Judith Mackay

Judith Mackay OBE, SBS, JP, FRCP (Edin), FRCP (Lon), is the director of Asian Consultancy on Tobacco Control, a senior policy advisor to the World Health

Organization, and special advisor to the Global Centre for Good Governance in Tobacco Control. She is a British medical doctor and has been living in Hong Kong since 1967, where she initially worked as a hospital physician. Since 1984, she has concentrated on public health, especially tobacco control. She has published over 250 papers and addressed 600 conferences on tobacco control. Her particular interests are tobacco and women, tobacco control in low- and middle-income countries, new tobacco products, and challenging the tobacco industry. She is the author or co-author of a dozen health atlases—portraying global health statistics in a colourful, graphic format—on health, sex, tobacco, cardiovascular disease, cancer, oral health, and global adult tobacco surveys. These have been translated into many languages. She is an honorary professor at the School of Public Health, the University of Hong Kong, and at the Chinese University of Hong Kong. She has received honorary degrees from the University of Edinburgh and Shue Yan University in Hong Kong. She is an honorary fellow of the Hong Kong College of Cardiology and the Hong Kong College of Community Medicine. In addition to many international and national awards ranging from the WHO Commemorative Medal and the *TIME* 100 World's Most Influential People Award to the BMJ Group's first Lifetime Achievement Award, she has been identified by the tobacco industry as one of the three most dangerous people in the world.

Renu Singh

Renu Singh is a political scientist in the Department of Social and Political Sciences at Bocconi University and a research fellow at the DONDENA Centre for Research on Social Dynamics and Public Policy. She is also a scholar at the O'Neill Institute for National and Global Health Law at Georgetown, a DAAD research ambassador for the Deutscher Akademischer Austausch Dienst/German Academic Exchange Service, an executive board member of the International Studies Association's Global Health Studies Section, and a faculty affiliate at the Hong Kong University of Science and Technology's Institute for Emerging Market Studies. Previously, she was a research assistant professor in the Division of Public Policy and an Institute for Advanced Study junior fellow at HKUST, a Fulbright fellow at the Hertie School in Berlin, and a DAAD scholar at the Helmholtz Zentrum München and the Max Planck Institute for Social Law and Social Policy in Munich. Her research is motivated by an interest in the relationship between political institutions, public opinion, and policy change in the context of public health policy, science policy, and global health security and governance. Her work has been published in *BMJ Global Health, International Studies Quarterly*, the *Journal of Health Politics, Policy and Law, Cleaner and Responsible Consumption, The Washington Post, Foreign Policy Magazine, The Conversation*, and the *Carnegie Endowment*, among others. She has also provided commentary and political analysis on health policy issues for several organisations, including CNN International, DAAD, Institut Pasteur, the Woodrow Wilson International Centre for Scholars, and the Physicians Association for Nutrition. She has a BA in political science and a BS in microbiology from the University of Massachusetts, Amherst, an MS in public policy and administration from the London School of Economics, and an MA and PhD in government from Georgetown University.

ManMohan S. Sodhi

ManMohan S. Sodhi, FIMA, FORS, is a professor in the Operations and Supply Chain Management group at the Bayes Business School (formerly Cass) of City, University of London. His research centres on risk and sustainability in the supply chain, and he has been recognised as a leading scholar globally based on his publications and citations. He received his PhD in management science from the Anderson School at UCLA in 1994. Subsequently, he taught operations management at the Ross School at the University of Michigan in Ann Arbor, where the Sloan Foundation funded his research on the trucking industry. He did a BTech in mechanical engineering at IIT-Delhi. Before joining Bayes, he was vice president at a software company based in San Jose. Previously, he worked as director for enterprise e-business strategy at Scient and as a manager in the Supply Chain Practice at Accenture. He has worked with clients in various industries, including consumer electronics, commodity and speciality chemicals, petroleum products distribution, hospitality industry procurement, and airlines.

Christopher S. Tang

Christopher Tang is a University Distinguished Professor and the Edward W. Carter Chair of Business Administration at the UCLA Anderson School of Management. Known as a world-renowned thought leader in global supply chain management, he has published 6 books, 30 book chapters, over 100 online blogs, and over 160 research articles in various leading academic journals. He has also written articles for the *Wall Street Journal, Financial Times, Barron's, Fortune, Forbes, Bloomberg Law, China Daily, Los Angeles Times*, and others. He has consulted with numerous global companies including Amazon, HP (California, Singapore, South Korea), IBM (New York, San Jose), Nestlé (USA), GKN (UK), and Accenture. He also taught courses at Stanford University, University of California at Berkeley, Hong Kong University of Science and Technology, National University of Singapore, MIT (Zaragoza), and London Business School. He is the former editor of the *Journal of Manufacturing and Service Operations Management* and has also served on the editorial board for *IIE transactions, Journal of Operations Management, Management Science, Operations Research, Production and Operations Management*, and others. He has been elected as a lifetime fellow by the Institute of Operations and Management Sciences, the Production and Operations Management Society, and the Manufacturing and Service Operations Management Society. He received his BSc (first class honours in mathematics) from King's College London, and his MA (in statistics), MPhil (in administrative science), and PhD (in management science) from Yale University.

1
Introduction

Christine Loh and Judith Mackay

COVID-19 provided a unique opportunity for the world to pull together in fighting a common enemy but it was squandered by bickering and sometimes violent disagreements among people, between people and their governments, and among governments. Moreover, it brought to light and called into question gross inequalities, styles of leadership, the favouring of hospital services while disregarding and undervaluing home-care services, the moral and social positioning favouring health over wealth or vice versa, individualism versus collective responsibility, the disregard of science amid changing public sentiments the unseemly rush to queue up for the not-yet-available vaccine, and the disproportionate economic burden upon the poor. As this book went to press at the end of 2022, COVID-19 still lingered in many parts of the world and was spreading in a major wave in China.

Yet some light of good shone through, with so many examples of people getting it close to right, of humanitarianism, of selfless devotion to duty, of families coming closer, and of the environment taking a breather—skies clearing and birds singing—albeit for a relatively short period.

COVID-19 was the most acute mortality shock since World War II. In 2020, it took the world seven months to record the first million COVID-19 fatalities. Within another five months, another million people died from the disease. Since then, a million people have died from the disease approximately every three months. The global death count reached five million at the end of October 2021. By the end of September 2022, the global confirmed death toll from COVID-19 had pushed pass 6.5 million people. Experts believe the true number of fatalities was probably much higher—an estimated 18 million died as a result of COVID-19 by end-2021.[1] There are at least three reasons for the discrepancy: jurisdictions counted COVID-19 deaths in different ways; there was a lack of testing for COVID-19 in many places; and record keeping, and death registrations were inadequate in some jurisdictions.

---

1. David Adam, 'COVID's True Death Toll: Much Higher Than Official Records', *Nature*, 10 March 2022.

These numbers, while large, cannot convey the many forms of suffering people from all walks of life experienced, starting with the dread of themselves or a family member catching COVID-19. Losing a family member is one of the most traumatic experiences one can have—COVID-19 deaths changed the lives of very many people all over the world. 'Long COVID' continues to affect some survivors of the infection. The sense of fear, loss of control, and helplessness amid lockdowns, massive business closures and lay-offs, and social isolation affected mental health on an incalculably large scale. School closures stunted the education of children all around the world, especially those from low-income households. In late February 2022, cases spiked in places that had previously managed to control the disease, reminding the world that the pandemic was not over after three years. Moreover, COVID-19 exacerbated the suffering of those who were poor and vulnerable, highlighting the depth of socio-economic inequalities around the world. One area of inequality was the availability of vaccines. Vaccines became available in rich economies by early 2021. By the end of May 2022, while nearly 66 per cent of the world population had received at least one dose of a COVID-19 vaccine, representing nearly 12 billion doses, but only 16.2 per cent of people in low-income countries had received at least one dose.[2]

Governance in the Time of Pandemic

Governance is of paramount importance in fighting pandemics. The COVID-19 crisis had enormous social and economic repercussions. It became clear that public governance mattered immensely. Governance arrangements played a critical role in how countries responded, and they remain crucial in the recovery process and in strengthening resilience against future epidemics and pandemics.

Trust in government was probably the single greatest identifiable factor for jurisdictions that performed better. The role of government in promoting confidence through clear, consistent, and compelling communication, as well as public trust in the government's ability to organise society to fight the pandemic, including getting people vaccinated when vaccines became available, was essential to success, which was by no means easy as there were several 'waves' of outbreaks and troublesome variants to deal with. Each jurisdiction evolved its own formula—there was a diversity of global responses to the same disease—that reflected their respective attitudes, basic public health practices, and local systems and cultures. What COVID-19 showed was that controlling an infectious disease was as much a socio-political undertaking as a scientific one, and missteps were costly not only in terms of public health, but also in social, economic, and political terms.

---

2.   Our World in Data, 'Coronavirus (COVID-19) Vaccinations', https://ourworldindata.org/covid-vaccinations.

Global Pandemic Unpreparedness

SARS-CoV-2, a highly transmissible virus of relatively low virulence, was enough to cause enormous global havoc for an extended period of time that had not ended when this book went to press. Had it been more lethal, the world would have been in greater trouble still. The WHO and health experts had warned continuously that governments needed to be prepared for a pandemic because it was just a matter of time before the world would face a highly transmissible and virulent disease. There were many scary forerunners—SARS, Ebola, Zika and MERS were recent epidemics. In 2009–2010, the swine flu, or H1N1, did become a pandemic, and subsequent studies over the years suggested that between 151,700 to 575,400 people globally may have died from it. Together, these recent outbreaks should have highlighted the need for effective national and international preparedness, but they may have contributed to a sense of complacency as the epidemics were controlled, and the H1N1 pandemic was considered manageable.

Dealing with outbreaks

While COVID-19 is not influenza, it has influenza-like transmissibility characteristics. The basics of dealing with influenza-like outbreaks are well-known. Information and good public messaging are crucial, because the authorities and the public need to cooperate to fight contagion. Containment measures to cut transmission consist of ramping up testing and contact tracing to find out where and how the virus is circulating, isolating those infected, and quarantining contacts. Mitigation measures, also referred to as public health and social measures—wearing face masks, social distancing, frequent handwashing, closing schools and businesses, work-from-home rules, and lockdowns—help to slow the spread and require public cooperation. When an infectious disease has ballooned, the ability to increase surge capacity to treat those needing hospital care becomes vital. Those working in healthcare need to be adequately protected from infection, with adequate supplies of protective gear such as gloves, gowns, shoe covers, head covers, masks, respirators, eye protection, face shields, and goggles. The higher the number of infections, even if mild, the greater the need for care, as there will be an increased number of severe cases. Fatalities rise if the hospital system is overwhelmed. Effective pharmaceutical interventions—vaccines and drugs—result in fewer infected people becoming very ill, but they cannot eradicate the pathogen. Before vaccines and drugs are available, containment and mitigation measures are what it takes to deal with the disease. Even with pharmaceuticals, those measures are still needed for various reasons: vulnerable groups (the elderly and those who are immunologically compromised) need protection, the disease may wane and wax again, pharmaceuticals are effective only for a limited period of time, and pharmaceuticals may not be widely distributed and used. COVID-19 tested every jurisdiction on how they managed outbreaks. Moreover, the single-minded effort needed to fight a pandemic means other illnesses have to wait to be treated, and deaths from those illnesses because patients could not access healthcare are part of the overall public health burden.

Understanding COVID-19

Infectious diseases differ greatly. The threats of a new disease are not immediately knowable. SARS-CoV-2, the new coronavirus that became known as the disease COVID-19, was particularly confounding as it had many manifestations. It humbled even renowned experts. It took time for it to reveal itself—its relatively low virulence, high transmissibility, victims of preference, symptomatic and asymptomatic natures, variable incubation periods, lengthy persistence, re-infections, and 'long-haul' impact on many patients were all part of its distinctive character. Animals were not spared. In late 2020, outbreaks of COVID-19 in people in Denmark and the Netherlands were linked to farmed mink, resulting in mass culls. In 2021, pet hamsters in Hong Kong were found to carry the virus.

There was a lot to discover about COVID-19, and more will unfold in time. As SARS-CoV-2 continued to spread, it evolved, which helped it to survive and gave rise to variants that were more or less transmissible and more or less deadly. Just to complicate things further, variants have subvariants, and some were more able to evade vaccines and antiviral drugs. The Omicron variant that emerged in late 2021, for example, has many sub-lineages—BA.1, BA.1.1, BA.2, BA.2.12.1, BA.2.75, BA.2.75.2, BA.3, BA.4, BA.4.6, BA.5, BA.5.1.7, BF.7, XBB, BQ1 and BQ1.1 and there could be new descendants. The Delta variant was more transmissible than the ancestral strain, and the subvariant BA.2 was a further 30 per cent to 60 per cent more transmissible than Delta, albeit less deadly.

While the emergence of variants is not surprising in populations with high levels of immunity from vaccinations and prior infections, the speed at which variants have evolved has surprised some. There is much more about COVID-19's evolution and the implications for protection from vaccination or previous infections that still needs to be discovered. New variants waves could still come and are a reason for caution. COVID-19 may eventually become 'endemic' and cause periodic outbreaks, like the seasonal flu, but when this book went to press, it had yet to become predictably endemic. Moreover, endemicity does not necessarily mean a disease is mild. What drives the evolution of viruses is transmission, and the variants that infect more people will thrive. Vaccinated, asymptomatic individuals can still carry a high viral load and therefore spread the virus. Experts warn that because most COVID-19 transmission happens while people have no or few symptoms, severity is not a driver of evolution, but instead a byproduct of whichever mutations improve transmission and how they interact with existing levels of immunity. For the Alpha and Delta variants that came before Omicron, it led to greater severity, while Omicron had less severity, but this was an evolutionary accident. The next variant could easily be more severe again.

The desire and need to understand COVID-19 were strong. Its emergence led to a torrent of studies and publications. Scientists, mathematicians, clinicians, medical doctors, economists, and other scholars published what they learnt as quickly as possible to help each other understand the many aspects of the virus, as well as to help authorities deal with the disease. The body of work on COVID-19 is very large. The earliest studies were on treating patients in hospitals and mortality in China. Other early studies focused on how SARS-CoV-2 spread in confined spaces and outdoor environments. There were studies using modelling to make predictions that could help control spread. There were also many studies on diagnostics and testing, the effectiveness of various mitigation measures, impacts on mental health and social and ethnic aspects, the impact on the economy, and much more. Scientific research traced the virus's path around the world. Publications from authors in mainland China and Hong Kong peaked first, and as the virus caused havoc in Italy, the number of papers from scientists there increased. One of the first and most cited papers about COVID-19 was the 24 January 2020 publication in *The Lancet* reporting on about 41 people hospitalised in Wuhan. The paper should have warned health authorities around the world that the new coronavirus was going to be challenging and ought not be dismissed as 'just like the flu'.

According to the scientific publication *Nature*, around 4 per cent of the world's research output was devoted to COVID-19 in 2020. London's Royal College of Physicians noted there were 125,000 articles published in the first ten months of the pandemic on COVID-19, of which 30,000 (around 25 per cent) were in online pre-print form that had not yet gone through a formal peer-review process. There was a sharp rise in sharing advanced outputs through pre-prints, as the scientific community felt there was great urgency to understand COVID-19. Experts also created online portals to keep track of data relating to COVID-19 cases and fatalities for each country, apart from the WHO dashboard, the best-known being the Johns Hopkins Coronavirus Resource Center.

One issue that remains unsettled is the origin of SARS-CoV-2. The definitive answer may not be known for a long time, considering that the origin of the 2003 SARS coronavirus has still not been definitively determined, although it is believed to have come from bats, most likely through an intermediate wild animal species such as the civet cat that was sold for human consumption in wet markets in China. The hunt for SARS-CoV-2's origin will continue, as knowledge is important to help head off future diseases. There are competing narratives. It has a close similarity to some bat coronaviruses, and there could have been other intermediate animals before the virus spilled over to humans. The spill-over may have happened in Huanan Seafood Market in Wuhan, which housed all kinds of wildlife. Scientists are continuing to investigate and publish their research. The second hypothesis is that the virus leaked from the Wuhan Institute of Virology, which is one of the few high-biosecurity laboratories in the world that collects and studies bat coronaviruses to identify those that might pose a pandemic threat. The second hypothesis has raised wider questions about how bio-laboratories that work on vaccine research or even bioweapons are managed, not just in China, but elsewhere in the world including the United States. A variation of the second hypothesis is that the virus resulted from laboratory research and experimentation, and it was likely created in the United States with American biotechnology and know-how that had been made available to researchers in China.[3] As both versions of the second hypothesis relate to a laboratory leak, and China had also suggested that the virus could have come from the United States, the origin of COVID-19 has become a part of the wider conflict between the United States and China in their power contest. In other words, the pursuit of science in this case has been unhelpfully mixed with politics. We will have to wait for further research and debate for greater clarity.

Phases of COVID-19

From the initially reported outbreak at the end of 2019 in the city of Wuhan in China to the summer of 2022, the world had to deal with phases of containment and relaxation, with waves of re-infections and the emergence of variants, and with vaccinations and 'living with COVID', each of which proved extremely challenging for decision-makers. The authorities' responses varied in the early months of outbreaks. Despite the severity of the outbreak in China, some acted aggressively right from the start, while others took considerable time to get organised, notably the United States and the United Kingdom. Some jurisdictions did better in the earlier phases of the pandemic—for example, Hong Kong, Taiwan, South Korea, Australia, and New Zealand—but the highly transmissible Omicron variant that emerged in late 2021 resulted in explosions of cases in the first half of 2022 in those previously low-infection jurisdictions, even as cases eased in North America and Europe (although COVID cases started to rise again from the summer of 2022; and by the end of the year, they faced a 'tripledemic' alongside influenza and other respiratory infections). By November 2022, mainland China saw a massive explosion of Omicron. It is doubtful whether any jurisdiction may be said to have gotten every step correct—a sobering thought. There is no place for politicising and moralising public health or pointing fingers at others—there are many lessons for collective learning.

Living with COVID

It is premature to speculate on what 'living with COVID' will entail, as the future path of the epidemic is unknown. Some major historical epidemics, such as the Black Death in the Middle Ages, burnt out within five or so years, but then periodically resurfaced over the next few centuries, killing large numbers of people with each wave. Some epidemics, such as smallpox, were eradicated by vaccines, but primarily because there was

---

3.   Neil L. Harrison and Jeffrey D. Sachs, 'Did US Biotechnology Help to Create COVID 19?', Project Syndicate, 27 May 2022.

no animal reservoir—one reason it is extraordinarily difficult to eradicate rabies, which is endemic in wildlife populations. Polio is on the verge of eradication by vaccination but not gone. Cholera has been eradicated in higher-income regions, but is still a persistent killer in low-income countries lacking adequate sewage treatment and access to clean drinking water. Transmission of HIV/AIDS has been reduced by barrier methods of sexual behaviour, and by ensuring uncontaminated blood transfusions; deaths have been reduced by treatment protocols. Influenza continues to sweep the world annually, and twice each year, vaccine authorities have to make educated guesses as to what the upcoming strains will be and produce a vaccine to target them.

There are different definitions of the transition from the pandemic to the endemic phase, and eliminating the disease is not feasible for any country with open borders.[4] The WHO has yet to declare an end to the 'emergency phase' of COVID-19. In March 2022, the International Health Regulations Emergency Committee on COVID-19, looking at the criteria needed to declare the public health emergency of international concern as terminated, noted that: 'As of now, we are not there yet.'[5] It is unknown where COVID-19 will be in a year's time, never mind in ten or 100 years. It does not bode well for the hope of total eradication that this virus, like the flu virus, rapidly mutates and has been detected in non-human animals. The best hope is that 'living with COVID' will most resemble 'living with the flu' and require only occasional public health interventions during the largest outbreaks.

Potential vs. performance

The Global Health Security Index (GHSI), first published in October 2019, warned the world was poorly prepared for epidemics and pandemics. The GHSI was the result of a partnership among Johns Hopkins Center for Health Security, the Nuclear Threat Initiative, and The Economist Intelligence Unit, and was funded by several philanthropic foundations to create 'a comprehensive assessment of countries' health security and considers the broader context for biological risks within each country, including a country's geopolitical considerations and health system and whether it has tested its capabilities to contain outbreaks'.[6] It uses six categories, 34 indicators, and 85 subindicators, covering prevention, detection and reporting, rapid response, health system robustness (including equipping healthcare workers with personal protective equipment or PPE), compliance with international norms, and risk environment. The GHSI surveyed and assessed 195 countries and ranked them in each of the six categories, and

---

4.   Sarun Charumilind, Matt Craven, Jessica Lamb, Adam Sabow, Shubham Singhal, and Matt Wilson, 'When Will the COVID-19 Pandemic End?', McKinsey, 1 March 2022, https://www.mckinsey.com/industries/healthcare-systems-and-services/our-insights/when-will-the-covid-19-pandemic-end.

5.   Thomas Mulier, Andy Hoffman, and John Lauerman, 'WHO Exploring When and How to Declare End of Covid Emergency', *Bloomberg Asia Edition*, 12 March 2022, https://www.bloomberg.com/news/articles/2022-03-11/who-is-exploring-when-and-how-to-declare-end-of-covid-emergency.

6.   GHS Index 2019, https://www.ghsindex.org/wp-content/uploads/2019/10/2019-Global-Health-Security-Index.pdf.

then gave an overall score to each country before ranking them according to it. The overall picture was highly concerning—'no country is fully prepared', and only 19 per cent of countries scored well on detection and reporting capabilities, whereas fewer than 5 per cent had the ability to rapidly respond and mitigate. The average global score was only 40.2 out of 100; and even for high-income countries, the average score was only 51.9.[7]

The GHSI 2019 was right that the world was unprepared. In the GHSI 2021 report, the global preparedness average score fell from 40.2 out of 100 in 2019 to 38.9, in the light of COVID-19. What was confusing about the GHSI was that the rankings did not reflect what happened on the ground. The United States had the best overall score among all the countries in 2019 with 83.5, followed by the United Kingdom with 77.9. The surprise was the strengths of the United States and the United Kingdom proved superficial when put to the test by the pandemic. They both had extremely high infections and fatalities. The GHSI 2021 report acknowledged their performance was poor. Nevertheless, it continued to rank the United States at the top position, while the United Kingdom dropped to seventh place. New Zealand's rank improved from 39th in 2019 to 13th in 2021 due to its quick decision to close its border in 2020. However, cases skyrocketed in February 2022 after the rankings were published. Likewise, South Korea, which did well to control COVID-19 in 2020, also saw record cases in early 2022. The same thing happened in Hong Kong, an autonomous sub-national part of China that was not covered by the GHSI. China is an outlier among countries in terms of how it mobilised resources to fight the outbreak domestically. It seems the GHSI categorisation system cannot account for China's efforts, which were very different but succeeded in keeping cases and fatalities relatively low.

The GHSI 2021 report explained its ranking system as follows:

> Even as many countries proved they could ramp up new capacities during the emergency—including setting up labs and creating cohorts of contact tracers to follow the spread of COVID-19—some responses were crippled by long-unaddressed weaknesses, such as lack of healthcare surge capacity and critical medical supplies. *Some countries found that even a foundation for preparedness did not necessarily translate into successfully protecting against the consequences of the disease because they failed to also adequately address high levels of public distrust in government and other political risk factors that hindered their response. Further, some countries had the capacity to minimize the spread of disease, but political leaders opted not to use it, choosing short-term political expediency or populism* over quickly and decisively moving to head off virus transmission.

Those factors do not excuse but may explain why countries that received some of the top marks in the 2019 GHS Index responded poorly during the COVID-19 pandemic. As a measure of health security, *the Index assigns the highest scores to countries with the most extensive capacities to prevent and respond to epidemics and pandemics.* With its vast wealth and scientific capacities, the United States was ranked first in the 2019 GHS Index and again in the 2021 edition, although in both cases, the highest position

---

7.   Ibid.

Table 1.1: GSHI rankings and scores in 2019 and 2021 (selected countries)

Country	2019 Overall GHSI Rank and Score	2021 Overall GHSI Rank and Score
United States	1 (83.5/100)	1 (75.9/100)
United Kingdom	2 (77.9/100)	7 (67.2/100)
Australia	4 (75.5/100)	2 (71.1/100)
Canada	5 (75.3/100)	4 (69/8/100)
Thailand	6 (73.2/100)	5 (68.2/100)
Sweden	7 (72.1/100)	10 (64/9/100)
South Korea	9 (70.2/100)	9 (65.4/100)
France	11 (68.2/100)	14 (61.9/100)
Germany	14 (66.0/100)	8 (65.5/100)
Japan	21 (59.8/100)	18 (60.5/100)
Singapore	24 (58.7/100)	24 (57.4/100)
Italy	31 (56.2/100)	41 (51.9/100)
New Zealand	35 (54.0/100)	13 (62.5/100)
Vietnam	50 (49.1/100)	65 (42.9/100)
China	51 (48.2/100)	52 (47.5/100)

was still measured to have critical weaknesses. Despite its ranking, the United States has reported the greatest number of COVID-19 cases, and its response to the pandemic has generally been viewed as extremely poor. *The result highlights that although the GHS Index can identify preparedness resources and capacities available in a country, it cannot predict whether or how well a country will use them in a crisis.* The GHS Index cannot anticipate, for example, how a country's political leaders will respond to recommendations from science and health experts or whether they will make good use of available tools or effectively coordinate within their government. The Index does, however, provide evidence of the tools that countries have and the risks they need to address to protect their communities. Countries that fail to use those tools or address those risks to thereby enable an effective response should be held accountable.[8]

In other words, the GHSI ranked countries against each other according to their potential capacities—not performance—in preparedness. The discrepancy between potential versus reality arises from a scoring system based on assessing technical infrastructure and universalised templates, which naturally favoured high-income developed economies. Scholars had criticised the GHSI's scoring system as being biased because

---

8.   Italics added for emphasis. GHS Index 2021, https://www.ghsindex.org/wp-content/uploads/2021/12/ 2021_GHSindexFullReport_Final.pdf.

it equates capacity with a country's wealth rather than the quality of decision-making.[9] The response to COVID-19 showed the importance of political and social features, as individual countries drew on their unique capabilities to create their responses when facing a fast-moving public health emergency, with China being a good case study. It may make more sense to change the GHSI to assess changes over time for an individual country rather than ranking them against each other, to avoid misperception between potential and actual performance.

Contagion Politics

The GHSI 2019 report noted that knowing the risk was not enough, and that 'political will is needed to protect people from the consequences of epidemics, to take action to save lives, and to build a safer and more secure world'. The 2021 report, quoted above, reemphasised this point. COVID-19 showed the importance of the political and social features of a jurisdiction, as each had to draw on its capabilities and capacities to respond to the contagion.

Trust in government and society

While the GHSI cannot predict how well a country would do in an epidemic or pandemic because it does not account for the consequences of poor leadership and dysfunctional political environments, other research suggests trust was possibly the most useful predictor of performance. A study published in *The Lancet* pulled together data from 177 countries and territories from January 2020 to September 2021 and found that trust in government and society stood out as the best predictor of how a country performed against the spread of infections.[10] Other factors, such as systems of government, governance styles, availability of universal healthcare, extent of inequality, belief in science, and even the degree of pandemic preparedness did not show a strong linkage to performance. The identification of trust as a key factor goes some way towards explaining why high-income countries such as the United States and the United Kingdom did poorly, as trust in government and among citizens in those jurisdictions were at an all-time low when COVID-19 struck. In other high-income societies, such as the Scandinavian countries, trust in government and among citizens was high, as was also the case with China,[11] Thailand, Vietnam, and Singapore. On the whole, Asia-

---

9. Matthew M. Kavanagh and Renu Singh, 'Democracy, Capacity, and Coercion in Pandemic Response: COVID-19 in Comparative Political Perspective', *Journal of Health Politics Policy and Law* 45, no. 6 (2020): 997–1012.

10. COVID-19 National Preparedness Collaborators, 'Pandemic Preparedness and COVID-19: An Exploratory Analysis of Infection and Fatality Rates, and Contextual Factors Associated with Preparedness in 177 Countries, from Jan 1, 2020, to Sept 30, 2021', *The Lancet* 399, no. 10334 (2022): 1489–14512, https://doi.org/10.1016/S0140-6736(22)00172-6.

11. In China, the trust level in the central authorities is high. Chapter 10 notes trust level among citizens is considered low, however.

Pacific jurisdictions were performing better than Western ones in terms of cases and fatalities as of the time this book went to press. Trust in government and in society appeared to determine people's willingness to follow government guidance and rules in observing mitigation measures, such as masking, social distancing, and vaccination.

The vaccines that became available by early 2021 in developed economies using the new Messenger RMA (mRNA) and viral vector technologies have been shown to be highly effective in preventing severe illness and death. While initially appearing to have lower effectiveness against infection, inactivated vaccines have also proved to confer a high level of protection against severe disease. Nevertheless, sizable numbers of people in jurisdictions where those vaccines were available and free of charge—such as the United States and Hong Kong—chose not to get vaccinated. As COVID-19 vaccines were rolled out, research showed the roles that trust, belief in conspiracy theories, and the spread of misinformation through social media played in impacting vaccine hesitancy.[12] In the United States, where trust was low, the choice to get vaccinated also appeared to be driven by a partisan divide rooted in party politics and political ideology. A key factor for the high fatalities in Hong Kong when the Omicron variant broke through in 2022 was the result of its failure to get the elderly vaccinated (which led to high death rates among them). Moreover, general complacency because the city had been previously successful in containing COVID-19, extremely dense living conditions, and also low trust in government that affected people's decision to get vaccinated were also factors. The experience makes it clear that governments must focus on vulnerable groups as a priority.

The Lancet's findings on trust can be examined alongside surveys from other organisations that carried out periodic trust scoring. Of the countries noted in Table 1.1, eleven were part of the annual 28 countries surveyed by the Edelman Trust Barometer,[13] as shown in Table 1.2. The barometer surveyed how the general population felt about their government, business, media, and NGOs. A score below 50 denotes low trust, a score between 50 and 60 indicates that the population is neutral on trust, and a score above 60 reveals high trust. The results of the OECD 2020 survey on trust in government among its member countries correlated with the Edelman barometer for the Organisation for Economic Co-operation and Development (OECD) countries. It showed that the level of trust in government was high in Sweden (above 70) and New Zealand (above 60), but scores for the United Kingdom, France, Italy, the United States, and Australia were all below 50. Japan was an outlier here, as cases and fatalities were relatively low despite having low trust in government.[14]

---

12. Jeffrey V. Lazarus, Scott C. Ratzan, Adam Palayew, Lawrence O. Gostin, Heidi J. Larson, Kenneth Rabin, Spencer Kimball, and Ayman El-Mohandes 'A Global Survey of Potential Acceptance of a COVID-19 Vaccine', *Nature Medicine* 27 (2021): 225–228; and Will Jennings, Gerry Stoker, Hannah Bunting, Viktor Orri Valgarðsson, Jennifer Gaskell, Daniel Devine, et al., 'Lack of Trust, Conspiracy Beliefs, and Social Media Use Predict COVID-19 Vaccine Hesitancy', *MDPI* 9, no. 593 (2021): 1–14.

13. Edelman is a public relations and marketing consultancy that has conducted trust surveys for 22 years. The 2022 report surveyed more than 36,000 respondents with at least 1,150 respondents per country.

14. OECD, 'Trust in Government', 2022, https://data.oecd.org/gga/trust-in-government.htm.

Table 1.2: Edelman Trust Barometer 2021 and 2022

Country	2021 Trust Level General Population	2022 Trust Level General Population
China	72/100	83/100
Singapore	68/100	66/100
Thailand	61/100	66/100
Australia	59/100	53/100
Canada	56/100	54/100
Germany	53/100	46/100
Italy	52/100	53/100
France	48/100	50/100
United States	48/100	43/100
South Korea	47/100	42/100
United Kingdom	45/100	44/100
Japan	40/100	40/100

Public trust in the media provides yet another lens to look at trust in society. The Reuters Institute Survey of 46 countries in 2021 found that people turned to trusted news organisations to get information during the pandemic, but there was a great diversity in the level of media trust across countries. Not surprisingly, trust was higher in well-known news media versus social media. The level of trust in media among Scandinavian countries was relatively high at 50–65 per cent. France had one of the lowest trust levels among European countries. In Asia, Thailand and Singapore had the highest levels of media trust. Canada's media trust level was 45 per cent, but the United States had the lowest level at 29 per cent among the countries surveyed. China and Italy were not included in that survey.[15]

'Infodemic', Sensationalism, and Conspiracies

The COVID-19 pandemic has been accompanied by an 'infodemic'—an overabundance of information—both online and offline, some accurate and some not, that made it hard for people to find trustworthy sources. While technology and social media played a vital role in keeping people informed, sharing information, and taking collective action, 'misinformation' appeared alongside 'disinformation'. Misinformation applies to incorrect statements often spread unwittingly by people who may believe

---

15. Nic Newman, Richard Fletcher, Anne Schulz, Simge Andı, Craig T. Robertson, and Rasmus Kleis Nielsen, 'Digital News Report 2021', Reuters Institute, https://reutersinstitute.politics.ox.ac.uk/sites/default/files/2021-06/Digital_News_Report_2021_FINAL.pdf.

Table 1.3: Reuters Institute Survey 2021

Country	Media Trust Level (%)
Germany	53
Thailand	50
Singapore	45
Canada	45
Australia	43
Japan	43
United Kingdom	42
South Korea	32
France	30
United States	20

they are true. Disinformation, by contrast, involves deliberate falsehoods spread to manipulate behaviour and public opinion by sowing confusion and division. Both are harmful.

The WHO was explicit about the harm:

> Mis- and disinformation can be harmful to people's physical and mental health; increase stigmatisation; threaten precious health gains; and lead to poor observance of public health measures, thus reducing their effectiveness and endangering countries' ability to stop the pandemic.
>
> Misinformation costs lives. Without the appropriate trust and correct information, diagnostic tests go unused, immunisation campaigns (or campaigns to promote effective vaccines) will not meet their targets, and the virus will continue to thrive.
>
> Furthermore, disinformation is polarising public debate on topics related to COVID-19; amplifying hate speech; heightening the risk of conflict, violence and human rights violations; and threatening long-terms [sic] prospects for advancing democracy, human rights and social cohesion.[16]

Mis- and disinformation can be hard to distinguish, and falsehoods were spread by a whole host of people, including political leaders, media, well-known figures, and even health professionals. For example, a research team at Cornell University analysed 38 million English-language reports on the pandemic in 2020 and found US President Donald Trump (2017–2021), in the context of COVID-19 misinformation, made up

---

16. See World Health Organization, 'Managing the COVID-19 Infodemic: Promoting Healthy Behaviours and Mitigating the Harm from Misinformation and Disinformation', Joint statement by WHO, UN, UNICEF, UNDP, UNESCO, UNAIDS, ITU, UN Global Pulse, and IFRC, 23 September 2020, https://www.who.int/news/item/23-09-2020-managing-the-COVID-19-infodemic-promoting-healthy-behaviours-and-mitigating-the-harm-from-misinformation-and-disinformation.

the largest single component of inaccurate information.[17] It was understandable that people had many questions about the disease, and experts needed time to understand the many manifestations of SARS-CoV-2. The WHO created the Information Network for Epidemics, an online portal, to provide updated information about COVID-19 in April 2020. The WHO and other public health institutions fought an uphill battle against mis- and disinformation in the 'fake news', 'post-truth', and 'alternative facts' era.

Worse, the global media's sensational reporting of COVID-19 sowed doubts, distrust, and division. Scholars have observed that contemporary opinion discourse in global media was often sensationalised and played a not inconsiderable role in stoking outrage, ridicule, mockery, insult, moral indignation, and *ad hominem* attacks on people with different views,[18] which spread like wildfire through social media.

Conspiracy theories proliferated during the pandemic, and their rapid spread through the press and social media among various segments of society all over the world jeopardised the public health response, for example by undermining people's motivation to socially distance and get vaccinated. At the heart of conspiracy theories is distrust. COVID-19 made people feel insecure and not in control, which in turn created the perfect circumstances for conspiracy theories. Scholars observe that most of the conspiracy theories stemmed from existing tensions between groups with different values and views, and as the pandemic continued, conspiracy theories further fuelled and deepened those tensions.[19]

The 'Freedom Convoy' protest provides a good illustration of the problem. In late January 2022, as Omicron was levelling off in Canada and COVID-19 measures were easing, large numbers of lorry drivers and others blocked roads and camped outside Parliament in Ottawa for over three weeks to oppose a vaccine mandate for lorry drivers. They also blocked US border crossings. While the Canadian government was preparing to get tough with protesters, certain segments of the Republican Party and sympathetic media organisations in the United States that were against COVID-19 restrictions threw their weight behind the truckers, describing them as 'heroes' fighting for freedom.[20] The Canadian protests were eventually curtailed when the Emergencies Act was invoked for the first time in Canada's history, allowing police to imprison the generally peaceful protesters and their supporters and freeze their bank accounts. The protests in Canada inspired convoys of vehicles in France, the Netherlands, and New Zealand to protest COVID-19 restrictions in their own countries. American lorry

17. Cornell, Alliance for Science, 'Cornel Study Suggests President Trump Played Leading Role in the COVID Misinformation "Infodemic"', October 2020, https://allianceforscience.cornell.edu/wp-content/uploads/2020/10/Cornell-misinformation-studypresser.pdf.

18. Jeffrey M. Berry and Sarah Sobieraj, *The Outrage Industry: Political Opinion Media and the New Incivility* (New York: Oxford University Press, 2014).

19. Karen M. Douglas, 'COVID-19 Conspiracy Theories', *Group Processes & Intergroup Relations* 24, no. 2 (2021): 270–275, https://doi.org/10.1177/1368430220982068.

20. 'How American Right-Wing Funding for Canadian Trucker Protests Could Sway US Politics', *PBS*, 17 February 2022, https://www.pbs.org/newshour/world/how-american-right-wing-funding-for-canadian-trucker-protests-could-sway-u-s-politics.

drivers and others organised their own ..'People's Convoy' to drive to Washington DC to protest against COVID restrictions and vaccine mandates. Those protests pulled together many strands of distrust and discontent that coalesced into general resistance against COVID-19 measures and the authorities.

Social Contracts

There may be another factor alongside trust that is also important. Similar cultural influences may explain why the East and Southeast Asian jurisdictions did better on the whole than their Western counterparts in dealing with COVID-19, irrespective of their varying levels of trust in their respective governments (Japan and South Korea were found to have low trust by the Edelman Trust Barometer). This phenomenon has been described as a paradox.[21] A useful frame to understand these Asian cultures is through the lens of how they see the 'social contract' between the state and its people. The term 'social contract', a Western coinage, broadly involves an implicit agreement by the people to follow policies and rules set by the government because they are for the greater good of society.[22] East Asian cultures are influenced by Confucian thinking, which has a deep sense of people living together like within a family set-up with each member having separate roles. The sovereign and subjects relate to each other like in a family, each having their respective responsibilities. Laypeople regard political leaders and bureaucrats as parental officials who should care for them, and rulers commit to serving the people as their children (*zimin* 子民). These deep-rooted sentiments continue to also influence relationships within society—everyone has an obligation to others. This is best demonstrated by the willingness of Asians to wear facemasks and increase social distancing as part of collective social behaviour to beat an infectious disease. Therefore, whatever might be the level of trust the Japanese and South Korean public might have in their respective governments, they observed their social obligations within their societies.

Purpose of This Book

It is not possible for this book to cover the many socio-economic and political issues that arose from the COVID-19 pandemic. No one publication could do so, as the impacts were so wide. This book seeks to fill in gaps in the overall deliberation about COVID-19. This book has two segments. The first eight chapters focus on the general good governance conditions needed to manage infectious diseases. Governance impacts preparedness, as well as how efforts are sustained over time. This book starts at the multi-lateral level in discussing the role of the United Nations and its agencies,

---

21. Yves Tiberghien, *The East Asian COVID-19 Paradox* (Cambridge: Cambridge University Press, 2021).

22. The idea of a social contract that binds individuals in a polity was developed during the Enlightenment by Thomas Hobbes (1588–1679) and others who articulated the social contract hypothesis in terms of individuals giving up their liberty to the sovereign on the condition that their lives were safeguarded by sovereign power.

especially the crucial role played by the WHO. Other publications have tended to focus on the response of specific countries, neglecting the multi-lateral efforts that have been so important, especially for low-income countries. Alongside governance at the international level was the opportunistic lobbying by certain industries, especially tobacco, for industry advantage, a topic that has so far not been covered in COVID-19 literature and is addressed in this book. Another important factor that has a governance perspective is vaccines. While there were important scientific and technological breakthroughs in the development of COVID-19 vaccines, questions about the risks and efficacy of the different vaccines played a role in people's unwillingness to get vaccinated. A contribution in this book shows all the vaccines created using different technologies are helpful and there is no reason to refuse any of them should they be available. However, making vaccines widely available around the world remained a challenge at the time this book went to press. An important factor influencing governance and how political leaders of different countries responded to COVID-19 had much to do with the nature of the respective social contracts in different countries. The use of the notion of the social contract as a frame in this book to assess the different COVID-19 responses is an original contribution to the overall deliberation about the pandemic. Governance involves not only how decisions were made about fighting the pandemic but also what to do about the collapsing economy. This first part of the book discusses in lay terms the mathematical concepts and modelling used to help governments think about their public health responses, as well as the decisions governments made to boost their economies. The final chapter of this part of the book includes a discussion about PPE—so important during any infectious disease outbreak—and the governance dimension related to good PPE supply chain management.

The second part of this book has four chapters with a geographical focus on specific countries and regions using the lens of good governance, political trust, and the social contract to compare their responses. The two major powers and largest economies (making up about 45 per cent of global Gross Domestic Product) are China and the United States. Their political, socio-economic, organisational, and cultural systems could not be more different. Their respective responses from the start of the COVID-19 outbreak to the summer of 2022 were also very different. This book provides a comparison of the influencing factors that resulted in these responses. Despite fatigue, grumbles, and protests in late 2022, the case of the Chinese people is unique in COVID literature during the pandemic in their overall response to lockdowns and stringent restrictions, which were influenced by their generally high trust in the central government, political values, and sense of obligation to obey regulations, how neighbourhoods are organised, and the impact of possible deterrence and sense of fairness. A discussion about China would not be complete without an account of the Greater China region, covering Hong Kong, Macao, and Taiwan. Singapore is also mentioned in this part of the book. A discussion about Europe helps to provide a fuller picture of the pandemic response of Western cultures, which had some similarities to that of the United States but were very different from the Asian response.

The authors have diverse expertise that includes public health, epidemiology, health policy, mathematics, economics and finance, business, supply chains, law, government institutions, and politics, which give this book a wide angle of interpretations. All but one of the authors are from Hong Kong or based in Hong Kong, and are also actively engaged internationally on the subjects they wrote about. They understand global conditions, and this perspective comes through in their writing about the pandemic. Chapter 13, the concluding chapter, is a collaboration of all the contributing authors, summarising their observations and recommendations.

Chapter 2 by Judith Mackay discusses the WHO. While the WHO (and many other UN agencies) played a critically important role internationally during the pandemic, there has yet to be a deeper reflection on that role, and in general on how wide the scope of the WHO should be in the future. Should there be an international treaty on pandemics; stronger, more reliable funding with less reliance on private funding; sanctions against countries that fail to comply with a WHO mandate; or more open governance of the WHO itself? This chapter opens up these debates.

Chapter 3 by Judith Mackay deals with the negative influence of commercial determinants of health upon government health policies during COVID-19. Remarkably little has been written about the influence of unhealthy commodity industries, such as Big Tobacco, Big Food, Big Soda, Big Alcohol, and others—all of which contribute to the global burden of non-communicable diseases, which in turn influence COVID-19 outcomes. These industries have taken advantage of COVID-19 to attempt to influence governments, politicians, and the media, and to position themselves as health partners.

Chapter 4 by Benjamin J. Cowling reviews the rapid development and deployment of COVID-19 vaccines and their effectiveness against infection and severe disease. While high-income countries had rapid access to vaccines from early 2021, there was a lack of equitable distribution to lower-income locations. The emergence of variants alongside observations of waning immunity led to the rollout of booster doses. This chapter also explores the future of COVID-19 vaccines and vaccine strategies.

Chapter 5 by Michael Edesess discusses the mathematics related to COVID-19. Understanding the spread of COVID-19 was particularly important in 2020, as experts and governments tried to devise plans to fight the new virus. The power of exponential spread was not always well-understood—many decision-makers acted too slowly—even though the concept is taught at the school level. Shockingly, COVID-19 fatalities decreased life expectancy in many countries. Chapter 5 provides an easy-to-read account of complex mathematical concepts and relates them to experiences readers may remember.

Chapter 6 by Renu Singh explains the theory behind and application of the notion of the 'social contract' to public health and healthcare policy, with a specific focus on COVID-19. Social contract theory centres on the relationship between individuals and society, with the exact definition varying among different regions, based on how they perceive the responsibilities and freedoms of individuals and of government.

Chapter 7 by Michael Edesess and Christine Loh discusses the economic and social consequences of COVID-19. The pandemic exacerbated inequalities around the world, with the most vulnerable bearing the biggest brunt. The authors reflect upon the enormous aid packages provided by the rich governments of the world in 2020 to demobilise economies, and the fact that those massive bailouts essentially enhanced the fortunes of the relatively well-off while doing too little to alleviate the suffering of the poor, while also privatising gains and socialising risks. The authors use the medical phenomenon of 'long COVID' to describe the lasting effects of the pandemic on the global economy as activity resumed in 2022, but they had to contend with rising geopolitical tensions between democracies and autocracies and the war between Russia and Ukraine, which further divide the world into two broad camps of rich and middle- and low-income economies with their very different interests – the latter want peace to pursue development.

Chapter 8 by Christopher S. Tang and ManMohan S. Sodhi discusses how COVID-19 affected the world as a public health crisis. Hospitals and the general public experienced severe shortages of medically necessary item including PPE and ventilators, revealing vulnerabilities in the supply chains of essential products. The authors identified the causes of the shortages and used the United States as the reference country to observe the challenges of managing PPE stockpiles.

Chapter 9 by Christine Loh compares how China and the United States dealt with COVID-19 at a time of increasing geopolitical rivalry. China is where the new coronavirus SARS-CoV-2 was first reported. China developed its own unique method to deal with the disease by calling upon the country's capacities and capabilities to mobilise resources on a massive scale. The chapter explains why China adopted the world's toughest containment and mitigation methods, and held onto them, and contrasts that with how the United States, considered the most advanced economy and considered the best-prepared for a pandemic, reacted to COVID-19. The contrast helps to explain fundamental differences in the governance structure, systems, cultures, and social contracts of the two jurisdictions. Chapter 9 should be read with Chapters 10 and 11 to gain a comprehensive picture of the COVID-19 response from Greater China.

Chapter 10 by Hualing Fu contains a detailed description of the neighbourhood structure and how it is managed in mainland Chinese cities, and the various roles played by local community units in fighting COVID-19. The ability and speed of the Chinese authorities to mobilise resources and manpower to contain outbreaks had much to do with the existence of that structure. China's anti-pandemic measures and 'stay at home' orders were enforced within neighbourhood structures all over the country. This chapter discusses how community mobilisation formed the core of the Chinese containment strategy and was the most crucial aspect of enabling China to contain COVID-19. The success, in turn, helped legitimise the existing social and political system. This localised governance system is in fact a unique public-private partnership under the leadership of the ruling party at the grassroots level, and while the poorly coordinated lockdown in Shanghai in April–May 2022 created widespread public complaints there, stretching local governance to a near breaking point, the neighbourhood structure remained intact while the local authorities worked to mend relations with residents, often through the same neighbourhood organisations.

Chapter 11 by Richard Cullen reviews how Hong Kong has managed its response to COVID-19 and includes some comparative discussion of the other Greater China jurisdictions of mainland China, Macao, and Taiwan, as well as the predominantly Chinese polity of Singapore. Hong Kong succeeded in keeping COVID-19 at bay for two years, with low infections and fatalities. That changed swiftly and dramatically with the Omicron onslaught in February 2022. The Hong Kong government called upon the mainland authorities for assistance, which provided a fascinating glimpse of the interaction between the mainland Chinese and Hong Kong governance systems. This chapter also explains key aspects of the contrast between Hong Kong and Singapore in their handling of COVID-19.

Chapter 12 by Renu Singh unpacks the application of the social contract to public health and healthcare policy in the European context. Europe has a unique relationship between government and citizens, given the fact that most jurisdictions not only have relationships with and expectations of their own local and national governments, but also the European Union (whether or not they are members of the supranational organisation itself). Despite the harmonisation of a number of policies at the European Union level, in the context of COVID-19 and health policy, much of the response involved predominantly national-level decision-making, ranging from some of the most stringent policies administered by Italy in early 2020 to the more laissez-faire policies of the United Kingdom. Chapter 12 explores COVID-19 responses in these three cases – the European Union, Italy, and the United Kingdom – through this framework, discussing why certain policy approaches were adopted as well as the public's reaction to these measures.

Chapter 13, the concluding chapter, is an effort by all the authors to collectively summarise their observations and recommendations.

One of the most remarkable things—perhaps the most remarkable thing—about the COVID-19 experience was the disparity between the assumed and the actual performance of countries in the pandemic. The rich countries with established and expensive health systems were among the worst performers in the number of cases and fatalities, whereas a number of emerging economies did much better. Those who acted quickly and decisively made a difference. The political will to act reflected how the notion of the 'social contract' was understood in different countries and cultures. The ability to act showed the capacity and capability of a jurisdiction to mobilise resources to fight outbreaks. Research showed the degree of public trust in government and within society made a difference too. Those jurisdictions with higher political and/or social trust did better. On the whole, Asia-Pacific jurisdictions did better because of the higher focus on community wellbeing and lesser assertion of individualist preferences. The results show that controlling an infectious disease is at least as much a social undertaking as a scientific, medical, and capital-intensive one.

2

The UN, WHO, and COVID-19

Judith Mackay

The United Nations played an important role in the COVID-19 pandemic in terms of socio-economic and political influence on governance, performance, and trust. The UN played an important global role in fighting the pandemic. At its headquarters in New York, a response strategy was rapidly adopted. Many UN agencies and related multilateral bodies were called into action since the pandemic affected so many aspects of life for people all over the world, especially those in low- and middle-income economies that did not have the means to absorb the shock.

The UN strategy had three components—to provide immediate relief, to help countries restructure, and for countries to be more resilient in their preparedness going forward. First, the World Health Organization (WHO) developed a Strategic Preparedness and Response Plan (SPRP 2019 and updated in 2021) and guided its implementation, playing a large-scale, coordinated, and comprehensive global role. Second, the UN made a wide-ranging effort to address the devastating socio-economic, humanitarian, and human rights impacts of the crisis, with a focus on saving lives and keeping vital services accessible, households afloat, businesses solvent, supply chains functioning, institutions strong, and public services delivered. This included immediate support to the most vulnerable people in the most vulnerable countries, with life-saving assistance through a Global Humanitarian Response Plan. It also included the call for a stimulus package amounting to at least 10 per cent of global Gross Domestic Product (GDP), as well as support for low-income countries, including a debt standstill, debt restructuring, and greater support through international financial institutions. Preventing and responding to the increased levels of violence against women and girls was also critical. Third, it began preparing for the recovery process because emerging from the pandemic was an opportunity to address the climate crisis, inequalities, exclusion, gaps in social protection systems, and the many other fragilities and injustices that the pandemic exposed. Instead of going back to unsustainable systems and approaches, the UN promoted its Sustainable Development Agenda—a 15-year plan to achieve specific goals—as the guide to recovery.

The UN's Massive Efforts

The magnitude of the UN efforts can be shown using a few examples. The UN produced policy briefs on key thematic areas in relation to COVID-19, such as women and gender equality, mental health, human rights, food security, decent work, education, cities, tourism, and universal healthcare coverage.[1] The UN Secretary-General, António Guterres, launched the US$2 billion Global Humanitarian Response Plan for the most vulnerable.[2] In March 2020, he called for a global cease-fire, urging warring parties in all corners of the world to pull back from hostilities to better enable tackling COVID-19.[3] In May 2020, he co-convened with nearly 50 heads of state and government and leaders of the International Monetary Fund (IMF), World Bank, Institute for International Finance, Organisation of Economic Co-operation and Development, special envoys of the UN, the African Union and others a 'High-Level Event on Financing For Development in the Era of COVID-19 And Beyond'. They created six work-streams to address problems related to liquidity, debt, action by private creditors, external finance, ending illicit financial flows, and rebuilding according to the UN 2030 Sustainable Development Goals (UNSDGs), which have 17 components.

Although the role of the WHO was very much in the public eye, other UN organisations and agencies played critical roles too. In fact, all units of the UN, except the very few that relate to weather and warfare were active in fighting COVID-19. Their actions had gone largely unnoticed (especially in high-income countries). These global institutions were active in responding to COVID-19, and they continue to be important in its aftermath. Table 2.1 shows the many UN-related bodies and their roles. The WHO, United Nations Development Programme (UNDP), and the World Bank played major roles, but very few UN agencies did not take specific and targeted actions.[4]

Three additional examples provide a more detailed perspective to illustrate how key UN agencies dealt with COVID-19, which set the stage for their involvement with other epidemics and pandemics that may arise in the future.

United Nations Development Programme

The UNDP is the technical lead in the UN's socio-economic recovery programme and the UN core agency for the UNSDGs.[5] The UNDP was and remains concerned that the severe economic and social consequences of the pandemic, including lockdowns, represented a massive setback for achieving the UNSDGs, especially in the areas of

1. United Nations, 'United Nations Comprehensive Response to COVID-19: Saving Lives, Protecting Societies, Recovering Better', June 2020, https://www.un.org/sites/un2.un.org/files/2020/07/un_comprehensive_response_to_covid-19_june_2020.pdf.
2. United Nations Development Programme (UNDP), 'COVID-19 Pandemic', accessed 13 September 2022, https://www.undp.org/coronavirus.
3. United Nations, 'United Nations Comprehensive Response to COVID-19'.
4. Ibid.
5. UNDP, 'COVID-19 Pandemic'.

Table 2.1: COVID-19 response of UN funds and programmes, specialised agencies, other entities and bodies, and related organisations

Abbreviated Name	Full Name	COVID-19 Responses, Including Working with Member States, to:
Funds and Programmes		
UNDP	UN Development Programme	Lead the UN's socio-economic response to COVID-19 as part of its mission to strengthen governance, eradicate poverty, reduce inequality, and build resilience to crises and shocks [see details below].
UNEP	UN Environment Programme	Educate frontline decision-makers on how to deal with COVID-19 medical waste. Help nations incorporate pandemic waste strategies into crisis preparedness and response.
UNFPA	UN Population Fund	Distribute personal protective equipment for health workers and support health systems where needed.
UNHABITAT	UN Human Settlements Programme	Help governments at city level prepare for, prevent, respond to, and recover from the COVID-19 pandemic.
UNICEF	UN Children's Fund	Advise on/provide health and nutrition, education, child protection, water, sanitation and hygiene, social protection, humanitarian response, and gender. Leader in COVAX facility.
WFP	World Food Programme	Adapt its emergency food response to include COVID19 issues.
Specialised Agencies		
FAO	Food and Agriculture Organization	Assess and respond to COVID-19's potential impact on people's lives and livelihoods, global food trade, markets, food supply chains, and livestock.
ICAO	International Civil Aviation Organization	Develop COVID-19-19 Recovery Platform to collate the forecasts, guidance, tools, and resources for national regulators.
IFAD	International Fund for Agricultural Development	Address immediate impacts and put in place the building blocks to support post-crisis recovery.
ILO	International Labour Organization	Address COVID-19 work issues and promote human-centred recovery.
IMF	International Monetary Fund	Provide financial assistance and debt service relief to member countries facing the economic impact of COVID-19.

Table 2.1 (continued)

Abbreviated Name	Full Name	COVID-19 Responses, Including Working with Member States, to:
IMO	International Maritime Organization	Address significantly impacted shipping industry and seafarers. Urge member states to designate seafarers as key workers, so they can travel between the ships that constitute their workplace, and their countries of residence.
ITU	International Telecommunication Union	Address communication issues for work, school, and families.
UNESCO	UN Educational, Scientific and Cultural Organization	Promote global solidarity through education, for example distance learning, open science, and knowledge.
UNIDO	UN Industrial Development Organization	Launch COVID-19 Industrial Recovery Programme (CIRP), to provide targeted support to national governments for restructuring their post-COVID-19 industrial sectors.
UNWTO	UN World Tourism Organization	Develop the UNWTO COVID-19 dashboard, the first comprehensive tourism recovery tracker worldwide, on country measures to support travel and tourism, restart tourism, and accelerate recovery.
UPU	Universal Postal Union	Monitor disruptions to the global postal supply chain and seek to identify possible ways to mitigate its impact—particularly with regard to the widespread restrictions and cancellations of passenger flights.
WHO	World Health Organization	Lead health agency on COVID-19. COVAX partner (see details below).
WIPO	World Intellectual Property Organization	Launch support measures to help leverage IP, creativity, innovation, and entrepreneurship to build back better post-pandemic through contributing to job creation, investment, enterprise growth, and socio-economic development.
WMO	World Meteorological Organization	
WB	World Bank	Help low and middle-income countries strengthen their pandemic response, increase disease surveillance, improve public health interventions, and help the private sector continue to operate and sustain jobs (see below).

Table 2.1 (continued)

Abbreviated Name	Full Name	COVID-19 Responses, Including Working with Member States, to:
Other Entities and Bodies		
UNAIDS	UN AIDS	As with HIV/AIDS, encourage governments to respect the human rights and dignity of people affected by COVID-19, e.g., equitable access to medicines, vaccines, and health technologies.
UNHCR	UN High Commissioner for Refugees	Provide a comprehensive protection and assistance response to people forced to flee who are disproportionately affected by COVID-19. Advocate for their inclusion in vaccination plans and work to address their growing needs in education, mental health and psychosocial support, child protection, and prevention and response to sexual and gender-based violence.
UNIDIR	UN Institute for Disarmament Research	
UNITAR	UN Institute for Training and Research	Assist in adult e-learning.
UNOPS	UN Office for Project Services	Fund country COVID-19 response projects, providing infrastructure, procurement, and project management services.
UNRWA	UN Relief and Works Agencies (for Palestinian refugees)	Raise funding to mitigate the worst impacts of the pandemic on registered Palestine refugees in the Middle East, with a special focus on health, cash assistance, and education.
UNSSC	UN System Staff College	
UNU	UN University	
UN Women	UN Women	Address gender-based COVID-19 violence: prevention and awareness-raising, support for rapid assessments, access to essential services, including helplines and shelters, addressing violence against women in public spaces, and support women's groups.
Related Organisations		
CTBTO	Preparatory Commission for the Comprehensive Nuclear Test Ban	

Table 2.1 (continued)

Abbreviated Name	Full Name	COVID-19 Responses, Including Working with Member States, to:
IAEA	International Atomic Energy Agency	Provide detection equipment, reagents and laboratory consumables, and biosafety supplies such as personal protection equipment and laboratory cabinets for the safe handling and analysis of COVID-19 samples.
IOM	International Organization for Migration	Track and protect migrants and host communities during COVID-19.
OPCW	Organisation for the Prohibition of Chemical Weapons	
UNFCCC	UN Climate Change	
WTO	World Trade Organization	Deal with IP rights regarding COVID-19 vaccines. Publishes WTO-IMF Vaccine Trade Tracker (see details below).
ITC	International Trade Centre	
Office of UN		
UNODC[i]	UN Office on Drugs and Crime	Address new waves of crime that exploit COVID-19, such as counterfeit medical products, fraud, and cyber-crime.

Source:
i. Organization of the United Nations Office on Drugs and Crime, 'Secretary-General's Bulletin', 15 March 2004, https://undocs.org/ST/SGB/2004/6.

poverty, decent work, education and health, and particularly areas affecting the poor and vulnerable, including women, daily wage labourers, informal sector workers, and migrant workers.[6] Every day, people lost jobs and income, with no way of knowing when normality would return.[7] Small island nations, heavily dependent on tourism, had empty hotels and deserted beaches. COVID-19 impacted travel for more than two years, which could potentially leave deep and longstanding economic scars.

The UNDP was able to draw upon its long experience with other epidemics— Ebola, HIV/AIDS, SARS, tuberculosis, and malaria.[8] In close coordination with the WHO, it responded to large numbers of requests from countries to help them prepare for, respond to, and recover from the COVID-19 pandemic, focusing particularly on the most vulnerable.[9] The immediate work of the UNDP was to help countries respond to the pandemic.[10] The next phase was to help decision-makers look beyond recovery towards 2030 and make better choices and manage complexity and uncertainty in four main areas: governance, social protection, green economy, and digital disruption.[11]

The Global Dashboard for COVID-19 Vaccine Equity, a joint initiative of the UNDP, the WHO, and the University of Oxford, found that inequality is a risk to economic recovery and that low-income countries would add US$38 billion to their 2021 GDP forecast if they had the same vaccination rates as rich countries.[12]

The World Bank

The World Bank mounted the largest crisis response in its history to help low- and middle-income countries strengthen their pandemic responses throughout the three stages of relief, restructuring, and resilient recovery. The World Bank was concerned with the steep increase in debt caused by COVID-19, especially in low- and middle-income countries. It projected that 800 million people would be unable to meet their basic needs. It estimated that 97 million people were pushed into poverty in 2020, an unprecedented increase. The International Labour Organization estimated that 205 million people would be unemployed in 2022, up from 186 million in 2019.[13] Globally, labour market recovery from the pandemic stalled during 2021.[14] Working hours in high- and upper-middle-income countries tended to recover in 2021, while both

---

6. UNDP, 'Responding to the COVID-19 Pandemic: Leaving No Country Behind', 23 March 2021, https://www.undp.org/publications/responding-COVID-19-pandemic-leaving-no-country-behind.
7. UNDP, 'COVID-19 Pandemic'.
8. Ibid.
9. UNDP, 'COVID-19 UNDP's Integrated Response', 15 April 2020, https://www.undp.org/publications/COVID-19-undps-integrated-response.
10. UNDP, 'COVID-19 Pandemic'.
11. Ibid.
12. Ibid.
13. Ibid.
14. International Labour Organization (ILO), 'ILO Monitor: COVID-19 and the World of Work, Eighth Edition Updated Estimates and Analysis', 27 October 2021, https://www.ilo.org/wcmsp5/groups/public/---dgreports/---dcomm/documents/briefingnote/wcms_824092.pdf.

lower-middle- and low-income countries continued to suffer large losses. Large and widening disparities emerged between richer and poorer economies.[15]

The World Bank took broad, fast action to help low- and middle-income countries strengthen their pandemic responses, increase disease surveillance, improve public health interventions, and help the private sector continue to operate and sustain jobs.[16] By early 2022, the World Bank had committed over US$157 billion to fight the health, economic, and social shocks that developing countries were still facing. The financing addressed the health emergency, strengthened health systems, protected the poor and vulnerable, supported businesses, created jobs, and aimed to jump-start a green, resilient, inclusive recovery.[17]

In addition, the World Bank partnered with COVID-19 Vaccines Global Access (COVAX) on a new financing mechanism that let COVAX make advance purchases—beyond the fully subsidised doses they were receiving from donors—to help speed up the vaccine supply.[18] Further funds helped low- and middle-income countries finance the purchase and distribution of COVID-19 vaccines, tests, and treatments for their citizens.

The World Trade Organization

The World Trade Organization (WTO)-IMF Vaccine Trade Tracker provides data on the trade and supply of COVID-19 vaccines by product, economy, and arrangement type, including intellectual property (IP) rights by country.[19] The WTO is the UN agency responsible for dealing with IP rights regarding COVID-19 vaccines.

One problem was that the head of the WTO, charged with bringing order to international trade relations, Director-General Roberto Azevêdo, announced in May 2020 that he would step down on 31 August 2020, cutting his second term short by exactly one year. This added another element of uncertainty to the COVID-19 pandemic.[20] It took some time to appoint a replacement. Dr Ngozi Okonjo-Iweala of Nigeria secured the support of the United States for Director-General of the WTO, and assumed office on 1 March 2021, becoming both the first woman and the first African to hold the position.

15. Ibid.
16. The World Bank, 'World Bank Group's Operational Response to COVID-19 (Coronavirus)—Projects List', 24 September 2021, https://www.worldbank.org/en/about/what-we-do/brief/world-bank-group-operational-response-COVID-19-coronavirus-projects-list.
17. The World Bank, 'How the World Bank Group Is Helping Countries Address COVID-19 (Coronavirus)', 10 January 2022, https://www.worldbank.org/en/news/factsheet/2020/02/11/how-the-world-bank-group-is-helping-countries-with-COVID-19-coronavirus.
18. The World Bank, 'World Bank Group's Operational Response'.
19. World Trade Organization (WTO), 'COVID-19: Measures Regarding Trade-Related Intellectual Property Rights', accessed 7 August 2022, https://www.wto.org/english/tratop_e/covid19_e/trade_related_ip_measure_e.htm.
20. Jack Ewing, 'W.T.O. Chief Quits Suddenly, Adding to Global Turmoil', *New York Times*, 14 May 2020, https://www.nytimes.com/2020/05/14/business/wto-chief-roberto-azevedo.html.

In 2021, India and South Africa submitted a plan to the WTO to allow countries to use existing IP to develop and manufacture vaccines and other medical products during the pandemic. This had the support of more than 100 nations, including China, but a handful of opponents from wealthy nations, including the United States, blocked it. Proponents of the IP waiver say removing barriers around existing vaccine technology would give countries the ability to produce vaccines for themselves or import them from anywhere that they could be made, as opposed to waiting for aid or limited purchase agreements to come through.[21] IP waivers fall under trade talks because the WTO has an agreement requiring countries to adopt and enforce these rules domestically. The WTO meetings to discuss this further in November 2021 were postponed due to COVID-19.[22] At a meeting of the Council for Trade-Related Aspects of Intellectual Property Rights (TRIPS) on 9–10 March 2022, members agreed to keep open two related agenda items on the WTO response to allow the Council to be reconvened at short notice when and if convergence is within reach.[23] In May 2022, the WTO director put forward the outcome document that emerged from the informal process conducted with the Quad (the European Union, India, South Africa and the United States) for an IP response to COVID-19.[24] At the 12th Ministerial Conference of the WTO in Geneva in May 2022, the proposed TRIPS agreement was opposed by the European Union, United Kingdom, United States and Switzerland, insisting that it would undermine pharmaceutical research. The final compromise deal will let governments compel companies to share their vaccine recipes for the next five years. The agreement fell short of the demand by India and South Africa to exempt all COVID-19 vaccines, treatments and diagnostics, though there will be a review in six months. Instead, governments can issue compulsory licences to domestic manufacturers but must compensate the patent holders.[25] Campaigners were disappointed with the result. Oxfam said: 'This is absolutely not the broad intellectual property waiver the world desperately needs to ensure access to vaccines and treatments for everyone, everywhere. This so-called compromise largely reiterates developing countries' existing rights to override patents in certain circumstances. And it tries to restrict even that limited right to countries which do not already have the capacity to produce COVID-19 vaccines. Put simply, it is a technocratic fudge aimed at saving reputations, not lives.'[26]

21. Simone McCarthy, 'A Year on, Proposal to Waive IP for Covid-19 Vaccines Is Still in Limbo', *South China Morning Post*, 5 October 2021, https://www.scmp.com/news/china/science/article/3151236/year-proposal-waive-ip-covid-19-vaccines-still-limbo.

22. World Economic Forum (WEF), 'What to Expect from the Next WTO Conference', https://www.weforum.org/agenda/2021/11/what-to-expect-from-the-next-wto-conference.

23. WTO, 'Members Updated on High-Level Talks Aimed at Finding Convergence on IP COVID-19 Response', 10 March 2022, https://www.wto.org/english/news_e/news22_e/trip_10mar22_e.htm.

24. WTO, 'Quad's Outcome Document on IP COVID-19 Response Made Public', 3 May 2022, https://www.wto.org/english/news_e/news22_e/trip_03may22_e.htm.

25. Andy Bounds, 'WTO Agrees Partial Patent Waiver for Covid-19 Vaccines', *Financial Times*, 17 June 2022, https://www.ft.com/content/9cfa15b6-dab8-4cc6-9ab4-c192c6ad0e0b.

26. Oxfam, 'WTO Agrees on Deal on Patents for COVID Vaccines—But Campaigners Say This Is Absolutely Not the Broad Intellectual Property Waiver the World Desperately Needs', 17 June 2022, https://www.oxfam.org/en/press-releases/wto-agrees-deal-patents-covid-vaccines-campaigners-say-absolutely-not-broad.

The World Health Organization

Before understanding the WHO and COVID-19, it is necessary to understand the WHO itself—what it can and cannot do, its funding sources and how they affect the WHO. The WHO is a specialised agency of the UN that is concerned with international public health. It was established on 7 April 1948, with headquarters in Geneva, Switzerland. There are currently 192 member states, 6 regional offices, and 141 country offices predominantly in low- and middle-income countries. It employs about 8,000 doctors, scientists, epidemiologists, managers, and administrators worldwide.

The Objective of the WHO in the WHO Constitution of 1948 is the attainment by all peoples of the highest possible level of health.[27] The functions are clearly laid out in Article 2:

1. to act as the directing and coordinating authority on international health work;
2. to establish and maintain effective collaboration with the UN, specialised agencies, governmental health administrations, professional groups and such other organisations as may be deemed appropriate;
3. to assist governments, upon request, in strengthening health services;
4. to furnish appropriate technical assistance and, in emergencies, necessary aid upon the request or acceptance of governments;
5. to provide or assist in providing, upon the request of the UN, health services and facilities to special groups, such as the peoples of trust territories;
6. to establish and maintain such administrative and technical services as may be required, including epidemiological and statistical services;
7. to stimulate and advance work to eradicate epidemic, endemic and other diseases;
8. to promote, in cooperation with other specialised agencies where necessary, the prevention of accidental injuries;
9. to promote, in cooperation with other specialised agencies where necessary, the improvement of nutrition, housing, sanitation, recreation, economic or working conditions and other aspects of environmental hygiene;
10. to promote cooperation among scientific and professional groups which contribute to the advancement of health;
11. to propose conventions, agreements and regulations, and make recommendations with respect to international health matters and to perform such duties as may be assigned thereby to the WHO and are consistent with its objective;
12. to promote maternal and child health and welfare and to foster the ability to live harmoniously in a changing total environment;
13. to foster activities in the field of mental health, especially those affecting the harmony of human relations;

---

27. Constitution of the World Health Organization, 1948, https://apps.who.int/gb/bd/PDF/bd47/EN/constitution-en.pdf.

14. to promote and conduct research in the field of health;
15. to promote improved standards of teaching and training in the health, medical and related professions;
16. to study and report on, in cooperation with other specialised agencies where necessary, administrative and social techniques affecting public health and medical care from preventive and curative points of view, including hospital services and social security;
17. to provide information, counsel and assistance in the field of health;
18. to assist in developing an informed public opinion among all peoples on matters of health;
19. to establish and revise as necessary international nomenclatures of diseases, causes of death, and public health practices;
20. to standardise diagnostic procedures as necessary;
21. to develop, establish and promote international standards with respect to food, biological, pharmaceutical and similar products; and
22. generally to take all necessary action to attain the objective of the WHO.

The WHO was created to coordinate health affairs within the UN system. Its initial priorities were malaria, tuberculosis, venereal diseases, and other communicable diseases, plus women and children's health, nutrition, and sanitation. In more recent years, it has addressed non-communicable diseases (NCD), climate change, and disease and drug classification. From the start, it worked with member countries to identify and address public health issues, support health research, and issue guidelines. The work of the WHO is predominantly in low- and middle-income countries, so many in high-income countries may be less aware of the globally important scope and reach of the WHO. In addition to governments, the WHO coordinates with other UN agencies, donors, non-governmental organisations and the private sector.

The World Health Assembly is the decision-making body of the WHO and reviews its work, sets new goals, determines the policies of the WHO, appoints the Director-General, supervises financial policies, and reviews and approves the proposed budget. The assembly is held annually in Geneva, Switzerland.

Investigating and managing disease outbreaks is the responsibility of each individual country, although originally under the International Health Regulations (IHR)—an overarching legal framework that defines countries' rights and obligations in handling public health events and emergencies that have the potential to cross borders—governments were expected to report cases of some contagious diseases such as plague, cholera, and yellow fever. A revised version refrains from mentioning specific diseases and takes an 'all hazards' approach that includes not only pathogens, known and novel, but also other events that may constitute a Public Health Emergency of International Concern (PHEIC), such as chemical spills.

WHO decisions are made through the consensus of its member countries, principally at the annual World Health Assembly. The WHO's function is to act as the global organisation and secretariat to coordinate and recommend the implementation of these decisions. The WHO has no authority to tell countries what to do or punish countries for failing to take measures. For example, decisions about membership or attendance for Taiwan lie solely with member states, not with the WHO.

The Secretariat of the WHO can sometimes respond quickly with technical advice, but requires the consensus of its member states for other decisions. This can seem unwieldy, cumbersome, and time-consuming, but the WHO must be cautious so that it is regarded as a reliable and trusted agency by member countries. Rarely, if ever, has the WHO had to retract a guidance, guideline, or recommendation, which are regularly revised to reflect evolving evidence—which sometimes means that earlier pieces of guidance or a recommendation are updated and changed. The WHO spends enormous amounts of time reading, learning, and absorbing the best and most recent robust evidence available and bases its global guidance on that, to reflect updated peer reviews and retractions, and with the expectation that each region and member state will adapt guidance to local circumstances in order to be most effective.

The WHO gets its funding from two main sources: member states assessed contributions—countries' membership dues, based on a percentage of GDP—cover less than 20 per cent of its total budget;[28] and funding from voluntary contributions largely from member states, as well as from other UN organisations, inter-governmental organisations, philanthropic foundations, the private sector, and other sources.[29] For some years now, the WHO's biggest financial backers have not been member states, but private entities.[30] Some of this funding is earmarked by the donor, while some is 'flexible funding.'

Deplorably, in 2020, 151 member states collectively owed the WHO nearly half a billion US dollars in unpaid dues—about 20 per cent of its annual budget. The sheer size of the dues of the two major debtors, the United States and China, highlighted the WHO's reliance on its largest members.[31] This precarious funding system illustrates its dependence on alternative funding, and in addition being beholden to any strings attached.

In spite of being seriously under-funded, the WHO has attained a number of signal achievements over the years, most prominently its vaccine programme, which is a widely agreed global health and development success story. The programme has proved effective against more than 20 life-threatening diseases. It currently prevents 2–3 million deaths every year from diseases like diphtheria, tetanus, pertussis, influenza, measles, and polio, in addition to having led to a steep reduction in river blindness and the eradication of smallpox.

---

28. World Health Organization (WHO), 'How WHO Is Funded', https://www.who.int/about/funding.
29. Ibid.
30. European Parliament, 'Private Financing of the World Health Organisation', 21 January 2020, https://www.europarl.europa.eu/doceo/document/E-9-2020-000327_EN.html.
31. Ben Parker, 'WHO's Members Owe It More Than $470 million', *The New Humanitarian*, 30 April 2020, https://www.thenewhumanitarian.org/maps-and-graphics/2020/04/30/world-health-organisation-funding.

The WHO has been criticised, however, for being slow to react when HIV/AIDS exploded across the world, and more recently with COVID-19 hit. This chapter explores whether the latter is true and whether the WHO is fit for purpose in the new era of the predominance of NCD, even while the world is still beset by infectious disease pandemics.

WHO Response to COVID-19

The WHO led the UN health response to COVID-19, harnessing the world's technical and operational expertise to translate knowledge into coordinated action. This included the SPRP 2019 and 2021. The WHO is the leader of the global Incident Management Support Team, the UN Crisis Management Team, the founder of the Access to COVID-19 Tools Accelerator,[32] and a partner in COVAX.

On the ground, the WHO response to COVID-19 included distributing medical supplies; training health workers; building testing and tracing capacities; preventing the spread of the virus, particularly among vulnerable populations, including in camps, prisons, and detention centres; disseminating information widely about prevention and containment measures; and supporting national response planning and decision-making.[33]

Early days

On 30 December 2019, the day before the WHO was formally alerted by China that atypical pneumonia cases had emerged in Wuhan, the Program for Monitoring Emerging Diseases (ProMED),[34] a programme of the International Society for Infectious Diseases had already picked up the information from Weibo, a Chinese social media platform. ProMED was launched in 1994 as an Internet service to identify unusual health events related to emerging and re-emerging infectious diseases, and toxins affecting humans, animals, and plants. ProMED is the largest publicly available system conducting global reporting of infectious disease outbreaks. It is an essential source of information used daily by international public health leaders, government officials, physicians, veterinarians, researchers, private companies, journalists, and the general public, providing timely reporting of important emerging pathogens and their vectors using a One Health approach. One Health is an approach to designing and implementing programmes, policies, legislation, and research in which multiple sectors communicate and work together to achieve better public health outcomes. The areas of work in which a One Health approach is particularly relevant include food safety,

---

32. WHO, 'Strategy and Planning', https://www.who.int/emergencies/diseases/novel-coronavirus-2019/strategies-and-plans.
33. United Nations, 'United Nations Comprehensive Response'.
34. Maryn Mckenna, 'How ProMED Crowdsourced the Arrival of COVID-19 and SARS', *Wired*, 23 March 2020, https://www.wired.com/story/how-promed-crowdsourced-the-arrival-of-covid-19-and-sars.

the control of diseases that can spread between animals and humans, and combatting antibiotic resistance.

On 31 December 2019, the WHO Country Office in Beijing noticed a media statement by the Wuhan Municipal Health Commission on its website about cases of 'viral pneumonia' in Wuhan. On 1 and 2 January, the WHO requested information from the Chinese authorities. China responded on 3 January. One day after being alerted on 1 January 2020, the WHO activated its Incident Management Support Team; put the organisation on an emergency footing for dealing with the outbreak; then informed its own regional and national offices; issued a Global Outbreak Report; shared information on its International Health Regulations Event Information System, which is accessible to all member states; and on 5 January 2020, issued its first Disease Outbreak News report, the first of many. The WHO then promptly established a dedicated COVID-19 website for advice, technical guidance, response, and research.[35] It eventually included every conceivable aspect of COVID-19, ranging from international data, research, dashboards, and situation reports to myth-busting,[36] advice to the public, and a Q&A Section. The WHO's SPRP 2019 coordinated action at the national, regional, and global levels to overcome the ongoing challenges, address inequities, and plot a course out of the pandemic.[37]

On 30 January 2020, the WHO declared a PHEIC—the highest level of alert—for only the 6th time since the alarm system originated in 2005.[38] A PHEIC is defined as an extraordinary event that constitutes a public health risk to other states through international spread and requires a coordinated international response. It is an ill-defined process whereby the WHO Director-General convenes Emergency Committees to provide their advice on whether an event constitutes a PHEIC.

Table 2.2 shows the times when PHEIC had been declared. At that point, all member states should have taken note to act.

The WHO was not starting from scratch to fight the outbreak. There were a host of existing committees and departments with decades of experience of emergencies, infectious disease outbreaks, health systems, vaccines, health promotion, treatments including drug therapies, law and economics, and more—all relevant to COVID-19's emergence. The WHO already had a dedicated department—the Immunization, Vaccines and Biologicals Department—ready to deal with epidemics.[39]

---

35. WHO, 'Fighting Misinformation in the Time of COVID-19, One Click at a Time', 27 April 2021, https://www.who.int/news-room/feature-stories/detail/fighting-misinformation-in-the-time-of-COVID-19-one-click-at-a-time; WHO, 'Corona Virus Disease (COVID-19)', https://www.who.int/health-topics/coronavirus#tab=tab_1.

36. WHO, 'Fighting Misinformation'.

37. WHO, 'Coronavirus (COVID-19) Pandemic', https://www.who.int/emergencies/diseases/novel-coronavirus-2019; WHO, 'Strategy and Planning'.

38. Amy Maxmen, 'Why Did the World's Pandemic Warning System Fail When COVID Hit?', Nature, 23 January 2021, https://www.nature.com/articles/d41586-021-00162-4.

39. WHO, 'Immunization, Vaccines and Biologicals Department of WHO', accessed 13 September 2022, https://www.who.int/teams/immunization-vaccines-and-biologicals/about.

Table 2.2: WHO public health emergencies of international concern (PHEIC) [i]

Year	Infection	Location and Spread
2009	H1N1 (swine flu)	Originated in Mexico and spread to the United States
2014	Polio	Reappeared in Afghanistan, Pakistan, and Nigeria
2014	Ebola virus infections	Spread throughout Guinea, Sierra Leone, and Liberia
2016	Zika virus epidemic causing microcephaly and other neurological disorders	The Americas
2019	Ebola outbreak	Spread in a conflict zone in the Democratic Republic of the Congo.
2020	COVID-19 pandemic	

Source:

i. Amy Maxmen, 'Why Did the World's Pandemic Warning System Fail when COVID Hit?', *Nature*, 23 January 2021, https://www.nature.com/articles/d41586-021-00162-4.

Table 2.3 outlines the most important WHO milestones in the early months of the pandemic. It provides a record to judge whether the WHO did its job of alerting the world about the emergence of a new infectious disease. The key takeaways from the table are that, given the circumstances, the WHO took action quickly, shared action quickly, and produced advice and guidelines quickly.

Challenges and Criticisms of the WHO

The WHO had to weather myriad issues relating to political personalities on a global scale, domestic politics of member countries, and increasingly fraught geopolitics. The WHO had hoped the world would pull together, but instead, it became even more divided. Some specific criticisms are outlined below.

Did the WHO fail to prepare the world for COVID-19? [40]

COVID-19 could not have been more predictable. Throughout history, nothing has killed more humans than viruses, bacteria, and parasites. Humans inhabit a planet dominated by micro-organisms. More than six distinct influenza pandemics and epidemics have struck in just over a century. Ebola viruses have spilt over from animals about 25 times in the past five decades. And at least seven coronaviruses, including SARS-CoV-2,

---

40. Matt Ridley, 'WHO Has Good Intentions but It Must Answer Serious Questions before It Is Trusted with Leading a COVID-19 Inquiry', *Telegraph*, 3 April 2020, telegraph.co.uk/news/2020/04/03/whohas-good-intentions-must-answer-serious-questions-trusted.

Table 2.3: Timeline summary on WHO's COVID-19 response, December 2019–April 2020

31 December 2019	WHO's Country Office in Beijing noted a media statement by the Wuhan Municipal Health Commission from its website on cases of 'viral pneumonia' in Wuhan. The Country Office notified the IHR focal point in the WHO Western Pacific Regional Office (WWPRO).
	WHO's Epidemic Intelligence from Open Sources (EIOS) platform also noted a media report on ProMED about the same cluster of cases of 'pneumonia of unknown cause' in Wuhan.
1 January 2020	WHO requested information from the Chinese authorities on the reported cluster of cases in Wuhan. WHO activated its IMST, as part of its public health emergency response framework, which ensures coordination of activities and response across the three levels of WHO (headquarters, regional, country), putting the organisation on an emergency footing for dealing with the outbreak.
2 January 2020	WHO Country Office wrote to China's National Health Commission, offering WHO support, and repeated the request for further information. WHO informed Global Outbreak Alert and Response Network (GOARN) partners about the cluster of pneumonia cases in China. GOARN partners include major public health agencies, laboratories, UN agencies, international organisations, and NGOs.
3 January 2020	Chinese officials provided information to WHO on the cluster of cases of 'viral pneumonia of unknown cause' identified in Wuhan.
4 January 2020	WHO tweeted that there was a cluster of pneumonia cases in Wuhan but there were no deaths, and that investigations to identify the cause were underway.
5 January 2020	WHO shared detailed information about a cluster of cases of pneumonia of unknown cause through the IHR Event Information System, which is accessible to all member states. It provided information on the cases and advised member states to take precautions to reduce the risk of acute respiratory infections.
	WHO issued its first of many Disease Outbreak News reports. This is a public, web-based platform for the publication of technical information addressed to the scientific and public health communities, as well as the global media. The report contained information about the number of cases and their clinical status; details about the Wuhan national authority's response measures; and WHO's risk assessment and advice on public health measures. It advised that 'WHO's recommendations on public health measures and surveillance of influenza and severe acute respiratory infections still apply'.[i]

Table 2.3 (continued)

9 January 2020	WHO reported that Chinese authorities determined that the outbreak was caused by a novel coronavirus. WHO convened the first of many teleconferences with global expert networks, beginning with the Clinical Network.
10 January 2020	The Director-General spoke with China's Head of the National Health Commission. He also shared information with the Director of the Chinese Center for Disease Control and Prevention (CCDC).
	WHO issued a comprehensive online package of technical guidance with advice to all countries on how to detect, test, and manage potential cases.
11 January 2020	Chinese media reported the first death from the novel coronavirus.
	WHO tweeted that it had received the genetic sequences for the novel coronavirus from China and expected these to be made publicly available soon.
10-12 January 2020	WHO published a comprehensive package of guidance documents for countries, covering: <ul><li>Infection prevention and control</li><li>Laboratory testing</li><li>National capacities review tool</li><li>Risk communication and community engagement</li><li>Disease Commodity Package (v1)</li><li>Disease Commodity Package (v2)</li><li>Travel advice</li><li>Clinical management</li><li>Surveillance case definitions</li></ul>
13 January 2020	The Ministry of Public Health in Thailand reported an imported case of lab-confirmed novel coronavirus from Wuhan, the first recorded case outside China.
14 January 2020	WHO suggested there could be human-to-human transmission.
19 January 2020	WWPRO tweeted that, according to the latest information received and WHO analysis, there was evidence of limited human-to-human transmission.
20-21 January 2002	WHO conducted the first mission to Wuhan and met with public health officials to learn about the response to the cluster of cases of novel coronavirus.
22 January 2020	WHO mission to Wuhan issued a statement saying that evidence suggested human-to-human transmission in Wuhan, but that more investigation was needed to understand the full extent of transmission.

Table 2.3 (continued)

23 January 2020	WHO Director-General convened an IHR Emergency Committee (IHREC), comprised of 15 independent experts from around the world charged with advising the Director-General as to whether the outbreak constituted a PHEIC. The IHREC was unable to reach a conclusion on 22 January based on the limited information available. The Director-General asked it to continue deliberations the next day. The Director-General held a media briefing to provide an update on the IHREC's deliberations. The IHREC met again on 23 January. Members were equally divided as to whether the event constituted a PHEIC, as several members considered that there was still not enough information. The IHREC advised it was ready to reconvene within 10 days. It formulated advice for WHO, China, other countries, and the global community. The Director-General accepted the advice and held a second media briefing, giving the IHREC's advice and what WHO was doing in response to the outbreak.
27-28 January 2020	A WHO delegation led by the Director-General arrived in Beijing to meet Chinese leaders, learn more about China's response, and offer technical assistance. The Director-General met with President Xi Jinping on 28 January, and discussed continued collaboration on containment measures in Wuhan, public health measures in other cities and provinces, conducting further studies on the severity and transmissibility of the virus, continuing to share data, and requested China to share samples with WHO. They agreed that an international team of leading scientists should travel to China to better understand the context, the overall response, and exchange information and experience.
30 January 2020	The WHO Director-General reconvened the IHREC, which advised the Director-General that the outbreak now met the criteria for a PHEIC. The Director-General accepted its advice and declared the novel coronavirus outbreak a PHEIC—WHO's highest level of alarm. At that time there were 98 cases in 18 countries except China. Four countries other than China had evidence (eight cases) of human-to-human transmission (Germany, Japan, United States, and Vietnam).
	The IHREC formulated advice for all countries and the global community, which the Director-General accepted and issued as Temporary Recommendations under the IHR. The Director-General gave a statement, providing an overview of the situation in China and globally; the statement also explained the reasoning behind the decision to declare a PHEIC and outlined the IHREC's recommendations.

Table 2.3 (continued)

24 February 2020	The Team Leaders of a WHO-China Joint Mission on COVID-19 held a press conference to report on the main findings of the mission. The mission warned that 'much of the global community is not yet ready, in mindset and materially, to implement the measures that have been employed to contain COVID-19 in China'.[ii] The Mission stressed that 'to reduce COVID-19 illness and death, near-term readiness planning must embrace the large-scale implementation of high-quality, non-pharmaceutical public health measures', such as case detection and isolation, contact tracing and monitoring/quarantining, and community engagement.
	Major recommendations were developed for China, countries with imported cases and/or outbreaks of COVID-19, uninfected countries, the public, and the international community. For example, in addition to the above, countries with imported cases and/or outbreaks were advised to 'immediately activate the highest level of national Response Management protocols to ensure the all-of-government and all-of-society approach needed to contain COVID-19'.
	In addition to the mission press conference, WHO published operational considerations for managing COVID-19 cases and outbreaks on board ships, following the outbreak of COVID-19 during an international voyage.
11 March 2020	At first, most cases were seen as being within China and among people who had travelled there, as well as those travellers' close contacts. While these cases were concerning, they did not suggest a pandemic, because there was not significant spread outside of China.[iii]
	On 11 March, WHO declared COVID-19 had reached the strict criteria to be labelled a pandemic.[iv] The Director General cautioned that 'Pandemic is not a word to use lightly or carelessly. It is a word that, if misused, can cause unreasonable fear, or unjustified acceptance that the fight is over, leading to unnecessary suffering and death.[v] Describing the situation as a pandemic doesn't change WHO's assessment of the threat posed by this virus. It doesn't change what WHO is doing, and it doesn't change what countries should do.'[vi]
13 March 2020	WHO, the UN Foundation and partners launched the COVID-19 Solidarity Response Fund to receive donations from private individuals, corporations, and institutions. In 10 days, it raised more than US$70 million from more than 187,000 individuals and organisations to help health workers on the frontlines to do their life-saving work, treat patients, and advance research for treatments and vaccines.

Table 2.3 (continued)

18 March 2020	WHO and partners launched the Solidarity trial, an international clinical trial that aimed to generate robust data from around the world to find the most effective treatments for COVID-19.
4 April 2020	WHO reported over one million cases of COVID-19 confirmed worldwide, a more than tenfold increase in less than a month.

Sources:

i. World Health Organization, 'Timeline—WHO's COVID-19 Response', accessed 21 September 2022, https://www.who.int/emergencies/diseases/novel-coronavirus-2019/interactive-timeline#!.

ii. World Health Organization, 'Timeline—WHO's COVID-19 Response', accessed 21 September 2022, https://www.who.int/emergencies/diseases/novel-coronavirus-2019/interactive-timeline#!.

iii. Jamie Ducharme, 'World Health Organization Declares COVID-19 a "Pandemic". Here's What That Means', Time, 11 March 2021, https://time.com/5791661/who-coronavirus-pandemic-declaration.

iv. Helen Branswell and Andrew Joseph, 'WHO Declares the Coronavirus Outbreak a Pandemic', Statnews, 11 March 20202, https://www.statnews.com/2020/03/11/who-declares-the-coronavirus-outbreak-a-pandemic.

v. 'WHO Director-General's Opening Remarks at the Media Briefing on COVID-19', 19 March 2020, https://www.who.int/director-general/speeches/detail/who-director-general-s-opening-remarks-at-the-media-briefing-on-covid-19-19-march-2021.

vi. https://www.who.int/director-general/speeches/detail/who-director-general-s-opening-remarks-at-the-media-briefing-on-COVID-19-19---11-march-2020.

have brought illness and death.[41] Centuries of history showed that such epidemics appear with recurring regularity, some killing as much as half the affected population.[42] Even the word 'influenza' relates to how pandemics were known to sweep the globe a few times every century; their viral origins yet to be discovered, these pandemics were attributed to the 'influence' of the stars.

Avoiding pandemics is, in practice, impossible. There were charges that the WHO had failed to prepare the world for another, inevitable, infectious disease epidemic. Given the recent epidemics of Ebola, Zika and SARS, should the WHO and individual countries not have been better prepared? Epidemiologists and researchers who specialise in biosecurity and public health have been outlining preparedness plans for at least 20 years. The core components consist broadly of surveillance to detect pathogens, data collection and modelling to see how they spread, improvements to public health guidance and communication, and the development of therapies and vaccines.[43]

In 1969, the WHO developed the IHR as a way of minimising the international spread of disease while interfering as little as possible in world trade, transportation, and travel. The IHR required that WHO be notified whenever cholera, plague, or yellow fever occurred, and published in *Weekly Epidemiological Record*. It also specified measures that countries should take with infectious diseases in general. Given today's vast number of global microbial threats, the regulations became outdated, and were revised in 2005. The revised IHR is now a formal framework for proactive international surveillance and response to any epidemic that begins to spread internationally.[44] Moreover, the WHO Health Emergencies Programme was established on 1 July 2016, at the request of the World Health Assembly.[45]

In 2017, the Wellcome Trust and the Bill and Melinda Gates Foundation launched the Coalition for Epidemic Preparedness Innovation (CEPI) at the World Economic Forum in Davos, Switzerland. Headquartered in Oslo, Norway, its aim was to develop vaccines to stop future epidemics. CEPI is an innovative global partnership between public, private, philanthropic, and civil society organisations, including the WHO.[46]

However, in spite of predictions and warnings, most national governments were ill-prepared for COVID-19.

41. Amy Maxmen, 'Has COVID-19 Taught Us Anything about Pandemic Preparedness?', *Nature*, 13 August 2021, https://www.nature.com/articles/d41586-021-02217-y.
42. Wikipedia, 'List of Epidemics', Wikipedia, accessed 13 September 2022, https://en.wikipedia.org/wiki/List_of_epidemics.
43. Maxmen, 'Has COVID-19 Taught Us Anything'.
44. Stanley M. Lemon, Margaret A. Hamburg, P. Frederick Sparling, Eileen R. Choffnes, and Alison Mack, *Ethical and Legal Considerations in Mitigating Pandemic Disease: Workshop Summary* (Washington, DC: National Academies Press), https://www.ncbi.nlm.nih.gov/books/NBK54171.
45. Felicity Harvey, Walid Ammar, Hiroyoshi Endo, Geeta Rao Gupta, Jeremy Konyndyk, Precious Matsoso, et al., 'Special Report to the Director-General of World Health Organization (PDF)', Independent Oversight and Advisory Committee for the WHO Health Emergencies Programme, 2018.
46. Coalition for Epidemic Preparedness Innovation (CEPI), 'Preparing for Future Pandemics', accessed 13 September 2022, https://cepi.net; Wikipedia, 'Coalition for Epidemic Preparedness Innovations', accessed 13 September 2022, https://en.wikipedia.org/wiki/Coalition_for_Epidemic_Preparedness_Innovations.

Did the WHO get its priorities wrong?

Some critics accused the WHO of having changed its initial focus on infectious diseases to spending too much time on NCDs and their risk factors like obesity, tobacco, poor food, lack of exercise, and climate change. Yet 60 per cent of deaths globally are now due to such diseases. Heart disease is no longer a disease of old men in high-income countries. Today, it affects the wealthy and the poor alike, and claims more lives in low- and middle-income countries than in high-income countries; over half the deaths from heart disease are in Asia.

Did the WHO act too slowly?

As outlined in Table 2.1, it is hard to see how the WHO could have acted any quicker on a report of a few respiratory cases from Wuhan, which might have been ordinary viral illnesses like flu. The main delays at the start of the pandemic were not by the WHO but were at the country level.

The WHO sounded its highest level of alarm on 30 January 2020, by declaring a PHEIC, signalling that a pandemic might be imminent. In hindsight, some epidemiologists believe it could have been issued sooner. Yet, even then, most of the world failed to act, and few governments heeded the WHO Director-General's call to governments to move fast with public health measures including testing, tracing and social distancing.[47] For example, the United States did not roll out testing across the country until late February 2020, did not bar large gatherings until March, and did not immediately introduce contact tracing.[48] By mid-March, COVID-19 had spread around the world.[49] As explained earlier, the WHO has no authority to compel countries to take action. A report in *Nature* in January 2021 noted that, in hindsight, the WHO should have declared a PHEIC about a week earlier than it did on 30 January 2020 but the largest failing, researchers agreed, was that so many countries, except in Asia, ignored it.[50]

There was also confusion around terminology. The precise term PHEIC and its importance are unfamiliar to most lay people. 'Pandemic' is not a defined declaration, and countries have not agreed to take any actions once the term is used.[51] In practice, the public, and even governments and politicians, mainly ignored the PHEIC declaration and only really took note when the WHO started using the term 'pandemic' on 11 March 2020, once it was already spreading in several continents.[52]

---

47. Maxmen, 'Why Did the World's Pandemic Warning System Fail'.
48. Ibid.
49. Ibid.
50. Ibid.
51. Ibid.
52. Ibid.; Helen Branswell and Andrew Joseph, 'WHO Declares the Coronavirus Outbreak a Pandemic', *STAT*, 11 March 2020, https://www.statnews.com/2020/03/11/who-declares-the-coronavirus-outbreak-a-pandemic.

Was the WHO's messaging contradictory?

Some critics claimed that once COVID-19 began its global sweep, there were contradictions and inconsistencies in the WHO statements and advisories, such as on wearing face masks and the means of transmission. In fairness, the WHO and the world were on shifting sands. It has been likened to flying an aeroplane while trying to build it. As explained in Chapter 1, COVID-19 was a new pandemic, and it took time for experts to understand its unique characteristics. Evidence evolved, sometimes on a daily basis, on almost every aspect of COVID-19, including masking, social distancing, vaccines, and treatment.

COVID-19 treatment is a good example of this. The WHO established the COVID-19 Solidarity Therapeutics Trial in 14,200 randomised hospitalised patients in 2,000 hospitals in 52 countries.[53] It was the largest global collaboration among member states, designed to provide robust results on whether a particular drug could save lives. It was discovered by trial and error that some drugs worked and some, even with the enthusiastic endorsement of famous figures, did not. Bit by bit, treatment protocols evolved, but these were unknown and unavailable at the start of the pandemic. Economists like John Maynard Keynes and Paul Samuelson, and also Winston Churchill, have been variously credited with saying 'When the facts change, I change my mind. What do you do, sir/madam?'

Was the WHO subservient to China?

The WHO's dealings with, statements about, and visits to China came under criticism. The United States used it as a reason to withdraw funding from the WHO. The WHO was accused of overly praising the Chinese government,[54] with the issue of Taiwan becoming entangled as well.

One accusation was that China was less than forthcoming, even obstructing any investigation of the origin of COVID-19. The origin of the COVID-19 virus outbreak is unresolved and may remain so for decades to come. Theories include that it originated in wildlife, including wildlife being sold at the Huanan Seafood Wholesale Market in Wuhan,[55] and that it was accidentally released from a research laboratory (see Chapter 1).[56] It is important to continue to investigate the origin, so as to better prevent other

53. WHO, 'WHO COVID-19 Solidarity Therapeutics Trial', accessed 13 September 2022, https://www.who.int/emergencies/diseases/novel-coronavirus-2019/global-research-on-novel-coronavirus-2019-ncov/solidarity-clinical-trial-for-COVID-19-treatments.

54. Kate Kelland and Stephanie Nebehay, 'Special Report: Caught in Trump-China Feud, WHO Leader under Siege', *Reuters*, 29 January 2020, reuters.com/article/us-health-coronavirus-who-tedros-special/special-report-caught-in-trump-china-feudwho-leader-under-siege-idUSKBN22R1IL.

55. 'More Evidence that Covid-19 Started in a Market, Not a Laboratory', *The Economist*, 5 March 2022, https://www.economist.com/science-and-technology/more-evidence-that-covid-19-started-in-a-market-not-a-laboratory/21807945.

56. Jon Cohen, 'Do Three New Studies Add Up to Proof of COVID-19's Origin in a Wuhan Animal Market?', *Science*, 28 February 2022, https://www.science.org/content/article/do-three-new-studies-add-proof-covid-19-s-origin-wuhan-animal-market.

epidemics in the future. Genetics may prove the answer. This is far from the first time that the origin of a virus has been questioned. Historically, when HIV/AIDS swept the world in the 1980s, various fringe and conspiracy theories arose to speculate on its origin. After decades of investigation, it is now thought to have crossed from chimpanzees to humans in the 1920s in what is now the Democratic Republic of Congo.[57]

The first field visit to Wuhan by the WHO international team studying the origins of SARS-CoV-2 was in February 2020. The team itself came under criticism as being selected in a hurry without the balance of most WHO committees, and one member was found to have competing interests. The visit yielded no definite conclusions on the origin of COVID-19. The WHO Director-General called for further studies and reiterated that all hypotheses remained on the table. In July 2021, the WHO established the Scientific Advisory Group for Origins of Novel Pathogens (SAGO), comprised of 26 experts from countries including China, the United States, India, and Kenya. SAGO produced a preliminary report in June 2022 calling for further studies.[58]

Other Issues of Importance

Vaccine inequity

Rich countries were able to pay for vaccines and poor countries could not. Some nations have given third booster doses while most of the world had yet to receive a single dose. COVAX is a worldwide initiative aimed at equitable access to vaccines directed by the global Vaccine Alliance (GAVI), CEPI, and the WHO. Its aim is to accelerate the development and manufacture of COVID-19 vaccines, and to guarantee fair and equitable access for every country in the world. From the start, the COVAX vaccine programme was (and still is) severely affected by vaccine inequity. The constant pleas of the WHO for vaccine support from high-income countries for low- and middle-income countries have fallen on deaf ears.

COVAX had allocated more than 2 billion COVID-19 vaccine doses by September 2022,[59] supplying these to over 140 countries,[60] but this is still totally inadequate. The WHO has repeatedly warned of the dire consequences of uneven vaccinations, including the emergence of variants. Its initial goal for every country to vaccinate 40 per cent

57. Wikipedia, 'Discredited HIV/AIDS Origins Theories', accessed 13 September 2022, https://en.wikipedia. org/wiki/Discredited_HIV/AIDS_origins_theories.

58. WHO, 'Scientific Advisory Group for the Origins of Novel Pathogens', accessed 13 September 2022, https://www.who.int/groups/scientific-advisory-group-on-the-origins-of-novel-pathogens-(sago); and WHO, 'Preliminary Report for the Scientific Advisory Group for the Origins of the Novel Pathogens', 9 June 2022, https://www.who.int/publications/m/item/scientific-advisory-group-on-the-origins-of-novel-pathogens-report.

59. COVAX Data Brief, 6 September 2022. https://www.gavi.org/sites/default/files/covid/covax/COVAX-data-brief_12.pdf.

60. 'Factbox: Vaccines Delivered under COVAX Sharing Scheme for Poorer Countries', Reuters, 7 October 2022, accessed 9 October 2022, https://www.reuters.com/business/healthcare-pharmaceuticals/vaccines-delivered-under-covax-sharing-scheme-poorer-countries-2022-01-03/.

of its population by the end of 2021 was not met.[61] Perhaps only when high-income countries have been fully vaccinated will it become easier to get them to share vaccines.

Another issue facing the WHO and COVAX was that of the tobacco industry and its forays into COVID-19 vaccines. The WHO Framework Convention on Tobacco Control (WHO FCTC) Article 5.3 specifically states:

> In setting and implementing their public health policies with respect to tobacco control, Parties shall act to protect these policies from commercial and other vested interests of the tobacco industry in accordance with national law.[62]

The tobacco industry has used COVID-19 to shift its image from vilified industry to trusted health partner, using the pandemic to maximise contact with policy-makers and health professionals;[63] as well as distributing ventilators, gels, personal protective equipment and free masks.[64] Philip Morris/Medicago are developing a COVID-19 vaccine with the unlikely support of the government of Canada.[65] Vaccines are also being produced by British American Tobacco's biotech subsidiary, Kentucky BioProcessing,[66] and others.

There are two issues—the first is that these vaccines are enabling the industry to gain publicity with slogans such as 'Tobacco to the rescue'.[67] The second is the access of the tobacco companies to the WHO, COVAX, and governments, in contradiction to WHO FCTC Article 5.3. This could lead to the unimaginable situation of GAVI, the WHO. and CEPI sitting in the same room and discussing public health with the tobacco industry. When these vaccines come onto the market, they will pose an ethical and health dilemma for the WHO and GAVI, and also for low- and middle-income countries short of vaccine supply. At the time of writing, WHO has formally rejected the Canadian vaccine, and it has not been approved by national regulators for distribution

61. McCarthy, 'A Year on'.
62. WHO, 'WHO Framework Convention on Tobacco Control Article 5.3'.
63. Campaign for Tobacco Free Kids (2020), 'Big Tobacco Is Exploiting COVID-19 To Market Its Harmful Products', https://www.tobaccofreekids.org/media/2020/2020_05_COVID-19-marketing; STOP, 'Trading "Philanthropy" for Favors: Tobacco Industry CSR During COVID-19', 17 August 2020, https://exposetobacco.org/news/ban-ti-csr/?utm_source=Stopping+Tobacco+Organizations+and+Products+%28STOP%29&utm_campaign=891101c19c-Stop_Newsletter_8.25.20&utm_medium=email&utm_term=0_a7474fe40f-891101c19c-354163305#utm_source=mailchimp&utm_medium=email&utm_campaign=COVID-19-accountability; Andrew Rowell, 'Coronavirus: Big Tobacco Sees an Opportunity in the Pandemic', The Conversation, 14 May 2020, https://theconversation.com/coronavirus-big-tobacco-sees-an-opportunity-in-the-pandemic-138188.
64. Alan Selby, 'Vape Firm Says Thank You to Frontline NHS Staff with Vouchers for E-Cigs', The Mirror, 11 August 2020, https://www.mirror.co.uk/news/uk-news/vape-firm-says-thank-you-22504039.
65. Philip Morris International, 'PMI Announces Medicago to Supply up to 76 Million Doses of Its Plant-Derived COVID-19 Vaccine Candidate', MarketScreener, accessed October 2020, https://www.marketscreener.com/quote/stock/PHILIP-MORRIS-INTERNATION-2836703/news/Philip-Morris-International-PMI-Announces-Medicago-to-Supply-Up-to-76-Million-Doses-of-Its-Plant-D-31601227.
66. Patricia Nilsson and Clive Cookson, 'BAT Joins Race to Develop COVID-19 Vaccine', Financial Times, 1 April 2020, ft.com/content/e3737752-6147-4c0e-82f2-e7df9eb9f6f8.
67. Ejinsight, 'How a Use for Tobacco Helps Accelerate COVID-19 Vaccine', 28 October 2020, https://www.ejinsight.com/eji/article/id/2617626/20201028-How-a-use-for-tobacco-helps-accelerate-COVID-19-accine.

in the United Kingdom, European Union or the United States. This subject is discussed in Chapter 3.

US withdrawal from the WHO

Matters came to a head in mid-2020 when then United States President Donald Trump announced he would end America's relationship with the WHO and withdraw funding. On 6 July 2020, the United States officially notified the UN Secretary-General of its intention to withdraw its membership. This was at the time the world and the United States were experiencing huge daily increases in the number of COVID-19 cases.[68] The United States reiterated accusations that the WHO was too lenient with China.[69] President Trump threatened to freeze WHO funding permanently, accusing the WHO of withholding critical information about the dangers of COVID-19.[70] None of the accusations was supported by facts.[71]

The decision would clearly damage the WHO. First, there was the loss of funding.[72] Second, it was an unwelcome distraction for an organisation trying to tackle one of the most serious threats in decades to global public health, including for Americans. In response, 750 US leaders from academia, science, and law urged the US Congress to block the president's action.[73] An article in *The Lancet* in August 2020 concluded that withdrawal would also harm the United States. Its withdrawal from the WHO would have dire consequences for US security, diplomacy, and influence. The WHO has unmatched global reach and legitimacy. The Trump administration was hard-pressed to disentangle the country from WHO governance and programmes. The Pan American Health Organization is among six WHO regional offices and is headquartered in Washington, DC. The United States is also a state party to two WHO treaties: the WHO Constitution, establishing it as the 'directing and coordinating authority on

---

68. Lawrence O. Gostin, Harold Hongju Koh, Michelle Williams, Margaret A. Hamburg, Georges Benjamin, William H. Foege, et al., 'US Withdrawal from WHO Is Unlawful and Threatens Global and US Health and Security', Comment, *Lancet* 396, issue 10247 (1 August 2020): 293–295, https://www.thelancet.com/journals/lancet/article/PIIS0140-6736(20)31527-0/fulltext.

69. Amy Maxmen, 'What a US Exit from the WHO Means for COVID-19 and Global Health', *Nature* 582, no. 17 (27 May 2020), https://www.nature.com/articles/d41586-020-01586-0.

70. Julian Borger, 'Caught in a Superpower Struggle: The Inside Story of the WHO's Response to Coronavirus', *Guardian*, 18 April 2020, https://www.theguardian.com/world/2020/apr/18/caught-in-a-superpower-struggle-the-inside-story-of-the-whos-response-to-coronavirus; Maxmen, 'What a US Exit from the WHO Means'.

71. Borger, 'Caught in a Superpower Struggle'.

72. McKee Martin, 'Coronavirus Has Killed 30,000 Americans, and All Trump Can Do Is Blame the WHO', *Guardian*, 16 April 2020, theguardian.com/world/commentisfree/2020/apr/16/coronavirus-30000-americans-trump-blame-who.

73. Lawrence O. Gostin, Matthew M. Kavanagh, John Monahan, Timothy Westmoreland, Eric A. Friedman, Charles Holmes, et al., 'Letter to Congress on WHO Withdrawal from Public Health, Law and International Relations Leaders', 30 June 2020, https://oneill.law.georgetown.edu/letter-to-congress-on-who-withdrawal-from-public-health-law-and-international-relations-leaders.

international health'; and the IHR 2005, the governing framework for epidemic preparedness and response'.[74]

> Various US institutions collaborating with WHO on vital work would be harmed if the
> relationship is severed. There are 21 WHO collaborating centres at the US Centers for
> Disease Control and Prevention (CDC) and three at the National Institutes of Health,
> focused on US priorities, including polio eradication, cancer prevention, and global
> health security. The Secretariat of the 44 WHO Collaborating Centers for Nursing and
> Midwifery is based in the USA.[75]

The UN Secretary-General said it was 'not the time' to cut funding or to question
errors. 'Once we have finally turned the page on this epidemic, there must be a time to
look back fully to understand how such a disease emerged and spread its devastation so
quickly across the globe, and how all those involved reacted to the crisis.'[76]

A formal notification to withdraw from the WHO requires one year before it
becomes effective. On his first day in office, Joseph Biden, who won the 2020 presidential
election, honoured a campaign promise to retract the withdrawal by his predecessor.[77]

> The WHO plays a crucial role in the world's fight against the deadly COVID-19
> pandemic as well as countless other threats to global health and health security. The
> United States will continue to be a full participant and a global leader in confronting
> such threats and advancing global health and health security.[78]

The WHO: The Way Forward

If not WHO, then who?

The WHO, over its over 70-year history, is the *only* global organisation with the
history, the reach, the experience, the in-country offices, the trust, the credibility and
the ability to coordinate global public health. Some governments around the world,
including in the United States, Australia, and the European Union, have called for the
WHO to be reformed or restructured amid criticism of its response to the COVID-19
outbreak.[79] Many agree that to improve the world's ability to respond to pandemics, the
WHO needs to be strengthened.

Suggestions have been made before and during the COVID-19 epidemic, and
include:

---

74. Gostin et al., 'US Withdrawal from WHO'.
75. Ibid.
76. Helen Davidson, '"Crime against Humanity": Trump Condemned for WHO Funding Freeze', *Guardian*,
    15 April 2020, https://www.theguardian.com/world/2020/apr/15/against-humanity-trump-condemned-
    for-who-funding-freeze.
77. Jenny Lei Ravelo, 'On His First Day in office, Biden Retracts US Withdrawal from WHO', *Devex*, 21 January 2021,
    https://www.devex.com/news/on-his-first-day-in-office-biden-retracts-us-withdrawal-from-who-98961.
78. Ibid.
79. Kate Kelland and Josephine Mason, 'WHO Reform Needed in Wake of Pandemic, Public Health Experts Say',
    Reuters, 13 January 2021, https://www.reuters.com/article/us-health-coronavirus-crisis-idUSKBN29I210.

1. **New treaty on pandemics:** The WHO could be strengthened through a new treaty on pandemics that countries would need to sign and ratify, akin to the existing WHO FCTC. In December 2021, the World Health Assembly agreed to kickstart a global process to draft and negotiate such a convention, agreement, or other international instrument under the Constitution of the WHO to strengthen pandemic prevention, preparedness, and response. Treaties take on average about a decade from conception to when they come into force, so it is hard to see how this treaty could be ready much before 2024. At the time of the May 2022 World Health Assembly, the idea drew vehement criticism on the basis that countries would have to cede their sovereignty to supranational governance, and even that democracy was under threat. This is untrue. Like the WHO FCTC, such a treaty would not have legal teeth for enforcement and compliance, and would rely on voluntary implementation by member states. The next steps will be a series of negotiations and a public consultation hearing, with a progress report to be delivered to the 2023 World Health Assembly, and an outcome document to the 2024 World Health Assembly.

2. **Larger, reliable, flexible/untied funding:**[80] For every US$1 invested in it, the WHO provides a return of US$35 in societal value.[81] A larger, reliable budget for the WHO would give the organisation greater autonomy. A wider and improved funding base would enable the WHO to be less reliant on its big country funders, in particular the United States and China,[82] and thereby avoid being dependent on fundraising amid a disaster.[83] In 2022, the Executive Board governing the WHO considered the most recent report of the Working Group on Sustainable Financing,[84] a Working Group set up under the Rules of Procedure of the Executive Board. The most recent discussions ended in a stalemate, not surprisingly, as this has recurred many times in the last two decades: every member state agreed that the WHO needs to be funded more sustainably and more flexibly, but there is no consensus on raising the needed contributions.[85] At the 2022 World Health Assembly, the member states of the WHO agreed to substantially improve the agency's financing model, giving it greater flexibility and enhanced capacity to fulfil its mandate. It is only the first step towards reform and investment, with many details to be worked out.

---

80. Claire Chaumont, 'Opinion: 5 Ways to Reform the World Health Organization', 5 August 2020, https://www.devex.com/news/opinion-5-ways-to-reform-the-world-health-organization-97843.

81. Alexandra Finch, Kevin A. Klock, Eric A. Friedman, and Lawrence O. Gostin, 'At Long Last, Member States Agree to Fix the World Health Organization's Financing Problem', 1 June 2022, https://www.thinkglobal-health.org/article/long-last-member-states-agree-fix-world-health-organizations-financing-problem.

82. Kelland and Mason, 'WHO Reform'.

83. Maxmen, 'Why Did the World's Pandemic Warning System Fail'.

84. WHO, 'Sustainable Financing: The Report of the Working Group', 10 January 2022, https://apps.who.int/gb/ebwha/pdf_files/EB150/B150_30-en.pdf.

85. WHO, 'Working Group on Sustainable Financing', 25 January 2022, https://apps.who.int/gb/ebwha/pdf_files/EB150/B150(2)-en.pdf.

3. **Stronger, enforceable sanctions:**[86] The WHO relies on consensus and diplomacy for the implementation of its recommendations. The IHR currently mandate that governments report any 'public health emergencies of international concern' and cooperate with the WHO, but the WHO has no legal ability to enforce this. There is a precedent with another UN-related organisation, the WTO, which has the ability to impose sanctions on its member countries when they fail to abide by its rules.[87] There are proposals to reform the IHR to include enforceable sanctions against countries that fail to comply with their mandate,[88] although this would probably not be acceptable to member states, especially large powers such as the United States, China, and India. Some member states might be glad to renegotiate the IHR, for a variety of conflicting agendas (perhaps to increase reporting requirements, reinforce the role of the WHO, shift other international/translational trade and travel obligations, and shift the requirements so that outbreaks do not shine lights on shortcomings), while others are reluctant to change the IHR for a variety of reasons (such as that the resulting instrument may be less effective, it would open up the difficult issue of state sovereignty, and negotiations would be time-consuming and expensive). At the moment, there does not seem to be any appetite to open the IHR to renegotiation, as reflected by member states deciding instead to establish a new negotiating body for a new pandemic-related international legal instrument, akin to the WHO FCTC. The WHO FCTC does not include enforceable sanctions but, like most UN Conventions, moves forward by consensus and holds regular Conference of Party Meetings with a regular reporting system where countries' progress (or lack of it) is published.

4. **More open governance:** There are recommendations that the governance of the WHO must be reformed to facilitate the inclusion of alternative voices, such as from civil society, and to better channel the influence of private philanthropists.[89] Appointing non-voting, non-state actors to the WHO's governing body is already under consideration.[90]

5. **More focussed mandate:** In theory, the WHO covers the broad remit of improving the health of all populations everywhere. Should the WHO examine the idea of focusing primarily on activities where it can bring the most added value?[91] It needs to be borne in mind that while new epidemics and their risk factors are complicated and lengthy, NCDs now cause 60 per cent of global deaths, and should not be ignored.

---

86. Chaumont, 'Opinion: 5 Ways to Reform'.
87. Ibid.
88. Ibid.
89. Ibid.
90. WHO, 'WHO Reform: Involvement of Non-state Actors in WHO's Governing Bodies Report by the Director-General', 4 January 2021, https://apps.who.int/gb/ebwha/pdf_files/EB148/B148_35-en.pdf.
91. Chaumont, 'Opinion: 5 Ways to Reform'.

6. **Bring in technical expertise from other sectors:** The WHO must maintain its technical focus but could broaden its expertise to include more input from political scientists, urban designers, lawyers, logisticians, philosophers, economists, and information technology specialists.[92]

7. **Improving the reporting system:** There are many practical suggestions regarding future pandemics. For example, countries with outbreaks might be more willing to share information if there was a gradient of warnings to the PHEIC, coded by colour, rather than an all-or-nothing decree.[93] There could be a more precise definition of a pandemic, and the obligation it would place upon all countries.

Reforms will not come immediately, if for no other reason than that the COVID-19 pandemic has not yet receded at the time of this book going to print. But if the discussion is delayed, then the danger is that the momentum and urgency might wane, as in the past. Panels were previously set up to assess failures in the response to the Ebola outbreak in West Africa in 2014–2016. One expert said: 'Less than 10 per cent of the recommendations were followed up on. We have an amazing talent to outrage ourselves about a situation, but when it comes time to deliver any change, there is very little traction, and people go back to doing whatever they had done before.'[94]

Could COVID-19 teach us to work differently?

---

92. C. Chaumont, 'Opinion: 5 Ways to Reform the World Health Organization, 5 August 2020, https://www.devex.com/news/opinion-5-ways-to-reform-the-world-health-organization-97843.

93. Maxmen, 'Why Did the World's Pandemic Warning System Fail'.

94. Ibid.

3

Good Governance Means Curbing Commercial Determinants of Health in the Time of COVID-19

Judith Mackay

> The tobacco industry has a well-documented history of deception and of capitalizing on humanitarian crises, and it is using the COVID-19 pandemic to attempt to improve its deteriorating public image. The tobacco industry has had no qualms about taking advantage of the COVID-19 pandemic by providing assistance to governments while continuing to interfere with the implementation of the WHO FCTC. But even during times of great need, we must remember the irreconcilable conflict between the interests of the tobacco industry and those of public health.
>
> —Dr Adriana Blanco Marquizo
> Head, Secretariat,
> World Health Organization Framework Convention on Tobacco Control[1]

Much has been written about government action during the COVID-19 pandemic, but remarkably little on another aspect—where the responsibility for action lies fully within the arena of government responsibility—private sector activities influencing commercial determinants of health (CDHs) during the pandemic. These CDHs are not new; sectors of the public health community have been battling them for decades. The tobacco industry was the first industry in modern history to be recognised as interfering with public health policy. More recently, similar tactics have been used by other industries, such as the fast food, alcohol, and sweetened beverages industries. This interference occurs at the international level and involves the infiltration of several United Nations organisations. It also occurs at the national level and includes attempts to influence governments, politicians, and the media.

Big Tobacco, Big Food, Big Soda, Big Alcohol, Big Gambling, Big Formula, Big Coal, and Big Oil—all of these industries contribute to the global burden of non-communicable diseases (NCD). Yet, these industries immediately devised remarkably similar strategies to capitalise on the COVID-19 pandemic. The Non-Communicable Disease Alliance and SPECTRUM Research Consortium crowd-sourced, mapped,

1.   Mary Assunta, 'Global Tobacco Industry Interference Index 2021', Global Center for Good Governance in Tobacco Control (GGTC), Bangkok, Thailand, November 2021, https://exposetobacco.org/global-index/.

analysed, and exposed industry COVID-19 practices from around the world that could ultimately increase NCD and worsen the severity of the pandemic.[2]

As early as September 2020, the initiative had already received 786 submissions from over 90 countries, with the most frequently cited countries being the United Kingdom and United States (each made 119 submissions), followed by Australia (56), India (43), Mexico (34), Brazil (29), and Jamaica (28). All of these examples involved governments, directly or indirectly. Numerically, alcohol and ultra-processed food and drinks products topped the list of reports (not necessarily indicating the order of seriousness), followed by tobacco, breast milk substitutes, fossil fuel and gambling.

The Non-Communicable Disease Alliance report, 'Signalling Virtue, Promoting Harm', raises concerns of 'corporate capture' of policy and public image during the pandemic, ironically by the very industries that are fuelling the burden of NCD worldwide and putting people at greater risk of severe COVID-19 outcomes. The report outlined four main strategies used by a multitude of industries—pandemic-tailored marketing campaigns and stunts, corporate social responsibility (CSR) programmes, shaping policy environments, and fostering partnerships with governments, international agencies and non-governmental organisations (NGOs).[3] The top activity was marketing and adapting advertising to the context of COVID-19, followed by CSR initiatives and involvement with policy, even though the latter might be more difficult to uncover. The irony is that most of these industries make people more vulnerable to COVID-19, yet these industries are positioning themselves as saviours. They are highly resilient industries. The Chairman and Chief Executive Officer of Coca-Cola said in March 2020: 'We do know that over 134 years of a business we've seen many types of crisis, be they military, economic, or pandemic, and the Coca-Cola Company has always emerged stronger in the end.'[4]

Detailed examples from the tobacco industry are given in this chapter. Outside the tobacco control community, there is little awareness of the sheer magnitude of the global scale of the malfeasance of the tobacco industry to derail tobacco control and undermine public health. The reality is that no government today can expect to pass effective tobacco control legislation or increase tobacco taxes without interference and legal or trade challenges mounted by the tobacco industry. What is mentioned in this chapter is but a fraction of the array of strategies that the tobacco industry has continuously used to impair public health over the past several decades.

2. NCD Alliance, 'Explore a Snapshot and Share Examples of Unhealthy Commodity Industries' Responses to COVID', 9 June 2020, https://ncdalliance.org/news-events/news/explore-a-snapshot-and-share-examples-of-unhealthy-commodity-industries-responses-to-COVID-19%C2%A0.
3. Jeff Collin, Rob Ralston, Sarah Hill, and Lucinda Westerman, 'Signalling Virtue, Promoting Harm: Unhealthy Commodity Industries and COVID-19', 2020, NCD Alliance, SPECTRUM, https://ncdalliance.org/sites/default/files/resource_files/Signalling%20Virtue%2C%20Promoting%20Harm_Sept2020_FINALv.pdf.
4. Motley Fool Transcribers, 'Coca-Cola Co (KO) Q1 2020 Earnings Call Transcript', 21 April 2020, https://www.fool.com/earnings/call-transcripts/2020/04/21/coca-cola-co-ko-q1-2020-earnings-call-transcript.aspx.

The World Health Organization (WHO) Report of the Committee of Experts on Tobacco Industry published in July 2000 stated:

> Evidence from tobacco industry documents reveals that tobacco companies have operated for many years with the deliberate purpose of subverting the efforts of World Health Organization to control tobacco use. The attempted subversion has been elaborate, well-financed, sophisticated and usually invisible.[5]

Australia faced three legal challenges when it pioneered the introduction of plain cigarette packaging—a constitutional challenge, a challenge via a bilateral investment treaty between Australia and Hong Kong, and a challenge through the World Trade Organization. Jane Halton, Australian Secretary of the Department of Health and Ageing, said in 2011:

> It is fair to say that we are being targeted by what can only be described as subversive and disgraceful tactics by the tobacco industry, including using every available vehicle and opportunity to try and intimidate and/or threaten us to withdraw the legislation.[6]

In 2021, during the COVID-19 pandemic, Hong Kong banned e-cigarettes and heated tobacco products. It was not the first jurisdiction to do so, but the government and the legislators came under intense pressure. One veteran legislator said he had never seen such massive lobbying of legislators on *any* topic—health or otherwise—during his two decades as a legislator.

Tobacco industry strategies have included tobacco advertising, promotion and sponsorship (which undermine government public health messages); discrediting proven science and economic data; manoeuvring to oppose the political and legislative process; exaggerating the economic importance of the industry; manipulating public opinion to gain the appearance of respectability; fabricating support through front groups; and intimidating governments with litigation of the threat of litigation or trade threats. These condemnations may seem harsh or even extreme, but the examples come from the WHO, hardly a radical body.[7]

Tobacco industry products are responsible for eight million deaths a year globally. More than seven million of those deaths are the result of direct tobacco use while around 1.2 million are the result of non-smokers being exposed to second-hand smoke. Tobacco kills at least half of its users. Over 80 per cent of the world's 1.3 billion tobacco users live in low- and middle-income countries.[8] While Big Tobacco makes its profits, it is governments or individuals who end up paying for the disease and death it causes.

---

5. Michael Eriksen, Judith Mackay, Neil Schluger, Farhad Islami Gomeshtapeh, and Jeffrey Drope, *The Tobacco Atlas*, 5th ed. (Atlanta, GA: American Cancer Society; and New York: World Lung Foundation, 2015). Available at http://tobaccoatlas.org.
6. Michael Eriksen, Judith Mackay, and Hana Ross, *The Tobacco Atlas*, 4th ed. (Atlanta, GA: American Cancer Society; New York: World Lung Foundation, 2012), Chapter 30. Also available at tobaccoatlas.org.
7. World Health Organization (WHO), World No Tobacco Day materials, 2012, https://www.euro.who.int/__data/assets/pdf_file/0005/165254/Tobacco-Industry-Interference-A-Global-Brief.pdf.
8. WHO, 'Tobacco: Key Facts', 24 May 2022, https://www.who.int/news-room/fact-sheets/detail/tobacco.

Tobacco is already responsible for health and productivity losses of around US$1.4 trillion every year. Health economists agree that tobacco is bad for the health and wealth of nations. COVID-19 and tobacco both exacerbate poverty.

The tobacco industry is rich and powerful: the combined revenues of the world's tobacco companies are close to a trillion US dollars. The profit equivalent is equal to the combined profits of Coca-Cola, Walt Disney, General Mills, FedEx, AT&T, Google, McDonald's, and Starbucks. The industry hardly fears governments because of its extensive resources and global market power.[9] For decades, the tobacco industry has attempted to intervene with public health policy, for example, by trying to prevent, delay or dilute the enactment of government tobacco control legislation and tax policy.

The actions of this predatory industry have long been incompatible with the WHO's first and only international convention—the Framework Convention on Tobacco Control (WHO FCTC), which came into force in February 2005. The WHO FCTC was, in its time, one of the fastest track United Nations conventions to be brought into force and ratified by the vast majority of countries in the world. By 2022, it had been ratified by 182 countries. Even during the drafting of the treaty 20 years earlier, it had been recognised that this treaty needed a unique article to rein in the tobacco industry. Article 5.3 of the WHO FCTC states:

> In setting and implementing their public health policies with respect to tobacco control, Parties shall act to protect these policies from commercial and other vested interests of the tobacco industry in accordance with national law.

In 2008, the WHO issued extensive Guidelines for Article 5.3,[10] emphasising that it applied to all branches of government—the executive, the legislature, and the judiciary.

Tobacco Industry in the Time of COVID-19

> The tobacco industry is unique in that even six decades after its product was found to be harmful and with the associated deaths mounting each day, it has remained recalcitrant and not taken any responsibility. This industry cannot be rehabilitated. It is in the hands of governments to stop it.
>
> —Mary Assunta, Global Center for Good Governance in Tobacco Control, 2022

Like many other background aspects of the COVID-19 epidemic, commercial interference in public health policy already existed. Governments should have anticipated that the industry would use its familiar tactics to exploit any epidemic and take immediate preventive action. Tobacco industry interference in public health is remarkably similar in countries around the world; it is the government response that varies. COVID-19 thus provides a litmus test in revealing responsible governance.

---

9. Eriksen et al., *The Tobacco Atlas*, 5th ed., Chapter 16, p. 48. Available at http://tobaccoatlas.org/ Data from 2013.
10. WHO Framework Convention on Tobacco Control, Article 5.3, Guidelines, 2008.

This chapter illustrates how the industry adapted the same interference strategies in the COVID-19 epidemic, strategies that would be expected to have a detrimental effect on both the pandemic and the tobacco epidemics.

These practices are well-documented and are published by the global tobacco industry watchdog Stopping Tobacco Organizations and Products (STOP) in a yearly series of Tobacco Industry Interference Indexes. The 2020 and 2021 editions of the Index both published exhaustive lists of tobacco industry interference during COVID-19.[11] The 2021 Index covered 80 countries and ranked them under several broad categories.

The Index examines several key areas affecting governance, with myriad examples from around the world:

1. The tobacco industry interfered in policy development and implementation.
2. The tobacco industry's pandemic-related CSR activities enhanced access to senior officials.
3. The tobacco industry received incentives that benefitted its business.
4. Inappropriate interactions occurred between governments and the industry.
5. Transparency and accountability decreased.
6. Public officials faced conflicts of interest.
7. Lack of government implementation of solutions to protect themselves from industry interference.

The study also concluded that in general non-parties languished behind parties to the WHO FCTC.

The Dominican Republic and Switzerland together occupied the worst category in allowing tobacco industry interference, followed by Japan, Indonesia, and Georgia. The United States was 11th worst, and China was 13th worst out of the 80 countries; however, China's score improved between 2020 and 2021, while the United States' score deteriorated. Brunei headed the table in a category of its own as the best at resisting tobacco industry interference, followed by New Zealand, the United Kingdom, France, Uganda, the Netherlands, Mongolia, Iran, and Kenya. As clearly shown in the indexes, the tobacco industry has exploited the pandemic to engage with governments to an extraordinary level, with government receipt and endorsement of charitable contributions (CSR activities) being the industry's key avenue to access senior officials, including several instances of the industry involving the prime minister's offices in various countries. The industry capitalised on the vulnerability of governments that faced a shortage of resources during the pandemic. Even in countries where health departments and ministries have a policy of not accepting donations from the tobacco industry, this was put aside during the pandemic.[12]

11. Mary Assunta, 'Global Tobacco Industry Interference Index 2019', GGTC, Bangkok, Thailand, November 2020, https://exposetobacco.org/wp-content/uploads/GlobalTIIIndex2020_Report.pdf, appendix A, p. 41.
12. Ibid.

The industry has engaged in the following activities during COVID-19:

1. Confusing the science[13]

Scientists with financial links to the tobacco industry published research related to COVID-19 without declaring their tobacco industry links. The research suggested that nicotine offers protection from COVID-19 infection. This hypothesis was published primarily on pre-print publishing platforms without peer review, such as Qeios, indicating that smokers were less likely to catch COVID-19.[14]

The Foundation for a Smoke-Free World, funded by Philip Morris International, published blogs and surveys on its website, including blogs that stated: 'there is currently no evidence that smokers who are diagnosed with COVID-19 are more likely to be hospitalized than non-smokers', and another that stated that 'more research needed' to be done before the public was warned about the potential risk factors tobacco products posed for COVID-19.[15]

In the United States, Bidi Vapor claimed on Instagram that 'A bidi stick a day keeps the pulmonologist away.'[16]

According to STOP, the studies have prompted a wide range of potentially misleading media reports with headlines, such as 'Smokers four times less likely to contract COVID-19', 'Smoking may lower coronavirus risk', 'Does nicotine help against the new coronavirus?', suggesting that smoking, and by implication nicotine, might reduce the risk of COVID-19. They led to some potentially dangerous misinterpretations. In France, the government issued a statement warning of misinterpretation, followed by an order limiting the sale of nicotine products to prevent panic buying and misuse. According to the Iranian Anti-Tobacco Association, the stories went viral in Iran, a country with high death tolls from COVID-19. The organisation reported that people were taking up smoking for the first time to protect themselves from COVID-19.[17]

The reality is that all forms of tobacco use are linked to COVID-19.[18] Smokers who develop symptomatic COVID-19 have almost three times the risk of dying than non-smokers.[19] People who vape and use waterpipes are at increased risk of contracting

13. Tobacco Tactics, 'COVID-19', accessed 13 September 2022, https://tobaccotactics.org/wiki/COVID-19/#database; STOP, 'Studies that Suggest Smoking and Nicotine Protect Against COVID-19 Are Flawed', New York, 28 April 2020 (and Iran), https://exposetobacco.org/news/flawed-COVID19-studies.

14. Tobacco Tactics, 'COVID-19'.

15. Ibid., https://tobaccotactics.org/wiki/COVID-19/#ttref-note-11, and https://tobaccotactics.org/wiki/COVID-19/#database.

16. Campaign for Tobacco-Free Kids (CTFK), 'Big Tobacco Is Exploiting COVID-19 to Market Its Harmful Products', 2020, https://www.tobaccofreekids.org/media/2020/2020_05_COVID-marketing.

17. STOP, 'Studies that Suggest'.

18. WHO, 'How to Protect Yourself', accessed 13 September 2022, https://www.who.int/southeastasia/outbreaks-and-emergencies/COVID-19/What-can-we-do-to-keep-safe/protective-measures/no-tobacco; Matthew L. Myers, 'Contrary to Recent Headlines, Evidence Indicates Smokers Are at Greater Risk, Not Protected, from COVID-19', Statement of Matthew L. Myers, President, Campaign for Tobacco-Free Kids, 24 April 2020, tobaccofreekids.org/press-releases/2020_04_24_tobacco-risk-COVID-19.

19. R. Peto, personal communication, January 2021, citing Million Women Study.

COVID-19 too. According to a Stanford University study, vapers have a five to seven times higher risk of contracting COVID-19.[20] Studies that suggest smoking and nicotine protect against COVID-19 are flawed.[21]

2. Attempting to shift its image to that of a trusted health partner

The tobacco industry has attempted to shift its image from vilified to trusted health partner, using COVID-19 to make and maximise contact with policy-makers and health professionals.[22] The industry has exploited the pandemic with a multi-pronged tactic to entice, persuade and coerce governments to adopt weaker public health policies. Many governments made vulnerable by the pandemic freely accepted and endorsed charity from the industry. Such donations often came with strings attached and compromising policies. Instead of removing benefits to the industry, many governments made decisions that benefitted the industry, particularly in lowering or not imposing taxes and delaying legislation or its implementation.[23]

The industry is providing resources to countries badly in need of them, framing itself as being 'part of the solution'—a classic tactic of the tobacco industry to get close to governments and enable it to interfere with, derail and undermine health policies. In reality, the industry is 'part of the problem' not 'part of the solution.' While governments have obligations under the WHO FCTC and also have the power to tighten regulations on the industry, unfortunately, the opposite seems to have happened during COVID-19. In many countries, governments have protected and even promoted the industry.[24] Although governments identified tobacco industry interference as a main obstacle to their efforts to implement tobacco control measures, many became vulnerable to the industry's tactics.[25] Many government officials even met with tobacco industry executives in a non-transparent manner and were persuaded to allow their business to function as 'essential' during the pandemic lockdowns.[26]

3. Promoting and selling more tobacco

Even in a pandemic, where all modes of tobacco use are a risk factor, the industry continued to produce and market its harmful products, often using social media influencers.[27] The industry also offered new and trendy tobacco products for approval and claimed

---

20. Erin Digitale, 'Vaping Linked to COVID-19 Risk in Teens and Young Adults', *Stanford Medicine*, 11 August 2020, https://med.stanford.edu/news/all-news/2020/08/vaping-linked-to-covid-19-risk-in-teens-and-young-adults.html.
21. STOP, 'Studies that Suggest'.
22. CTFK, 'Big Tobacco'.
23. Assunta, 'Global Tobacco Industry Interference Index 2019'.
24. Ibid.
25. Ibid.
26. Ibid.
27. CTFK, 'Big Tobacco'.

they were moving away from cigarettes. In reality, they were selling more cigarettes and simultaneously obstructing government regulatory efforts that would affect cigarette sales.[28] For example, British American Tobacco aggressively promoted its heated cigarette Glo in several countries with special discounts, contest prizes, and even offering branded face masks and hand sanitisers with purchase.[29]

4. Using CSR programmes

During the COVID-19 pandemic, the tobacco industry moved swiftly to step up its CSR activities, such as making donations to higher-risk communities, handing out personal protective equipment (PPE) to the health sector, and supplying medical equipment to hospitals.[30]

COVID-19-related tobacco industry CSR has been documented in dozens of countries, especially where the industry has subsidiaries and sells its products.[31] For example, the industry used COVID-19 opportunities for brand marketing, such as free masks bearing industry logos; and offering ventilators, gels, PPE and even cash, amid a flurry of publicity.[32] In Kazakhstan, British American Tobacco provided Glo-branded masks to more than a dozen Instagram influencers who posted photos wearing the masks, with captions advertising free Glo masks with the purchase of a Glo device.[33] The Korean tobacco company, KT&G, donated oxygen generators to Indonesia and Russia. The KT&G website stated: 'We fulfilled our corporate social responsibilities by providing COVID-19 diagnostic kits to Indonesia, Russia, and Turkey *where our overseas subsidiaries are located.*'[34] VPZ, the largest vape retailer in the United Kingdom, offered £100,000 in coupons for a free vaping device as a 'thank you' to National Health Service frontline staff.[35] Philip Morris International reported it donated over US$32 million across 62 markets in the first few months of the pandemic. In the countries surveyed, its CSR activities included the distribution of ventilators to the Czech Republic and hand sanitisers to Brazil, Indonesia, the Netherlands, and the Philippines. In India, ITC Limited (formerly known as the India Tobacco Company) partnered with the Government of Kerala, through its brand, Savlon, on a state-wide handwashing campaign called 'Break the Chain'.

28. Assunta, 'Global Tobacco Industry Interference Index 2019'.
29. CTFK, 'Big Tobacco'.
30. Assunta, 'Global Tobacco Industry Interference Index 2019'.
31. Tobacco Unmasked South Asia, 'Globally Reported Tobacco Industry Interference during COVID-19 Pandemic', accessed 13 September 2022, https://www.tobaccounmaskedsouth.asia/Globally_Reported_ Tobacco_Industry_Interference_during_COVID-19_Pandemic.
32. CTFK, 'Big Tobacco'.
33. Ibid.
34. KT&G, 'KT&G to Deliver Medical Oxygen Generators to Russia . . . Support for Overcoming COVID-1', 9 November 2021, https://en.ktng.com/ktngNewsView?cmsCd=CM0048&ntNo=483&rnum=450&src=&s rcTemp=&currtPg=1.
35. Alan Selby, 'Vape Firm Says Thank You to Frontline NHS Staff with Vouchers for E-cigs', *The Mirror*, 11 August 2020, https://www.mirror.co.uk/news/uk-news/vape-firm-says-thank-you-22504039.

5. Interfering with governments' COVID-19 responses

While publicising its charitable acts to resuscitate its image as being part of the solution, the tobacco industry was simultaneously lobbying governments not to impose restrictions on its business and even to declare tobacco as an 'essential' item during the pandemic.

In South Africa, for example, the tobacco industry challenged the government after it banned cigarette sales during lockdown. In Kenya, the government listed tobacco products as 'essential products' under the foods and beverages category during the COVID-19 pandemic, which meant logistics providers of those sectors were given protection and special permits to transport during the lockdown. In Jordan, three days into the complete lockdown, the government instructed city buses to deliver bread and other essentials directly to neighbourhoods, and the Minister of Labour announced the government would initiate the distribution of cigarettes to smokers as well. Jordan documented a more than 50 per cent increase in consumption of tobacco during the lockdown.[36]

6. Interfering more broadly with tobacco control policy

The industry used COVID-19 as an opportunity to block, amend, and delay broader tobacco control measures while governments were distracted.[37] In many countries that received charity from the industry, the report found the tobacco industry received tax benefits in the form of reduced taxes, no tax increases, or tax exemptions.[38] Her Royal Highness Princess Dina Mired of Jordan said tobacco companies 'preyed on governments during the pandemic'.[39]

7. Producing COVID-19 vaccines

Several tobacco companies are in the business of producing COVID-19 vaccines. These include the Philip Morris subsidiary Medicago's vaccines in Canada,[40] British American

36. Assunta, 'Global Tobacco Industry Interference Index 2019'.
37. Patricio V. Marquez, 'Tobacco Use and Coronavirus (COVID-19): A Deadly but Preventable Association', World Bank Blogs, 27 May 2020, https://blogs.worldbank.org/voices/tobacco-use-and-coronavirus-COVID-19-deadly-preventable-association; Tobacco Reporter, 'Sampoerna Suspends Operations After Covid Deaths', 1 May 2020, https://tobaccoreporter.com/2020/05/01/sampoerna-suspends-factory-operations-after-coronavirus-deaths.
38. Jenny Lei Ravelo, 'Tobacco Industry "Preyed On" Governments During COVID-19 — Report', Devex, 4 November 2021, https://www.devex.com/news/tobacco-industry-preyed-on-governments-during-COVID-19-report-101973.
39. Ibid.
40. Philip Morris International, 'PMI Announces Medicago to Supply up to 76 Million Doses of Its Plant-Derived COVID-19 Vaccine Candidate', accessed October 2020, https://www.marketscreener.com/quote/stock/PHILIP-MORRIS-INTERNATION-2836703/news/Philip-Morris-International-PMI-Announces-Medicago-to-Supply-Up-to-76-Million-Doses-of-Its-Plant-D-31601227.

Tobacco's biotech subsidiary Kentucky BioProcessing's vaccine,[41] and others. This was hailed by the industry with headlines such as 'Tobacco to the rescue' on the cover of the industry's own journal, with the subtitles 'The industry's remarkable efforts to develop a COVID-19 vaccine', 'The unlikely savior', and posing questions such as 'Does nicotine protect against the coronavirus?'

These vaccines are enabling the industry to gain enormous favourable publicity,[42] and eventually access to the WHO and governments, in direct conflict with WHO FCTC Article 5.3. The big concern is that these tobacco industry vaccines become part of the COVID-19 Vaccines Global Access (COVAX) distribution programme. The Philip Morris-Medicago vaccine is partly funded by the Canadian government, and Canada has offered the vaccine to COVAX, which is co-led by the Coalition for Epidemic Preparedness Innovations (CEPI), Vaccine Alliance (GAVI) and the WHO, alongside the key delivery partner United Nations International Children's Emergency Fund (UNICEF). COVAX aims to accelerate the development and manufacture of COVID-19 vaccines, and to guarantee fair and equitable access for every country in the world. The Canadian tobacco industry vaccine could lead to the unimaginable situation of GAVI, the WHO, CEPI, and UNICEF sitting in the same room and discussing public health with the tobacco industry. At a minimum, the distribution of all vaccines through COVAX should comply with both the WHO Framework of Engagement with Non-State Actors (FENSA)[43] and WHO FCTC Article 5.3 mentioned earlier: 'In setting and implementing their public health policies with respect to tobacco control, Parties shall act to protect these policies from commercial and other vested interests of the tobacco industry in accordance with national law.'[44]

There needs to be a firewall between the tobacco industry and COVAX, national governments, and the end recipients. All four of the founding partners of COVAX are committed to reducing the tobacco epidemic and protecting public health. Donors to COVAX include many of the 182 countries and regions that are parties to the WHO FCTC, as well as several foundations that have strong anti-tobacco policies, including the Bill and Melinda Gates Foundation. However, in March 2022, the WHO announced that it refused to approve Medicago's COVID-19 vaccine because of the pharmaceutical company's ties to the tobacco industry. At the time of writing, it has also not been approved by national regulators for distribution in the UK, EU or the US. The issue is not yet completely resolved, as the Canadian government and Medicago might attempt to sell or distribute directly to countries.

41. Patricia Nilsson and Clive Cookson, 'BAT Joins Race to Develop COVID-19 Vaccine', *Financial Times*, 1 April 2020, ft.com/content/e3737752-6147-4c0e-82f2-e7df9eb9f6f8.

42. 'How a Use for Tobacco Helps Accelerate COVID-19 Vaccine', *Ejinsight*, 28 October 2020, https://www.ejin-sight.com/eji/article/id/2617626/20201028-How-a-use-for-tobacco-helps-accelerate-COVID-19-accine.

43. WHO, 'Guide for Staff on Engagement with Non-State Actors', Framework of Engagement with Non-State Actors (FENSA), accessed 13 September 2022, https://www.who.int/docs/default-source/documents/fensa/fensa-guide-for-staff.pdf?sfvrsn=46b61881_2.

44. WHO Framework Convention on Tobacco Control, Article 5.3.

Actions to Minimise the Influence of the Tobacco and Other Industries during the Pandemic

1. World Health Organization

WHO Economic and Commercial Determinants of Health Programme

So concerned had the WHO become about the tactics of the unhealthy commodity industries, that in 2021 it introduced a new programme called the 'Economic and Commercial Determinants of Health.' The programme has four goals: to strengthen the evidence base; develop tools and the capacity to address commercial determinants; convene partnerships and dialogue; and raise awareness and advocacy. For example, this programme runs a series of webinars and discussions on CDH.

WHO defines CDH as private sector activities that affect people's health positively or negatively.[45] Although there are positive contributions to well-being by 'healthy' industries ranging from manufacturers of bicycles and other sports equipment to makers of motorcycle helmets or seat belts, most attention is on the unhealthy commodity industries: tobacco, ultra-processed foods, sugar-sweetened beverages, and alcohol, which lead to NCD such as high blood pressure, Type 2 diabetes, certain cancers, cardiovascular disease, and obesity.

The WHO is rightly concerned at how private enterprise now plays an increasing role in public health policy and regulations, and the COVID epidemic is a recent example of this. The tobacco industry and other corporations influence public health through political lobbying and funding, including donations to political parties, and by courting the media. More subtly, corporations influence the science through funding medical education and research, where data may be skewed in favour of commercial interests. They further shape preferences through corporate front groups, consumer groups and think tanks, and CSR programmes, allowing them to manufacture doubt and promote their own industry framings.

WHO Framework Convention on Tobacco Control

In the case of tobacco, it is shown that governments that followed the WHO FCTC Article 5.3 and its Guidelines are better able to safeguard their tobacco control efforts during the pandemic, while governments that did not follow Article 5.3 found their efforts being undermined, delayed, or defeated by the industry.[46] Government-wide implementation of Article 5.3 of the convention is one powerful means of protecting tobacco control policies from the influence of private industries.

---

45. WHO, 'Commercial Determinants of Health', 5 November 2021, https://www.who.int/news-room/fact-sheets/detail/commercial-determinants-of-health.
46. Assunta, 'Global Tobacco Industry Interference Index 2019'.

2. Government action

During the COVID-19 pandemic, several governments took action to protect public health. India and South Africa banned the sale of tobacco products during the pandemic, while in the Philippines, three municipalities banned the sale of cigarettes, Mexico prohibited the sale of e-cigarettes, and the United States listed vape, smoking and cigar shops as non-essential businesses that must close. Hong Kong banned new tobacco products.

To protect public health policy against tobacco and other harmful industries, especially during COVID-19, STOP advises that:

1. **The whole of government, not just the health sector, must curb interference in public health policy by the tobacco and other negative industries.** For example, a whole-of-government approach to implementing WHO FCTC Article 5.3 was done in Botswana, the Philippines, and the United Kingdom.

2. **Endorsement of tobacco industry activities must stop.** Governments must limit interactions with tobacco and other harmful industries to only when strictly necessary for regulation.

3. **Denormalise so-called socially responsible activities.** Governments must reject harmful industries' CSR activities as these are a form of promotion and compromise the integrity of government officials to regulate the products.

4. **Reject non-binding agreements with the tobacco industry.** There should be no collaboration between governments and the industry.

5. **Stop giving incentives to the tobacco industry.** The tobacco industry should not be granted incentives or any preferential treatment to run its business as incentives directly conflict with tobacco control policy.

6. **Governments must divest from the tobacco industry.** Governments should financially divest from the tobacco business to obtain independence from it and prioritise public health. State-owned tobacco enterprises should be treated like any other tobacco company.

7. **Require greater transparency for increased accountability.** Transparency when dealing with unhealthy industries will reduce interference. All interactions must be recorded and made publicly available.

8. **Implement a code to provide a firewall.** Governments should adopt a code of conduct with clear guidance on interactions with the tobacco industry. For example, the Philippines government has introduced a civil service Code of Conduct when dealing with the industry, but few countries have followed suit.

9. **Compel the tobacco industry to provide information about its business.** The tobacco industry should be compelled to disclose its expenditure on marketing, lobbying and philanthropic activities.

All of these recommendations apply equally to other unhealthy commodity industries. Tobacco control will never be successful unless the vectors—such as the tobacco industry—are exposed and curtailed. While NGOs and academia can research and expose the industry, it is the governments which are ultimately responsible for curtailing unhealthy industries and their influence on public health policy.

4

COVID-19 Vaccines and a Pathway out of the Pandemic

Benjamin J. Cowling

The development of COVID-19 vaccines occurred at lightning speed during the first year of the pandemic. Stringent public health and social measures had been used intermittently in most parts of the world in the first year of the pandemic, and vaccines represented a light at the end of the tunnel. That is because vaccines could be used to complement public health and social measures and reduce the impact of COVID-19 infections, with an expectation that they could eventually allow governments to relax all community-wide measures. However, expectations of vaccine performance had to be adjusted as the pandemic progressed and new SARS-CoV-2 variants emerged, while delays in the global sharing of vaccines led to discussions over equity. In the third year of the pandemic, it became clearer that repeated administration of COVID-19 vaccines will be key to protecting people, particularly older and more vulnerable individuals, as the disease continued to circulate globally into the summer of 2022.

A Brief History of Vaccines

Viruses such as SARS-CoV-2 require human or animal cells to reproduce and spread. When a person is infected with the SARS-CoV-2 virus, cells in their respiratory tract are invaded by the virus and used as virus-making factories to produce large numbers of copies of the virus. Those virus copies can then be emitted back out of the respiratory tract through breathing, talking, coughing, sneezing, vaping etc. and pass to another person. In this way, the virus propagates through a community.

Humans are born with an immune system that can fight off mild infections but can sometimes struggle to deal with more serious infections. Once the immune system notices that an infection is occurring, for example because cells are not performing their usual functions, an immune response is mounted with the aim of eliminating the virus from the body and repairing any damage that has occurred. A long-established observation in infectious diseases is that recovery from an infection can provide long-lasting immunity against re-infection. This long-lasting protection is due to the 'adaptive' component of our immune systems, including antibody-producing 'B cells' and killer 'T cells' that can hunt down and eliminate viruses and virus-infected cells. During infection, these cells learn to recognise the infecting pathogen and commit that recognition to a type of memory. One of the most important responses to a viral infection is the production by B cells of antibodies to that virus in case it is encountered again. Antibodies are small proteins that attach to the receptors on a virus surface and prevent the virus from being able to infect cells, as well as marking the virus as an intruder for other parts of the immune system to react to.

While immunity to common pathogens is clearly advantageous, acquiring that immunity through infection can be dangerous. Smallpox—caused by the virus *variola major*—killed 30 per cent of the people it infected, a remarkably high fatality rate. In China, an approach called variolation was used for many centuries to reduce the public health impact of smallpox. The dried scabs from smallpox survivors were collected and ground into a powder, which was then insufflated, i.e., blown up the nose. Another variolation approach spread from Turkey into Western Europe in the seventeenth and eighteenth centuries, which involved making superficial scratches or cuts in the skin and then exposing these either to scabs or contaminated clothes from an infected individual. The infections that resulted from variolation tended to be milder, although not without risk.

In the late eighteenth century Edward Jenner and other scientists noted the observation that milkmaids who contracted cowpox—an animal infection that was much milder in humans than smallpox—seemed to be immune to smallpox. Edward Jenner then demonstrated that deliberate infection with cowpox provided immunity to smallpox, and was safer than variolation. Since the pathogen causing cowpox was called *variolae vaccinae* (*vacca* is Latin for cow), Jenner named his procedure 'vaccination'. Interestingly, opposition to Jenner's vaccine grew into a huge anti-vaccination movement in the nineteenth century.[1] Ultimately, however, the mass global use of cowpox infection in the skin as a smallpox vaccine ultimately led to the eradication of smallpox by 1980.

While inoculation of one virus to provide immunity to another, more serious infection was the first approach to vaccination, it is not the most common. More than 20 vaccines are used worldwide to prevent human diseases caused by viruses, and most of these are made from either inactive viruses or non-infectious components of viruses.[2] Infection with attenuated (weakened) viruses has also been used as an approach to vaccination, most notably for polio. In more recent years, a new approach has been developed that involves genetically modifying one virus (including removal of disease-causing genes) and inserting part of the genetic code of a second virus. The first virus

1.　Jess McHugh, 'The World's First Anti-Vaccination Movement Spread Fears of Half-Cow Babies', *Washington Post*, 14 November 2021, https://www.washingtonpost.com/history/2021/11/14/smallpox-anti-vaccine-england-jenner.

2.　Brian Greenwood, David Salisbury, and Adrian V. S. Hill, 'Vaccines and Global Health', *Philosophical Transactions of the Royal Society of London. Series B, Biological Sciences* 366, no. 1579 (2011): 2733–2742, https://doi.org/10.1098/rstb.2011.0076.

is then used as a vector to carry the genetic material of the target virus and train our immune system to respond to future exposures to viruses with the same components. Because the vector virus is designed to be able to infect cells, it can also stimulate a robust cellular response in addition to the production of antibodies.

Rapid Development of COVID Vaccines

From the early days of the COVID-19 pandemic, it was clear that infections were so severe that unmitigated epidemics would lead to considerable loss of life. The three major toolboxes for mitigating viral epidemics and pandemics include (1) public health and social measures, (2) antiviral drugs and associated therapeutics for the treatment of infections, and (3) biological vaccines and prophylactics to prevent infections. Given that antivirals and vaccines were not initially available, most governments around the world could only rely on public health and social measures to suppress transmission in the early months of the pandemic.

The vaccine development cycle typically takes many years because of the sequence of steps required. The pre-clinical development of a candidate vaccine involves identifying a formulation of virus or virus components that could stimulate a protective immune response, as well as other necessary ingredients such as stabilisers and preservatives. Some vaccines also include chemicals known as adjuvants that can help to stimulate a stronger immune response to the vaccine. The clinical development process typically includes a series of trials in humans, starting with small trials to measure the immune response and common side effects, followed by larger trials to determine the effectiveness of the vaccine in preventing the disease of interest.

For COVID-19 vaccines, this cycle was compressed into less than a year, by speeding up the pre-clinical process and by moving through clinical trials at a record pace. Vaccine developers moved faster than usual, often running multiple trials in parallel, and setting up the next round of clinical trials while waiting for the previous round to finish in the expectation (or hope) that those results would be positive. Regulators such as the United States Food and Drug Administration provided rapid evaluation and emergency approvals. Vaccine manufacturing was also scaled up, often before the availability of clinical trial results and regulatory approval, taking the risk that the vaccine might not ultimately be approved. The rapid development of vaccines and scaling up of manufacturing capacity were generally supported by public funds. For example, the vaccines developed by Moderna and Johnson & Johnson were aided by American government funding under Operation Warp Speed.[3] The development of the

---

3. Lancet Commission on COVID-19 Vaccines and Therapeutics Task Force Members, 'Operation Warp Speed: Implications for Global Vaccine Security', *Lancet Global Health* 9, no. 7 (2021): E1017–E1021, https://doi. org/10.1016/S2214-109X(21)00140-6.

Oxford University/AstraZeneca vaccine was largely supported by funds from the UK government.[4]

Around 30 COVID-19 vaccines are being used around the world, from four major technology classes (Table 4.1). The mRNA vaccines developed by BioNTech/Pfizer/Fosun Pharma and Moderna could be considered the newest technology, since mRNA vaccines have never previously been used in mass vaccination campaigns, although mRNA vaccines for several other diseases have been tested in clinical trials.[5] This novel technology works by encoding the recipe for viral components, in this case, the spike protein of SARS-CoV-2, in mRNA form and using cellular machinery to adapt the recipe and produce spike proteins. In simple terms, injection with an mRNA vaccine allows our own cells to be used as factories for SARS-CoV-2 spike proteins, and our immune system can then mount an immune response to those spike proteins that will provide protection against future exposures. While live vaccines also use our own cells as factories to produce more viruses that our immune system can respond to, there is always a risk that a live virus vaccine might transmit infection between individuals, as has happened with the live oral poliovirus vaccine for example. Viral subunit vaccines such as the one produced by Novavax include individual viral spike proteins rather than complete viruses, and therefore do not infect cells but stimulate an immune response to those viral components.

The vaccines against COVID-19 provide two layers of defence in general. The first layer is protection against infection, mostly mediated by antibodies. The second layer is protection against severe disease, even if infection occurs. An infection in a vaccinated individual is sometimes called a 'breakthrough' infection, and breakthrough infections can tend to be milder in severity than infections in unvaccinated individuals because of this second layer of defence, mediated by T cells and other components of the immune system. Whereas SARS-CoV-2 variants have been able to escape the first layer of defence by evading antibodies against the original strain of the virus, the second layer of defence against severe disease has generally remained robust and provided sustained protection against severe COVID-19 in breakthrough infections.

There is a clear difference in the approaches taken in China, relying mostly on inactivated vaccines, compared to the approach in Europe and North America of using newer technologies to manufacture vaccines with higher efficacy against mild infection. All vaccine technologies were able to provide a high level of protection against severe COVID-19.

4. Samuel Cross, Yeanuk Rho, Henna Reddy, Toby Pepperell, Florence Rodgers, Rhiannon Osborne, et al., 'Who Funded the Research behind the Oxford–AstraZeneca COVID-19 Vaccine?', *BMJ Global Health* (2021) 6: e007321, https://doi.org/10.1136/bmjgh-2021-007321.
5. Norbert Pardi, Michael J. Hogan, Frederick W. Porter, and Drew Weissman, 'mRNA Vaccines—A New Era in Vaccinology', *Nature Reviews Drug Discovery* 17 (2018): 261–279, https://doi.org/10.1038/nrd.2017.243.

Table 4.1: Overview of COVID-19 vaccine technologies

	mRNA	Viral Sub-unit	Viral Vector	Inactivated Virus
Example vaccines by manufacturer	BioNTech (Pfizer), Moderna	Novavax	AstraZeneca, Johnson & Johnson, CanSino	Sinovac, Sinopharm, Covaxin
Doses required to be 'fully vaccinated'[a]	Two	Two	Two	Two (<60y) or Three (≥60y)
Advantages	Very strong immune response	Very strong immune response	Broader and more durable immune response (in theory)	More traditional manufacturing approach
Disadvantages	Complex to develop and manufacture, stronger side-effects	Complex to develop and manufacture	Complex to develop and manufacture	Weak and short-lived immune response
Initial efficacy estimates against symptomatic COVID-19 with ancestral strain in large clinical trials	90%–95%	96%	76%	51%–78%
Initial efficacy estimates against severe COVID-19 with ancestral strain in large clinical trials	>99%	>99%	>99%	>99%

a. The definition of 'fully vaccinated' varies in different locations, here we refer to the World Health Organization recommendations for primary vaccination series.

Global Vaccination Uptake and Impact

As of August 2022, more than 12 billion doses of COVID-19 vaccines have been administered worldwide, and more than 68 per cent of the world's population has received at least one vaccine dose. In many higher-income countries, more than 70 per cent of the population have received at least two doses of vaccine, with many locations achieving high coverage with booster doses.

Israel was one of the first countries to achieve high vaccination coverage, and in February 2021 reached two-dose coverage of 84 per cent among persons ≥70 years of age. Substantial reductions in severe disease particularly in older adults were clear evidence of the impact of the vaccination programme.[6] As vaccination coverage continued to increase in Israel, by the end of March, levels of infection had dropped to a point where public health and social measures could be relaxed.[7]

However, a gradual loss of vaccine performance had become apparent by mid-2021, attributable to two specific phenomena. The first phenomenon was waning in immunity after vaccination, recognised for many vaccines, but not initially for COVID-19 vaccines because the focus of the earliest trials was short-term protection within a few months of receipt of initial vaccine doses. The second phenomenon was the emergence of SARS-CoV-2 variants. The first of these was the Alpha variant, first identified in the United Kingdom, and included a number of mutations on the spike protein that allowed the virus to infect individuals who already had antibodies against the original virus either through vaccination or infection, because of a mismatch between the antibodies against the original virus and against the mutated Alpha variant. A number of other variants were detected, each of which had the capacity to evade antibodies from prior infections or vaccinations, the most recent variant being Omicron.

Notwithstanding waning immunity and the emergence of variants, vaccines have saved many lives already, and will save many more in the coming years. One study estimated that almost half a million lives have been saved in the first 11 months of the vaccination programme in the European Union.[8] Another study conducted over a similar period estimated that vaccines have prevented more than 1 million deaths in the United States.[9]

---

6.   Ehud Rinott, Ilan Youngster, and Yair E. Lewis, 'Reduction in COVID-19 Patients Requiring Mechanical Ventilation Following Implementation of a National COVID-19 Vaccination Program—Israel, December 2020–February 2021', *Morbidity and Mortality Weekly Report* 70, no. 9 (2021): 326–328, https://doi.org/10.15585/mmwr.mm7009e3.

7.   Stuart Winer, 'With Most Israelis Now Fully Vaccinated, Virus Spread Continues Sharp Drop-Off', *Times of Israel*, 25 March 2021, https://www.timesofisrael.com/with-most-israelis-now-fully-vaccinated-virus-spread-continues-sharp-drop-off.

8.   Margaux M. I. Meslé, Jeremy Brown, Piers Mook, José Hagan, Roberta Pastore, Nick Bundle, et al., 'Estimated Number of Deaths Directly Averted in People 60 Years and Older as a Result of COVID-19 Vaccination in the WHO European Region, December 2020 to November 2021', *Eurosurveillance* 26, no. 47 (2021): pii=2101021, https://doi.org/10.2807/1560-7917.ES.2021.26.47.2101021.

9.   Eric C. Schneider, Arnav Shah, Partha Sah, Seyed M. Moghadas, Thomas Vilches, and Alison Galvani, 'The U.S. COVID-19 Vaccination Program at One Year: How Many Deaths and Hospitalizations Were Averted?', Commonwealth Fund, 14 December 2021, https://doi.org/10.26099/3542-5n54.

However, vaccines have not been equally available everywhere in the world. The World Health Organization established the 'COVAX' programme to provide vaccines worldwide with costs varying by income status (see Chapter 2). The concept of this programme was to encourage higher and lower-income locations to purchase vaccines through the programme, as well as to receive donations, using the large programmatic budget as leverage to negotiate for discounts on vaccine purchases that could then be passed to the lower-income locations. Vaccines purchased through COVAX would then be distributed fairly to all participating countries. By mid-April 2022, the COVAX programme had shipped 1.4 billion vaccine doses to 145 countries, somewhat short of the initial aim of 2 billion doses by the end of 2021 but still a fantastic achievement.

While initial vaccine programmes aimed to provide adults (and, more recently, children) with two vaccine doses, the loss of immunity to infection with virus variants has led to third dose 'booster' programmes in many locations, and even more recently to fourth-dose campaigns. There is clear evidence that these additional doses provide improved protection against infection and severe disease. Where discussion remains is the optimal interval between booster doses, whether it be as short as 3 months, as long as 12 months, or perhaps somewhere in between.

Individual Immunity, Population Immunity, and Herd Immunity

As noted above, COVID-19 vaccines provide two layers of defence—against infection, and against the development of severe disease if we still get infected. For the ancestral strains of the virus, the mRNA vaccines were extremely effective in preventing even mild infections. If infection can be prevented, then there is of course no chance of severe disease occurring. With the emergence of virus variants, however, vaccine effectiveness against infection has declined, and the second layer of defence has come to the fore. In a recent study of Omicron BA.2 cases in Hong Kong, my colleagues and I estimated that two doses of the mRNA vaccine produced by BioNTech/Pfizer/Fosun Pharma provided adults 20–59 years of age with around 31 per cent protection against mild infection, but 95 per cent protection against severe disease. In comparison, two doses of the inactivated vaccine produced by Sinovac provided adults 20–59 years of age with around 18 per cent protection against mild infection, but 92 per cent protection against severe disease.[10] While it is not yet fully understood which exact immune mechanisms contribute to the different layers of protection, a common view is that antibodies play a major role in protection against infection, while cellular immunity has a greater role in protection from severe disease in breakthrough infections.

---

10. Martina E. McMenamin, Joshua Nealon, Yun Lin, Jessica Y. Wong, Justin K. Cheung, Eric H. Y. Lau, et al., 'Vaccine Effectiveness of One, Two, and Three Doses of BNT162b2 and CoronaVac against COVID-19 in Hong Kong: A Population-Based Observational Study', Lancet Infectious Diseases 22, no. 10 (2022):1435–1443, https://doi.org/10.1016/s1473-3099(22)00345-0.

Immunity can also be acquired through infection, of course, and there are ongoing scientific debates about which source of immunity might be stronger or more durable, depending as well on the sequence of vaccination first or infection first, and the types of vaccines. Where there is no debate is that vaccination is a safer process than natural infection, not only because of the risk of severe disease in natural infections but also because of the possibility of exacerbation of an underlying medical condition and the possibility of developing long-term symptoms after recovery ('long COVID').

The broad concept of 'population immunity' refers to the degree of immunity in the population as a whole, perhaps against infections, or perhaps measured against severe disease. For example, a population in which the vaccine coverage is very high is likely to have a high level of population immunity against severe disease, in the sense that rates of severe disease in any epidemic would be substantially reduced by the high vaccine coverage. Because the risk of severe disease is much higher in older adults than in younger individuals, it is possible that population immunity against severe disease could still be considered high in a population that has a high vaccine coverage in older adults but a low vaccine coverage in other groups. Immunity from natural infections should also be considered in an assessment of population immunity.

A more specific concept is 'herd immunity'. This is a technical term in the study of infectious diseases, referring to a level of population immunity against infection that is high enough to prevent an epidemic from occurring. An example of herd immunity for COVID-19 is when Israel achieved a high enough vaccine coverage—above 60 per cent, with a highly effective vaccine (the mRNA vaccine produced by BioNTech/Pfizer/Fosun Pharma)—that COVID-19 transmission ceased in the community in early 2021. Given that a small fraction of the population had likely been infected and had natural immunity, the herd immunity threshold was likely surpassed when somewhere between 60 per cent and 70 per cent of the population had immunity against infection.

For the newer variants of COVID-19, such as the Omicron variant, vaccines do not provide a high level of protection against infection, and herd immunity cannot be achieved by vaccination alone. Infections however do provide strong specific immunity—there are very few known cases of re-infection with the same strain of the virus—and many locations have now reached herd immunity against Omicron BA.1 and BA.2 following epidemics of these viruses in their communities. In fact, there are only two reasons why daily COVID-19 case numbers decline over a period of time. One reason is because of the implementation of public health and social measures, as happened around the world in 2020 bringing community epidemics under control. The other reason is that the herd immunity threshold has been surpassed (at around the time an epidemic curve peaks), and the virus essentially runs out of people to infect. It is important to recognise that not everyone would be infected in such a scenario, the cumulative proportion of the population infected in an epidemic would exceed the herd immunity threshold but would fall short of 100 per cent (see Chapter 5). In Hong Kong's large community epidemic of Omicron BA.2 in February, March and April 2022 my colleagues and I estimate that around two-thirds of the population was infected, while a further fraction of perhaps 15 per cent of the population already had immunity against infection provided by vaccination, with three doses of an mRNA vaccine providing a moderate level of protection against infection that was higher than the protection provided by two doses of that vaccine or two or three doses of an inactivated vaccine.

Looking into the future, it is unlikely that vaccines will be able to provide strong immunity against infection unless somehow the strains included in vaccines can keep up with viral evolution. New vaccine technologies might be able to provide stronger protection, but there is not likely to be any short-term change in the technologies used for COVID-19 vaccines. Infections do provide long-lasting immunity against re-infection with the same strain, and the large community epidemics of Omicron subvariants that have been occurring in early 2022 will ultimately confer herd immunity against those specific subvariants. However, that herd immunity against one subvariant would likely not translate to herd immunity against another, and that was why in April 2022, the world saw an increasing spread of the latest Omicron subvariants, such as BA.4 and BA.5.

As time goes on, population immunity against severe disease will tend to rise to higher and higher levels because of the infections that occur in community epidemics, aided by booster vaccines, particularly in high-risk groups. This means that COVID-19 will likely pose less of a threat to public health as time goes on. In Hong Kong's population of 7.4 million, seasonal epidemics of influenza cause between 500 and 1,000 deaths annually, far fewer than the 9,000 deaths and counting caused by Omicron in 2022. But in future years, the annual death toll of COVID-19 might reduce to a level more comparable to influenza.

Vaccine Recommendations and Mandates

When COVID-19 vaccines were first introduced, priority was generally given to individuals at the highest risk of severe disease, i.e., older adults and those with underlying medical conditions, as well as those at potentially higher risk of infection or with an important role in society such as healthcare workers and other key workers. Vaccines were subsequently made available to other age groups, and many countries now offer COVID-19 vaccines to children. While some aspects of vaccine recommendations can vary from one country to another, it is clear that COVID-19 vaccines have provided benefits to all age groups that have received them, and that re-vaccination from time to time will be recommended in the years to come.

Where controversy has arisen is in the use of coercive policies to increase vaccination uptake beyond what can be achieved voluntarily, with the recognition that higher vaccine uptake will reduce the health impact of COVID-19 epidemic waves in a community. For example, Israel introduced a 'green pass' that restricted the movements of unvaccinated individuals (noting that recovery from a documented infection was permitted as an alternative to vaccination).[11] In January 2022, Austria introduced a law requiring all adults to receive COVID-19 vaccination, but withdrew it in March.[12] As of April 2022, a number of countries only permit residents or visitors to arrive in the country if they are vaccinated. Vaccine mandates, or the implementation of vaccine passes or passports, have a number of ethical considerations.[13]

According to the World Health Organization, mandating vaccination or any other medical procedure requires strong justification such as an emergency situation. That is because vaccination is a medical procedure and requires an 'informed consent' process beforehand. Three key components of the informed consent process include (1) the consenting person is of sound mind; (2) the consenting person understands the risks and benefits of the procedure; and (3) the consenting person does so voluntarily. These principles are modified when applied to children or those unable to consent themselves for some reason. A well-informed person is fully entitled to refuse a medical procedure, even if it unequivocally offers more benefits than risks.

COVID-19 has been a clear public health emergency since the World Health Organization first declared the Public Health Emergency of International Concern on 30 January 2020 (see Chapter 2). Stringent public health and social measures were implemented around the world in the first year of the pandemic. Restriction of individual freedoms with a range of public health measures was justified based on the societal risk, and particularly the risk of substantial harm to the community if healthcare systems became overwhelmed with COVID-19 cases. Once vaccines became available, they presented an opportunity to protect individuals and healthcare systems even after the relaxation of those public health measures. That is because the immunity provided by COVID-19 vaccines, as well as any immunity in the population following previous infections, could substantially reduce the risk of severe COVID-19.

Given compelling evidence of the effectiveness of vaccines, most developed countries have been able to achieve high vaccination coverage in the segments of their population at the highest risk of severe COVID-19, namely the elderly and those with underlying medical conditions. In many cases, high coverage was achieved without a mandate. In circumstances where vaccine coverage had not reached high levels in high-risk subpopulations, a mandate could have been justified to protect the community as a whole, despite overriding individual freedoms. Differences in the social contract, discussed elsewhere in this book, would also play into the rationale for mandates in different locations. However, moving into 2022 there seems to be little justification for continuing vaccine mandates, vaccine passes or vaccine passports. Any need for them had passed.

11. Shelly Kamin-Friedman and Maya Peled Raz, 'Lessons from Israel's COVID-19 Green Pass Program', *Israel Journal of Health Policy Research* 10, no. 61 (2021), https://doi.org/10.1186/s13584-021-00496-4.
12. Geir Moulson, 'Austria Suspends Vaccine Mandate before Enforcement Starts', *AP News*, 9 March 2022, https://apnews.com/article/covid-health-europe-austria-e0ebc5d6fa43913c8361f718a3688fb3.
13. Mark A. Hall and David M. Studdert, '"Vaccine Passport" Certification—Policy and Ethical Considerations', *New England Journal of Medicine* 385 (2021): e32, https://doi.org/10.1056/NEJMp2104289.

Vaccines in the Era of COVID-19 'Epidemicity'

It is now clear that SARS-CoV-2 will not disappear but will continue to cause infections around the world in the coming years. Successive emergence of variants, most recently the Omicron variant, will likely continue as the virus evolves to escape population immunity. SARS-CoV-2 infections will occur in periodic epidemics, perhaps more likely in the winter months in temperate locations, and so the term 'endemic' may not be the right term as it means the virus would remain in a community year-round. It is possible that some parts of the world will see temporary disappearances of the virus, with travellers then introducing the latest strains that will go on to cause local epidemics. In that sense, 'epidemicity' might perhaps be a better word.

An interesting debate has revolved around the severity of infections, with Omicron often perceived as 'milder' than previous strains of SARS-CoV-2. However, this is not actually the case. In Hong Kong, unvaccinated adults infected with Omicron had roughly the same risk of severe disease or death as they did in early waves with the original strain of SARS-CoV-2.[14] In adults with pre-existing immunity, either from a prior infection or from vaccination, Omicron is a milder infection. As levels of immunity reach higher and higher levels, SARS-CoV-2 will appear to become a milder and milder infection whether or not there is any change in its intrinsic severity.

Given that most individuals around the world now have some degree of immunity from infections, vaccinations, or a combination of both, SARS-CoV-2 will pose less of a threat to public health and the integrity of healthcare systems than it did in the first two years of the pandemic. However, the danger has not completely passed. New variants will emerge and cause large numbers of infections. Even when most infections are mild, the small fraction of more severe cases can still be a large absolute number and pose challenges for weak healthcare systems as influenza does in some years. A priority now is to ensure that vaccination coverage remains high in vulnerable individuals, particularly older adults and those with underlying medical conditions.

Nevertheless, one major country, China, chose to maintain its control measures for COVID-19 into April 2022, despite achieving high vaccination coverage. In China, the 'Dynamic Zero COVID' approach has successfully minimised the number of infections, severe COVID-19 cases, and deaths during the first two years of the pandemic. There are two major components of this approach. The first is to keep infections out of the local community as much as possible, achieved through strict on-arrival quarantines not only for arrivals from outside China but also in some cases for inter-provincial travellers. The second is to identify any outbreaks as quickly as possible and respond as quickly as possible with very stringent measures to control the outbreak while it is still at a very early stage. At the time of writing in June 2022, a large outbreak in Shanghai had just been controlled although not eliminated through a prolonged lockdown of

---

14. Yonatan Mefsin, Dongxuan Chen, Helen S. Bond, Yun Lin, Justin K. Cheung, Jessica Y. Wong, et al., 'Epidemiology of Infections with SARS-CoV-2 Omicron BA.2 Variant, Hong Kong, January–March 2022', *Emerging Infectious Diseases* 28, no. 9 (2022): 1856–1858, https://doi.org/10.3201/eid2809.220613.

more than two months combined with frequent testing of the entire population. This has been extremely costly and disruptive to China's largest and wealthiest city. If outbreaks continue to occur in Chinese cities, it is unlikely that the local elimination policy can be sustained without enormous social and economic impact.

One of the reasons sometimes used to explain China's persistence with Dynamic Zero COVID is the relatively lower vaccine coverage in the elderly compared to other age groups. A number of factors have led to the relatively lower vaccination uptake in the elderly to date, perhaps one being the overall elimination strategy that minimises the risk of infection and therefore minimises the risk of severe COVID-19 even in unvaccinated individuals. Vaccines provide a pathway out of the pandemic, but high vaccine coverage in the elderly will be essential if China is to minimise the health impact of a transition away from its Dynamic Zero COVID strategy.[15]

Now that fourth doses are being administered in some locations, it would be a good time to review the optimal timing of vaccine doses. Administering vaccines 3–4 times per year is unlikely to be sustainable, but perhaps twice-annual vaccination for the highest risk could be weighed against annual vaccination, with advantages and disadvantages of both. Among the advantages of twice-annual vaccination would be the regular top-up in immunity, but its disadvantages would be the additional costs and perhaps only incremental benefits, especially if SARS-CoV-2 tends towards winter epidemics. Similar discussions have occurred for influenza vaccination. One final issue is whether there is any immunologic disadvantage of frequent vaccination, which remains a controversial topic for influenza vaccination.[16]

In conclusion, the rapid development of SARS-CoV-2 vaccines has already likely saved millions of lives worldwide and allowed safe relaxation of public health and social measures with minimal morbidity and mortality, particularly in parts of the world that were able to keep COVID-19 at bay for the first two years of the pandemic.

15. Jun Cai, Xiaowei Deng, Juan Yang, Kaiyuan Sun, Hengcong Liu, Zhiyuan Chen, et al., 'Modeling Transmission of SARS-CoV-2 Omicron in China', *Nature Medicine* 28, no. 7 (2022): 1468–1475, https://doi.org/10.1038/s41591-022-01855-7.
16. Mark G. Thompson and Benjamin J. Cowling, 'How Repeated Influenza Vaccination Effects Might Apply to COVID-19 Vaccines', *Lancet Respiratory Medicine* 10, no. 7 (2022): 636–638, https://doi.org/10.1016/S2213-2600(22)00162-X.

5

The Mathematics of COVID-19

Michael Edesess

Emerging infectious diseases represent major threats to public health. SARS-CoV-2, a novel coronavirus that became known as the COVID-19 disease, not only resulted in very high numbers of infections and deaths all around the world, but also led to huge economic losses and social disruptions that threatened global security. While every pandemic is unique—and COVID-19 certainly has a set of unique manifestations as noted in Chapter 1—when a new disease, or a new variant of an old one, bursts upon the scene, four questions urgently need answers:

- How does it spread and how fast will it spread?
- How many cases will require hospitalisation or other emergency medical attention, and when will these needs arise?
- How many deaths will there be?
- What can be done to change and improve the outcome?

Mathematics played an important role in helping policy-makers and healthcare professionals answer these questions when COVID-19 emerged. Mathematical modelling provided quick, approximate answers. Its predictions improved as more information was gathered that could be applied to help stem the course of the disease. Over the course of COVID-19, including its variants, mathematics contributed greatly to fighting the pandemic. Much learned research was produced all around the world, resulting in many publications on all aspects of the disease.

But mathematics helps in another way. When a disease first appears and begins to spread, the situation is like the proverbial 'fog of war'. Little is known and it is confusing to try to understand what really matters and what doesn't. Mathematical modelling requires attention only to those variables that actually affect the spread of the disease. It tends to focus on the things that matter and removes focus from those that do not, providing much-needed clarity. For example, as we will see, from a mathematical modelling standpoint, the only things that matter to the spread of disease are (1) the number of contacts per day between an infectious person and a susceptible person; (2) the probability that the disease will be transmitted during a contact; and (3) the number of days for which an infectious person is infectious. Focusing on those things, as a mathematical epidemiological model does, helps policy-makers determine what levers they need to push to affect the course of the disease.

While epidemics emerge at least every five years, few of them have caused the high level of global concern, strong action, and urgency that COVID-19 did. The reason is simple: COVID-19's combination of transmissivity and virulence led to high hospitalisations and deaths. Other epidemics were contained quickly, had low transmissivity or low virulence, died out on their own after an initial panic (such as severe acute respiratory syndrome or SARS), submitted to vaccines or pharmaceutical remedies, or became endemic in the global population with varying effectiveness of treatments and preventive measures (such as malaria or tuberculosis). What was unique about COVID-19 was that mathematical models predicted a very high level of severe cases, hospitalisations, and deaths in the tens of millions if immediate action was not taken. These predictions were taken very seriously in some countries and acted upon, and much less seriously in others, partly because in those countries the mitigating measures were not acceptable to many people and to the countries' leaders themselves. This difference in national action in response to the predictions, and the explanations for them, has widened the gulfs between governmental systems and social contracts, and even between social groups within nations. The key catalyst was the predictive models, upon which countries could either act firmly, rapidly, and decisively or in a more desultory manner, depending on their national philosophies and level of organisation.

How Fast Will It Spread?

At the beginning of any outbreak, the speed of spread is exponential. Exponential growth, a concept taught at school, starts slowly at first but then is extremely rapid. Exponential growth is often illustrated by the example of placing coins, or grains of rice, on a checkerboard with sixty-four squares. One coin is placed on the first square, two on the second, four on the third, and eight on the fourth. The number of coins placed on a square then continues to double on each square. Most people are completely surprised to learn that by the time the process gets to the 64th square, the number of coins placed on that square will be more than 18 million trillion, a number that can be written as the number 18 with 18 zeros after it. If they were grains of rice instead of coins, the quantity of rice placed on the last square would weigh more than 387 billion tonnes, about the weight of Mt. Everest.

In the case of the spread of disease, suppose for example that the number of COVID-19 infections doubles every five days. This was roughly the case before any measures were taken to stem the spread. As Figure 5.1 illustrates, what doubling every five days means is that if the disease began with one person, two people would have been infected in five days; four in ten days; sixty-eight people in a (30.5-day) month; 4,700 people in 2 months; 323,000 in 3 months; and 22 million in four months.

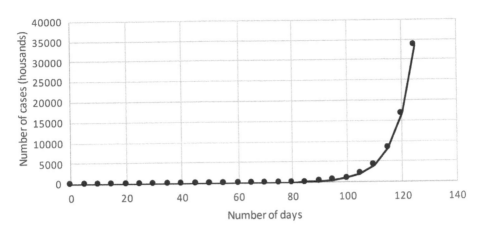

Figure 5.1: Exponential growth in case numbers

Suppose that 10 per cent of cases require hospitalisation. That would mean that at least two million hospital beds would be needed in four months—a tenth of the 22 million cases. If there were only 900,000 hospital beds available (approximately the actual number in the United States in 2021)[1] that would mean more than a million COVID-19 patients would not have hospital beds. Besides hospital beds, doctors and nurses are also essential, but there would be a shortage. There would be other patients that needed hospital beds and professional care for other serious medical problems. Such a situation would truly be a disaster. In addition to the deaths that would occur, what the healthcare community was most concerned about was extremely overburdened medical facilities, supplies, and service professionals. Using China as an example, there were only 6.41 public health professionals per 10,000 population at the end of 2019.[2] In other words, it could lead to the health system being totally overwhelmed.

There are only two solutions to such a situation, which should preferably be deployed concurrently: construct more hospitals and expand the number of health workers very quickly, and constrain the disease from spreading. Since there is a limit to building hospitals that quickly, measures had to be taken to stem the growth. It should be noted that China developed the *fangcang* cabin facilities that could be built rapidly, and healthcare professionals and personal protective equipment were mobilised and dispatched from other parts of the country to send to Wuhan and Hubei during the initial outbreaks (see Chapter 9), which helped the situation, but reducing the growth rate of COVID-19 remained the goal.

1. American Hospital Association, 'Fast Facts on U.S. Hospitals, 2022', accessed 13 September 2022, https://www.aha.org/statistics/fast-facts-us-hospitals.
2. Shuangyi Sun, Zhen Xie, Keting Yu, Bingqian Jiang, Siwei Zheng, and Xiaoting Pan, 'COVID-19 and Healthcare System in China: Challenges and Progression for a Sustainable Future', *Globalization and Health* 17, no. 1 (2021): 1–8.

The Urgency of Reducing the Rate of Growth

If the growth rate of the infectious disease could be cut in half, then in the example above, the number of hospital beds needed in four months would be only 470 (10 per cent of 4,700)—the same as the number required in two months under the fast-growth scenario—instead of two million. This shows what a huge impact reducing the rate of spread by half would make. If the disease continued to spread at the halved rate, there would still be a need for 2 million hospital beds in eight months instead of four. Perhaps by then, a medicinal cure or a vaccine would be found—or the disease might have dissipated on its own by mutation. That would be the hope. Meanwhile, the strain on hospitals, medical care workers, and equipment would have eased.

The Determinants of Spread

The answer to the following question is the key to determining how fast the disease will spread.

If a given person, let's call him Bob, has the disease and is infectious, how many other people will get the disease from Bob? The answer depends on the answers to three further questions:

- How many susceptible people (people who can catch the disease) does Bob interact with each day?
- How likely is it that each susceptible person will catch the disease from Bob when Bob interacts with them?
- For how many days is Bob infectious?

For example, suppose Bob interacts with an average of ten people a day, and they are all susceptible to the disease. Let's assume none of the ten people has had the disease and so have no immunity, and that there is as yet no vaccine or cure available. Suppose that each time Bob interacts with someone, let's say Alice, there is a one in 20 chance that Alice will catch the disease from Bob. That is, the probability that Alice will catch the disease from Bob during their interaction is 0.05. To put it another way, for every 20 susceptible people that Bob interacts with, one catches the disease.

And suppose further, for our example, that Bob is infectious for six days. Thus, Bob interacts with ten people each day for six days. With each interaction, there is a one in 20 chance that the person will get the disease. Multiplying these three numbers together shows how many people Bob will infect: 10 people/day, times 0.05 chance of infection, times 6 days = 3 people ($10 \times 0.05 \times 6 = 3$). The result of multiplying these three numbers together derives what is called R, the *reproduction number*—that is the average number of people each person with a disease goes on to infect. Hence, in this example, one infectious person will infect three more people—that is $R = 3$. If Bob was the *first* person to be infected, so that every person that Bob interacts with is susceptible to the disease, then R is designated $R0$ (pronounced R-zero or R-naught). $R0$ is called the *basic reproduction number*.

It is assumed in this example that once infected, the person will not be susceptible to it for the duration of the simulation period, which is usually no more than a few months. If Bob is not the first person infected, then some people he interacted with would have had the disease already and would not be susceptible any longer. When that happens, R becomes less than $R0$. More about that later.

R can also become less than $R0$ because measures are undertaken to stem the spread. Public policy is focused intensively on reducing R.

Measures to Stem the Spread of the Disease

Assuming no treatment or cure is yet available, the number of days for which the diseased person, Bob, is infectious cannot be changed. That leaves only two variables that can be altered to reduce the number of people Bob infects:

(1) the number of people Bob interacts with each day; and
(2) the probability that Bob gives the disease to a person when Bob interacts with them.

The number of people Bob interacts with each day can be reduced by isolating or quarantining Bob to keep him away from other people. The probability that Bob gives the disease to another person when he interacts with them can be reduced if Bob wears a mask and keeps a distance from the other person of at least one and a half metres.

Neither of these is an absolute guarantee, of course. A very strict quarantine, however—such as was adopted in mainland China—is almost an absolute guarantee that Bob would not interact with anybody while he is infectious, and therefore would not give them the disease.

Less strict isolation or quarantine policies, such as were practised in many countries during the COVID-19 pandemic, provide less of a guarantee that an infected person would not interact with other people, but they did reduce the number of interactions enough to have an important effect. Thus, if Bob can be induced or required to interact with only five people a day instead of ten, that will cut the growth rate in half and hugely slow the rate of spread.

In addition to the possibility of infection due to direct in-person interactions with infected persons, there is the possibility of catching it from touching viral residues on surfaces and then touching one's mouth, nose, or eyes. The risk of infection is reduced by sanitising surfaces and washing hands. The route of transmission via surfaces was regarded as important during the first six months of the COVID-19 outbreak but it was determined subsequently that the chances of contracting the coronavirus from surfaces were low, and the major transmission route by far was in-person interactions.[3]

---

3. U.S. Centers for Disease Control and Prevention, 'Science Brief: SARS-CoV-2 and Surface (Fomite) Transmission for Indoor Community Environments', https://www.cdc.gov/coronavirus/2019-ncov/more/science-and-research/surface-transmission.html.

Using the Reproduction Number to Predict the Spread

In the simplest possible form of the standard mathematical model, everyone is assumed to have the same R—that is each infected person is assumed to infect the same number of other people. An important additional number is the *generation time*. Generation time is the time from when a person gets infected until the next person that person infects becomes infected. The generation time for SARS and COVID-19 has been estimated at seven days. Hence, the first person infected, Bob, will infect three additional people in seven days. Each of those people will infect three more people in another seven days, for a total of nine people infected after 14 days (in addition to the original three). And after 21 days, 27 more people (3 × 9) will be infected.

Figure 5.2 shows the growth of infections over the course of four months if the population were always 100 per cent susceptible (or if the population were infinite).

Of course, the population is not infinite in real life, and will not always be 100 per cent susceptible either. The percentage of the population that is susceptible will decline over time, as people become infected and recover with immunity, or die as a result of being infected. When an increasing percentage of the population is no longer susceptible, the reproduction rate R declines because the number of susceptible people Bob or another infected person interacts with is less. This causes the number of infections to eventually peak, and then decline, as shown in Figure 5.3. Figure 5.3 assumes the total population is 330 million, like the population of the United States, and it is assumed that there are no cases brought in from outside the country.

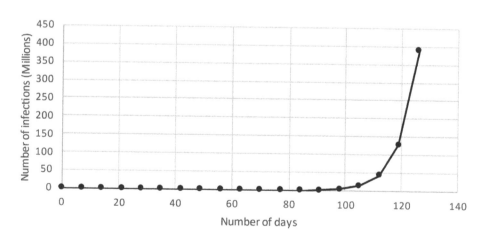

Figure 5.2: Growth of infections, infinite population

In Figure 5.3, the dashed line is the number of cases added each day, while the solid line is the number of active cases—that is, those that are still viral. If the hospitalisation rate is 10 per cent, then the number of people with the disease in hospital would be 10 per cent of the values on the solid line.

In Figure 5.4 the assumed population is 7.9 billion, which is the world's population today. With a larger population, it takes longer for the disease to peak—about four months in this example instead of three and a half.

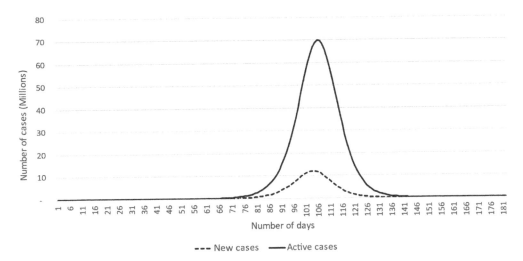

Figure 5.3: Predicted cases over time—United States size population

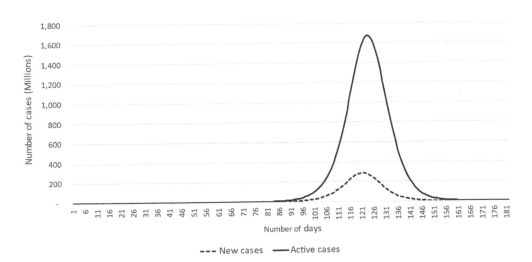

Figure 5.4: Predicted cases over time among world population (7.9 billion)

In Figure 5.5, the cumulative number of cases is also shown, as a dotted line. Figure 5.5 shows that in this model, if nothing were done to reduce the growth rate of the disease, ultimately almost six billion people would have contracted it, about 75 per cent of the world's population.

Figure 5.6 shows why the number of cases peaks and then declines. In addition to the number of daily new cases and currently viral cases over time, it also shows the R number, with its value on the right axis.

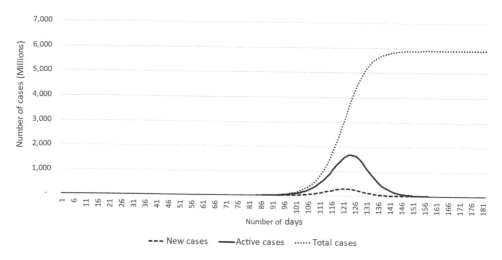

Figure 5.5: Predicted cases over time among world population (7.9 billion)

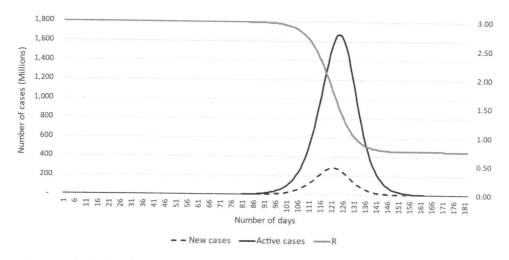

Figure 5.6: Predicted cases over time among world population (7.9 billion)

Notice how R declines as the disease catches fire in the population. At the beginning and for a long while, before exponential spread really takes off and the disease afflicts a large number of people, R has a value equal to or very close to its initial value of $R0 = 3$ (each infectious person infects three more people). As a larger and larger percentage of the population is infected and is no longer susceptible to infection, R declines because the number of susceptible people an infected person interacts with is now less.

Finally, as the rightmost part of Figure 5.5 shows, the disease no longer grows in the community, even though (in this example) 25 per cent of the population is still susceptible. This is known as *herd immunity* (see Chapter 4). What happens is that, as the number of people infected starts to decline, the percentage of the people they meet who are susceptible declines too. Eventually, they are unable to meet each other before the infected people are no longer infectious anymore, and the disease dies out.

The SIR Model

The graphs above are an example of the kind of output produced by the Susceptible-Infected-Removed (SIR) model. This is the standard model used by most mathematical modellers of the spread of disease. In this model, the population begins with all but one person, the first one infected, susceptible to the disease. Then, as the first infected person and gradually many infected people start to interact with the susceptible people there is a chance that a susceptible person will become infected. This chance is called the *transition rate* from susceptible to infected. It is often measured—or estimated—as a daily probability. Once infected, an infected person has a daily probability of transitioning to 'removed', which can mean either recovered or dead. In either case, that person is no longer in the susceptible pool.

The examples shown above are only illustrative and do not represent actual predictions that were made by any specific SIR models. But all predictive models will have the same pattern over time, at least in the absence of public policies to alter the predictions.

But All Rs Are Not the Same

Most SIR models do not make the simplistic assumption that every infected person has the same R. 'Compartmental' models place people into different compartments, at different times of day, in different locales and engaged in different kinds of activities, where they will have different Rs when they interact with other people within the compartment, and yet other different Rs when they interact with people in other compartments.

For example, in one model of the spread of influenza, people were put into these different compartments: child in household; adult in household; child in small play group; child in large day-care centre; child in elementary school; child in middle school; child in high school; adult in workgroup; adult in neighbourhood; and adult in community.[4] Different contact probabilities were assumed for each pair of possible contacts. For example, the probability of contact (per day) of two children in a household was 0.6 (60 per cent chance of contact), while the probability of contact of two children in a large day-care centre was only 0.15, or one-fourth as much. (A contact was defined as being within a specified distance of each other for a specified length of time.) Different probabilities of contact yield different Rs. The model also needs to make assumptions about how much time a child, for example, spends at the day-care centre (or school), how much time in the household, and how much in the neighbourhood or community. Many assumptions are needed to be fed into a full-scale, advanced SIR model. The assumptions are, of course, of necessity imprecise, but they are the best that can be made.

Running the SIR Model Base Case

Once all these assumptions are fed into the model, it can be run for a large population that is allocated to the various compartments (another set of assumptions, usually obtained from demographic data). Running the model entails beginning with one or only a few infected cases, then simulating the progress of the spread day by day after that. Each day, some proportion of the susceptible people will transition to infected, and then, some proportion of the infected people will transition to the removed category. This will provide how many of the population are still susceptible, infected, or removed on each future day.

The model will also make additional assumptions about how many of the infected will be hospitalised, and how many will die. These assumptions may be different for different age groups. Hence, the models can make a prediction not only about how many people will be infected on each day in the future, but how many will be hospitalised and how many deaths there will be.

Hypothesising Public Health Policies and Changing the Assumptions Accordingly

The mathematical modelling base case is run under the assumption that nobody changes the way they lived their lives before the disease started to circulate. This is of course not a realistic assumption, but it is standard practice for modelling. In reality, people would likely change their routines and their number of interactions with other people out of fear of the disease. However, that is not likely to reduce the spread enough. Up until March 2020, in the United States and the United Kingdom, the public policy approach was to do practically nothing.

---

4. Timothy C. Germann, Kai Kadau, Ira M. Longini, Jr., and Catherine A. Macken, 'Mitigation Strategies for Pandemic Influenza in the United States', *Proceedings of the National Academy of Sciences* 103, no. 15 (2006): 5935–5940 (supplemental materials).

This changed dramatically after the results of research by academics at Imperial College, London, were announced in mid-March 2020.[5] That research predicted 510,000 deaths in the United Kingdom and 2.2 million in the United States if nothing were done to mitigate the spread of COVID-19. That caused concern. The Imperial College study also explored how those numbers of deaths could be reduced if certain public policy interventions were adopted to contain the spread. Those interventions included: case isolation in the home; voluntary home quarantine; social distancing of those over 70 years of age; social distancing of the entire population; and closure of schools and universities.

Compared to measures that had already been taken in China beginning in late January, these were mild measures. In China, much stricter measures were taken to try to ensure that the disease did not spread any further at all, after the first few weeks of spread. These measures were notably successful, as discussed in Chapter 9.

In the Imperial College study, further assumptions had to be made about how much each of the potential policies to contain the spread of the disease would reduce the Rs. Then for each possible containment policy, and combination of policies, the Imperial College team reran the model. Figure 5.7 shows the predictions from the Imperial College study's results for several different policy measures and combinations thereof.

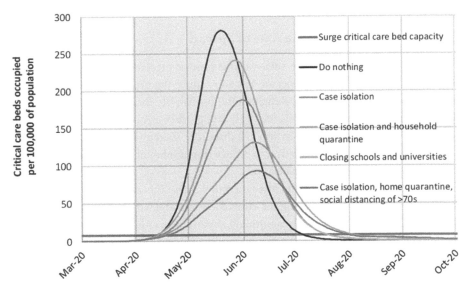

Figure 5.7: Mitigation strategy scenarios for the United Kingdom showing critical care bed requirements. Courtesy of Neil M. Ferguson et al.

5.   Neil M. Ferguson, Daniel Laydon, Gemma Nedjati-Gilani, Natsuko Imai, Kylie Ainslie, Marc Baguelin, et al., 'Report 9: Impact of Non-pharmaceutical Interventions (NPIs) to Reduce COVID-19 Mortality and Healthcare Demand', Imperial College COVID-19 Response Team, 16 March 2020.

The solid black ('Do nothing') line (line with the highest peak number of critical care beds) shows the unmitigated epidemic (base case). The light grey line (line with the second-highest peak) shows a mitigation strategy incorporating the closure of schools and universities; the line with the third-highest peak shows case isolation; the line with the fourth-highest peak shows case isolation and household quarantine; and the line with the lowest peak shows case isolation, home quarantine, and social distancing of those aged over 70. The shaded area indicates the 3-month period in which these interventions are assumed to remain in place.

In order to arrive at these predictions, the modellers had to make assumptions about how much each of the interventions would reduce the rate of spread. For example, they assumed that for 'case isolation in the home', symptomatic cases would stay at home for seven days and that this would reduce non-household contacts by 75 per cent during that period. They also assumed that 70 per cent of households would comply. For 'social distancing', they assumed that it would reduce contact rates by 50 per cent in workplaces and reduce other contacts by 75 per cent, but that as a result, it would increase household contacts by 25 per cent (because people would be at home more), and they assumed 75 per cent compliance with the policy.

Each of these assumptions for a mitigation policy changes the contact probability assumptions and the Rs when the model is run. This is how the alternative sets of predictions for different mitigation strategies are arrived at in the modelling process.

Interventions to Reduce the Rate of Spread

As mentioned before, there are two ways to reduce the rate of spread: reduce the number of contacts an infected person has and reduce the probability that the person contacted will catch the disease. Reducing the probability that a person will catch the disease from an infected person is relatively straightforward—wear a mask (and possibly other protective gear) and maintain a distance. Therefore, almost all of the intervention strategies have one objective: to reduce the number of contacts made between infected persons and susceptible persons.

The first priority is to identify infected individuals. This can be done by means of testing for COVID-19 and tracing the contacts of anyone who tests positive. Beyond that, it is all about isolating and quarantining anyone who either has tested positive for the virus or has been in contact with someone who tested positive, or even someone who was in contact with someone who was in contact with someone who tested positive—unless they have repeatedly tested negative. How effective these strategies are, depends on how strictly they are enforced, or adhered to.

Superspreaders

As noted above, not every infected person has the same R. As a matter of fact, studies have shown that the dispersion of Rs among infected individuals is very wide. This dispersion is measured by another letter of the alphabet, k. (Confusingly, a small k indicates wide dispersion—it has been estimated that k for COVID-19 has a low value of 0.1).[6] It has been found that some infected people, and some gatherings of people, contribute to the *overdispersion* of Rs. In other words, there seems to be a small percentage of the infected who have very high Rs, whether because they carry a high viral load or because they interact at close quarters with a large number of people. It appears that a small percentage of infected people do most of the spreading of the virus, while the much larger percentage spread it relatively little. For example, a two-and-a-half-hour chorus practice in the American state of Washington in May 2020, attended by sixty-one persons among whom there was one person infected with COVID-19, resulted in at least thirty-two additional cases and perhaps as many as 52, when secondary infections are considered.[7]

Both people and events that spread the virus unusually widely are referred to as *superspreaders*. The importance of the phenomenon of superspreading—both superspreading individuals and superspreading events—is that it has implications for contact tracing.

Contact tracing has typically been done when a person is confirmed to be infected. They are then questioned as to which other people they interacted with and what venues they have been to since they got infected. This way, people who may have caught the virus from them can be identified, tested, and isolated if infected. This is called *forward tracing*, because it identifies contacts going forward in time beginning with when the person became infectious.

The fact of superspreading events and people indicates that more cases can be winnowed out by doing *backward tracing*. This means that in addition to identifying with whom the infected person has interacted *since* becoming infectious, the investigation goes back to the event or person from whom the infected person contracted the disease. Because the infecting person or event may have been a superspreader, the backward tracing process seeks to identify who else may have contracted the virus from the superspreader.

Figure 5.8 shows why more cases of infection are discovered by doing both forward and backward contact tracing.[8] Black dots indicate detected cases, dark grey dots quarantined cases, and light grey dots undetected cases. This chart shows two infectious cases are discovered, 'Index case #1' and 'Index case #2' (dark grey dots to the left and right of chart A). They have a common source in a 'Primary case', but that primary case

6. Akira Endo, Centre for the Mathematical Modelling of Infectious Diseases COVID-19 Working Group, Sam Abbott, Adam J. Kucharski, and Sebastian Funk, 'Estimating the Overdispersion in COVID-19 Transmission Using Outbreak Sizes Outside China', *Wellcome Open Research* 5 (2020).

7. Lea Hamner, 'High SARS-CoV-2 Attack Rate Following Exposure at a Choir Practice—Skagit County, Washington, March 2020', *Morbidity and Mortality Weekly Report* 69 (2020).

8. See Akira Endo, Quentin J. Leclerc, Gwenan M. Knight, Graham F. Medley, Katherine E. Atkins, Sebastian Fun, et al., 'Implication of Backward Contact Tracing in the Presence of Overdispersed Transmission in COVID-19 Outbreaks', *Wellcome Open Research* 5, no. 239 (2020), https://www.ncbi.nlm.nih.gov/pmc/articles/PMC7610176.3.

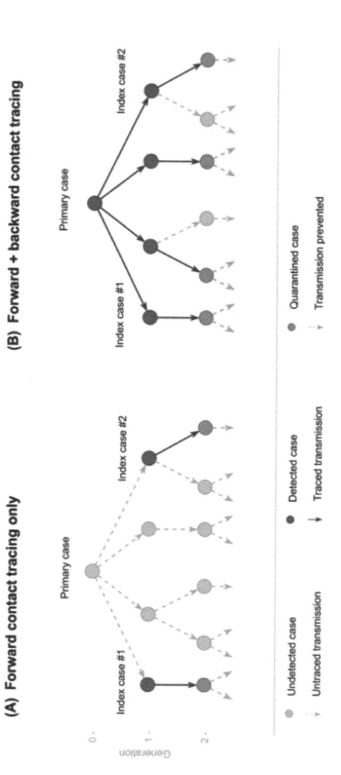

Figure 5.8: Forward and backward contact tracing. Courtesy of Akira Endo.

is initially undetected (light grey dot at the top of chart A). In (A), only forward tracing is conducted, identifying only two infected persons, while those coloured light grey are undetected. In (B), backward tracing is conducted in addition to forward tracing. Backward tracing identifies the primary case, which therefore has become a black dot, and then forward tracing from there identifies additional contacts that were made with potentially infectious people (there are still two light grey undetected cases in (B) because contact tracing is imperfect). Some of those additional contacts tested positive and are quarantined.

The Actual Pattern of Cases and Infections over Time

The results of simulations shown in Figures 5.3 through 5.7 do not represent what happens in the real world. They show only what will happen if a single course of action—or no action—is pursued without deviation. In the real world, actions taken in response to the disease change over time, and the disease can change too.

The best analogue to the spread of a disease is the spread of a wildfire. If the wildfire finds a patch of kindling or dry wood or dry shrubbery it can spread extremely quickly. If that fire is then put out but not completely extinguished, so that it smoulders for a while afterwards, its smouldering remains can again find or leap to another patch of kindling or dry wood or shrubbery. A fire that is not completely extinguished can even smoulder underground, undetected, and emerge at a distance to flare up very rapidly again. The spread of a viral disease is similar if it is not completely extinguished. If there are remaining viruses lurking in the population then it can flare up again, astonishingly quickly, just as it could at the onset of the disease.

China is the most prominent exception among countries. For other countries, the objective of their intervention measures was not to eradicate COVID-19 completely, but to 'flatten the curve', meaning to reduce the level of the predicted peak of cases, hospitalisations, and deaths. A key objective was to get the number of hospitalisations and the demand for intensive care units, ventilators, and other specialised equipment below what was expected to be available. Once that objective was achieved, the interventions were often eased up. However, that meant that the virus was still smouldering. Consequently, it could—and often did—leap into flame again. When that happened, interventions were re-imposed or tightened, with the result that the pattern of cases over time had multiple peaks. This pattern of interventions over time, in which initially a serious effort was made to suppress the virus, which was then slackened when it was successful, and then re-imposed when the virus flared up again, was called 'the hammer and the dance' by an early commentator on COVID-19, Tomas Pueyo.[9]

For example, Figure 5.9 shows the number of daily cases in France from March 2020 to December 2021.

---

9. Tomas Pueyo, 'Coronavirus: The Hammer and the Dance', 19 March 2020, https://tomaspueyo.medium. com/coronavirus-the-hammer-and-the-dance-be9337092b56.

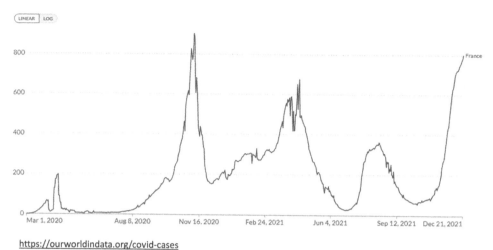

https://ourworldindata.org/covid-cases

Figure 5.9: Daily new COVID-19 cases in France per million people (seven-day rolling average) to December 2021. Courtesy of Our World in Data.

The peaks represent when the virus flared up. In this graph of actual cases over time, a trough does not represent when the virus dissipated due to herd immunity—as it did in the more theoretical Figures 5.3–5.6—but when government interventions that were tightened or imposed repeatedly in response to the peaks started to be loosened again. Also playing a role was the programme of vaccinations that began at the end of December 2020. In December 2021, Figure 5.9 shows, cases rose sharply because of a new Omicron variant.

Notice that although measures to reduce the rate of growth of cases, hospitalisations, and deaths are often referred to as strategies for 'flattening the curve', they do not, in fact, flatten the curve. The phrase 'flattening the curve' really refers to the attempt to reduce the heights of the peaks so that they do not exceed a nation's capacities, for example for hospital beds. Perhaps instead of the phrase 'flattening the curve', a more accurate phrase should be borrowed from the electric power industry: 'peak shaving'.

How Long Should Someone Who May Have the Disease Be Quarantined?

Some people are impatient with the length of time for which they need to quarantine, especially after returning from a foreign country. For example, in Hong Kong, many travellers returning from overseas were required to quarantine for 21 days at one stage, and then to be tested twice even after quarantine. If the period of time during which someone infected with the disease is infectious averages only several days, why does the quarantine period need to be so long?

The answer has to do with the mathematical concept known as 'fat tails'. Although the average infectious period may be only a few days, there will be variations. Some people will be infectious for longer times, some for shorter times. There will be a distribution of infectious periods, from only three or four days to weeks. Such distributions typically have 'fat tails'—that is, there will be very few people who will have much longer infectious periods than others (i.e., they will be way out on the right-hand tail of the infectious period distribution).

Suppose only one in 10,000 returnees from overseas is infectious for as long as 21 days. That means that if 10,000 people return, there is a good chance one will still be infectious in 21 days, and there is no way to know which one. That is too big a chance to take when a single carrier can ignite a flare-up that can spark exponential spread. If the goal is to ensure no spread, it is prudent to quarantine them all for 21 days. Even supposing that only 1,000 people return, then a chance of one in 10,000 is a chance of one-tenth in 1,000 or still a one-in-ten chance that of those 1,000 one will be infectious in 21 days and ignite exponential spread.

Estimating the Input Parameters to a COVID-19 Prediction Model

Modelling the course of a disease using a predictive simulation requires inputting to the model many assumptions, such as R0 numbers, hospitalisation rates, death rates, generation time, etc. These are called the *parameters* of the model. They can also include additional numbers, like the percentage of potentially susceptible people who have been vaccinated. And they can include assumptions about what percentage reduction in rates of personal contact will occur when certain mitigating measures are introduced, like school closures.

Because the spread of a disease is exponential in its early stages, decisions need to be made very quickly on whether to adopt policies to clamp down on the rate of growth. These decisions are made with the aid of the mathematical model's projections. For the models to make reasonably accurate predictions, they need reasonably accurate parameters to be input into them. Estimating those parameters in the beginning stages of a new and previously unknown disease, however, is difficult because little data is available.

To help understand the difficulty, consider this dilemma that arose around the end of 2021 and the beginning of 2022. The COVID-19 Omicron variant had just begun to spread rapidly, out-competing the previous variant, Delta, and accounting for the vast majority of COVID-19 cases. Figure 5.10 extends the Figure 5.9 graph of cases in France per million people through the end of the year 2021 and into the beginning of 2022.

Notice how the daily cases of Omicron had, within a space of only two to three weeks, shot up to be much greater than the highest rate before Omicron appeared. The

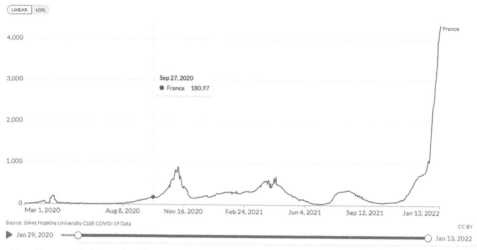

Figure 5.10: Daily new COVID-19 cases in France per million (seven-day rolling average) to mid-January 2022. Courtesy of Our World in Data.

R0 for Omicron was estimated to be as high as 10,[10] on par with the formerly rapidly spreading childhood diseases measles, mumps, and chicken pox (until almost all children were vaccinated for them). An *R0* of 10 implies a doubling of cases approximately every two days.

Early data indicated that the effects of Omicron were milder than previous variants, and it was less likely to require hospitalisation. But because it spread so much more rapidly it might require more hospital beds than previous variants, even though the ratio of hospitalisations to cases was lower. It should be noted that vaccination does not prevent infection, but it lowers the risk of the infected person becoming very sick. With Omicron, the rate of hospitalisation was much lower for those who had been vaccinated. The disease manifested itself as less severe in an infected person who had been vaccinated.

In the United States, there was a desire to estimate what percentage of vaccinated and unvaccinated people who caught Omicron would need hospitalisation. To gather the data needed for this estimate, before Omicron had already spread very widely, was extremely difficult. Hospitalisations lag case discoveries by about two weeks, so the empirical rate of hospitalisation would not be known until at least two weeks after Omicron's onset. Furthermore, Omicron first took hold in regions in the United States where the vaccination rate was high, such as New York, Massachusetts, and New Jersey,

---

10. Talha Khan Burki, 'Omicron Variant and Booster COVID-19 Vaccines', *The Lancet Respiratory Medicine* 10, no. 2 (2022): e17.

while the spread to regions with lower rates of vaccination, such as rural and Southern regions, took a week or two longer. Hence, it was difficult to estimate the hospitalisation rate for the unvaccinated until as much as a month after Omicron's onset, by which time it might have already peaked.

Estimating a Rate of Growth from Early Data

As an example of how a parameter can be inferred from a small amount of early data, suppose that a researcher, Molly, has only two weeks of data for the daily number of cases of a disease. Let us suppose that the number of cases can be assumed to grow exponentially for at least the next six weeks. How can Molly infer the rate of exponential growth, so that she can extrapolate that rate of growth from the first two weeks to the following six weeks?

Figure 5.11 shows the data for the first 14 days, while Figure 5.12 extends this graph to several possible hypothetical future paths with 14 per cent, 17 per cent, 20 per cent, and 23 per cent daily rates of growth of cases.

Which of these possible growth rates best fits the data we have, which is only for the first 14 days? Figure 5.13 shows 14 per cent, 17 per cent, 20 per cent, and 23 per cent daily rates of growth of cases for the first 14 days.

Figure 5.13 shows the 20 per cent growth rate fits the data best. (A statistical best-fit test would confirm this visual impression.) Therefore, our best-guess projection of future cases in the next six weeks is the 20 per cent growth case in Figure 5.12.

In practice, a modeller will show not only the best-guess projection but an error band with a range of possible projections. Obviously, which growth rate results from the fitting of the 14-day data to a growth rate makes a very big difference. As more data is gathered, the estimate will be revised.

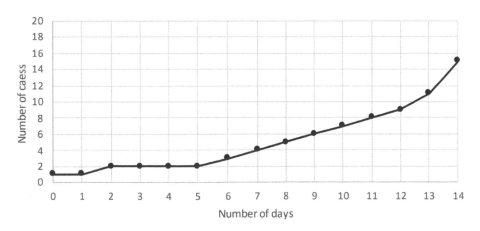

Figure 5.11: Cases for the first 14 days

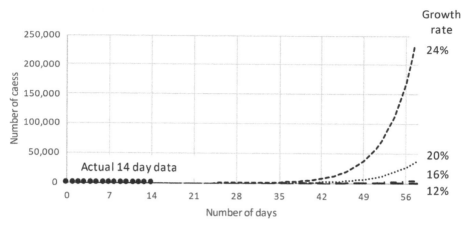

Figure 5.12: Projected cases for 8 weeks

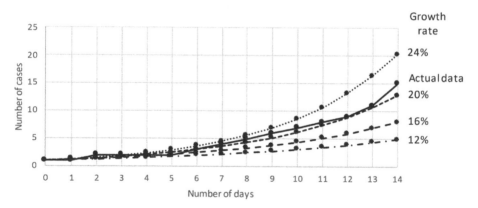

Figure 5.13: Cases for the first 14 days

If the model is an SIR model (which is more appropriate for making predictions of the spread of disease over a period of several months than an exponential model), then a similar approach can be taken to estimating R0 using early data. Several different R0s can be tried, and a simulation run for the first few weeks using each of those hypothetical R0s. Whichever of those simulations produces the closest match to the available data, the R0 that it uses can be adopted for further simulations extended into the future.[11]

Other parameters can be estimated in a similar manner, but a great deal of care is necessary because of the mismatches of data and timing. For example, one cannot

---

11. The actual methodology used is a little more complicated, but the principle is the same.

estimate the hospitalisation rate or the case fatality rate (the ratio of deaths to symptomatic cases) by dividing the daily or weekly hospitalisations or deaths by the daily or weekly cases for those same days or weeks. Hospitalisations lag the onset of cases—and therefore when the cases are reported—by roughly two weeks and deaths lag by roughly three weeks. Since during the interval between a reported case and a death the number of cases could have ballooned, the death rate could be wildly underestimated.

The Problem of Lag Time in Reporting

In the previous example, in order to project the number of cases into the future, it would be better to know the R number, the reproduction rate, on each day. This number can vary from day to day, depending on what social distancing measures are being imposed and adhered to. But the actual R number can only be measured after cases become symptomatic and are detected and reported, which can be more than a week after a carrier is infected and becomes infectious. Hence, R numbers can only be estimated several days after their impact on disease spread.

To estimate the R number in real time, the COVID-19 research team at the University of Hong Kong—which had made some of the first estimates of R0, in early 2020—used a novel method, a method that applies particularly well in Hong Kong. Most travellers in Hong Kong use public transportation—buses and the train system known as the MTR—and most of those pay by using an Octopus card, which is swiped on entry to a train station or bus. The Octopus card is also used for small purchases, such as at 7-11 stores.

The level of use of Octopus cards over time is a measure of the level of social mixing. The more the Octopus card is used, the more people are using public transportation and entering stores, and therefore the more they are making contact with one another. The University of Hong Kong researchers calculated the correlation of Octopus card use with past R numbers that had been observed after the fact in the population and found that the correlation was strong. Therefore, they estimated real-time R numbers by applying that correlation to the level of Octopus card use on a given day and even at a given hour. Using this estimated R number, they were able to make instantaneously updated projections of the subsequent spread of disease.

The Hong Kong team was challenged by the rapid spread of Omicron in February and March 2022 to estimate whether and how the spread could be contained. Because of the low percentage of vaccinations among the elderly in Hong Kong, as well as the close quarters in which people live, the challenge was great, especially in residential care homes for the elderly. Their modelling showed that the conclusion was inescapable that the spread would not be fully containable (that the R number could not be made to go below 1.5) even with the most stringent control measures that would be practicable in Hong Kong. But because of the rapid spread, more than half the population would be infected and infections would peak by April 2022; however, the risk of resurgences would linger.

Are the Statistics Really What They Seem?

Compounding the difficulty of estimating the parameters of COVID-19 is the fact that the statistics gathered from reporting, recording, or observation are often not what they seem to be. For example, when the Omicron variant broke out, it was found immediately that Omicron spread very quickly but it soon emerged that it caused a lower ratio of hospitalisations to infections, especially in people who were vaccinated. However, as there were so many Omicron infections, the number of hospitalisations was still high. *The New Yorker* magazine, however, noted that a lot of the hospitalisations attributed to Omicron, perhaps as many as half to two-thirds of them, were not due to Omicron at all:

> More than a hundred and fifty thousand Americans are currently hospitalised with the coronavirus—a higher number than at any other point in the pandemic. But that figure, too, is not quite what it seems. Many hospitalized *covid* patients have no respiratory symptoms; they were admitted for other reasons—a heart attack, a broken hip, cancer surgery—and happened to test positive for the virus. There are no nationwide estimates of the proportion of hospitalized patients with "incidental *covid*," but in New York State some forty per cent of hospitalized patients with *covid* are thought to have been admitted for other reasons. The Los Angeles County Department of Health Services reported that incidental infections accounted for roughly two-thirds of *covid* admissions at its hospitals.[12]

Even so, while the hospital admission was for another malady, affliction with the Omicron virus could have been a complicating factor, perhaps enough to drive the person admitted over the threshold for being admitted to a hospital.

It may seem a simple matter to determine how many deaths were caused by COVID-19—just add up all the deaths that were reported to be caused by it. But *The Economist* magazine notes that it is much more complicated than that:

> How many people have died because of the Covid-19 pandemic? The answer depends both on the data available, and on how you define 'because'. Many people who die while infected with SARS-CoV-2 are never tested for it, and do not enter the official totals. Conversely, some people whose deaths have been attributed to Covid-19 had other ailments that might have ended their lives on a similar timeframe anyway. And what about people who died of preventable causes during the pandemic, because hospitals full of Covid-19 patients could not treat them? If such cases count, they must be offset by deaths that did not occur but would have in normal times, such as those caused by flu or air pollution.[13]

---

12. Dhruv Khullar, 'Do the Omicron Numbers Mean What We Think They Mean', *The New Yorker*, 16 January 2022.
13. *The Economist*, 'The Pandemic's True Death Toll', 2 November 2021, https://www.economist.com/graphic-detail/coronavirus-excess-deaths-estimates.

These complicating factors have caused compilers of statistics to resort to other means to estimate the number of deaths due to COVID-19, and sometimes the number of hospitalisations.

One common means to estimate deaths that can be attributed to the virus is to compare the number of total deaths that occurred while the virus was raging with the number of total deaths 'that would have occurred anyway'. That is, it requires estimating a counterfactual: how many deaths would have occurred if there had been no virus?

For example, Figure 5.14 shows, as a wavy solid line, the number of deaths that would have been expected each week during the years 2018 through 2021 in the United States, extrapolated from the pattern of previous years' weekly deaths.[14] The pattern reflects the fact that more deaths occur during the winter months. The vertical bars are the number of deaths that occurred.

Notice that until April 2020, the number of actual deaths agreed fairly closely with the projected number of deaths from extrapolation. But for most weeks from April 2020 on, the number of actual deaths exceeded the number of projected deaths, in some cases by a wide margin. These excess deaths are very likely attributable to COVID-19. For most countries around the world, excess deaths calculated in this manner do not agree, in many cases not even closely, with the number of deaths reported to have been caused by COVID-19.[15] A March 2022, study in *The Lancet* said that while reported COVID-19 deaths worldwide as of the end of the year 2021 totalled 5.94 million, an estimated 18.2 million died worldwide because of the COVID-19 pandemic as measured by excess mortality—more than three times reported deaths (with a 95 per cent uncertainty interval from 17.1 to 19.6 million).[16] The COVID-19 pandemic has truly been a global tragedy.

Decline in Life Expectancy

Another way to measure the impact of deaths caused by the pandemic is to track life expectancy before the pandemic, and for the years 2020–2021 during the pandemic. It is possible, using mortality data on age at death during a particular year, to calculate life expectancy without having to follow a whole cohort of individuals for their entire lifetimes; in fact, it is much more accurate than following a whole cohort until each of their deaths because life expectancy changes over time.

The method is to calculate the percentage of individuals at each age who died during the year. For example, the data may show that 0.1 per cent of individuals aged zero to one died during the year, while 9 per cent of individuals aged 90 died during the

---

14. National Center for Health Statistics, 'Excess Deaths Associated with COVID-19', accessed 13 September 2022, https://www.cdc.gov/nchs/nvss/vsrr/covid19/excess_deaths.htm.

15. *The Economist*, 'Tracking Covid-19 Excess Deaths Across Countries', 20 October 2021, https://www.economist.com/graphic-detail/coronavirus-excess-deaths-tracker.

16. COVID-19 Excess Mortality Collaborators, 'Estimating Excess Mortality Due to the COVID-19 Pandemic: A Systematic Analysis of COVID-19-Related Mortality, 2020–21', *The Lancet* 399, no. 10334 (2022): 1513–1536.

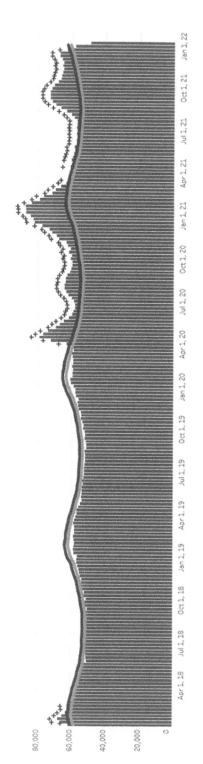

Figure 5.14: Number of actual deaths in the United States versus expected deaths

year. This enables the construction of an entire actuarial table of probabilities of death at each age, from which life expectancy can be calculated.

Not surprisingly, life expectancy declined in several countries. An important study,[17] not yet peer-reviewed at the time of this writing, calculated life expectancy for the three years 2019–2021 (2019 being before the pandemic, and 2020 and 2021 during the pandemic) for the United States and 19 peer countries including Austria, Belgium, Denmark, England and Wales, Finland, France, Germany, Israel, Italy, Netherlands, New Zealand, Northern Ireland, Norway, Portugal, Scotland, South Korea, Spain, Sweden, and Switzerland. The decline in life expectancy over the two years from 2019 to 2021 was by far the largest in the United States. Life expectancy in the United States declined by 2.26 years, from 78.86 years in 2019, before the pandemic, to 76.60 years two years later in 2021, comprising a 1.87-year reduction from 2019 to 2020 and a 0.39-year reduction from 2020 to 2021. By contrast, the other 19 peer countries averaged only a 0.57-year decrease from 2019–2020 and a 0.28-year *increase* from 2020–2021. Among the 19 peer countries, the greatest decline over those two years was 0.93 years, in England and Wales. Life expectancy in the United States was already below that of the peer countries before the pandemic; during the pandemic, the gap increased to more than five years. However, deaths from drug overdoses in the United States also increased by about 30,000 from 2019 to 2021,[18] which cannot be directly attributed to COVID-19; hence, the decline in life expectancy in the United States may slightly overstate the impact of COVID-19.

COVID-19's Last Gasp? Omicron in Shanghai

At the beginning of March 2022, the Omicron variant of COVID-19 began to spread in Shanghai, a city with a population of 25 million in a country of 1.4 billion. China had previously locked down very rapidly once the high transmissibility of the disease and its virulence became clear and henceforth maintained a 'zero-COVID' policy. With the exponential spread of the less virulent Omicron variant in Shanghai, the question arose as to whether the zero-COVID strategy should be maintained (now also called 'dynamic zero' to account for the fact that absolute zero is virtually impossible), or whether something more closely resembling a 'living with COVID' strategy should be initiated. A mathematical model documented by Chinese and US epidemiologists in the journal *Nature* helped to make the decision.[19]

The simple SIR model described earlier in this chapter had assumed that once a person had contracted the disease, they were no longer susceptible to it, at least not

---

17. Ryan K. Master, Laudan Y. Aron, and Steven H. Woolf, 'Changes in Life Expectancy between 2019 and 2021: United States and 19 Peer Countries', *medRxiv* 1 June 2022, https://doi.org/10.1101/2022.04.05.22273393.
18. National Center for Health Statistics, 'Provisional Drug Overdose Death Counts', accessed 13 September 2022, https://www.cdc.gov/nchs/nvss/vsrr/drug-overdose-data.htm.
19. Jun Cai, Xiaowei Deng, Juan Yang, Kaiyuan Sun, Hengcong Liu, Zhiyuan Chen, et al., 'Modeling Transmission of SARS-CoV-2 Omicron in China', *Nature Medicine* 28 (2022): 1468–1475.

for a long time. But experience showed that people could contract the disease more than once, even within relatively short periods of time. Consequently, the authors of the *Nature* article used an altered version of the model, instead of susceptible-infected-recovered they used a susceptible-latent-infectious-removed-susceptible model to indicate that a person could go from infected and infectious through recovery to susceptible again. The 'latent' phase indicates that an infected person can be asymptomatic in the early stage of the disease.

Running the model produced concerning results, even though Omicron was less deadly than previous COVID-19 variants. The authors reported that: 'We find that the level of immunity induced by the March 2022 vaccination campaign would be insufficient to prevent an Omicron wave that would result in exceeding critical care capacity with a projected intensive care unit peak demand of 15.6 times the existing capacity and causing approximately 1.55 million deaths.' The authors were, nevertheless, confident that continued access to vaccines and antiviral therapies, and implementation of non-pharmaceutical interventions—i.e., lockdowns, social distancing, isolation, and so on—would suffice to prevent overwhelming the healthcare system. Hence, China continued with its lockdown approach in Shanghai, even though the Omicron variant was less deadly and the lockdown was very painful (see Chapter 9).

Host-Parasite Coevolution and the Disease Endgame

As the disease continues to be endemic in the host population and evolves with COVID-19, the virus and its variants become more or less transmissible, and more or less virulent—where 'virulent' means harmful to the host's health or, simply, lethal. It would help to anticipate and plan for the virus 'endgame' if there were a mathematical model to predict how the relationship between virus transmissibility and virulence will evolve over time. Will the disease evolve to become like the common cold, which is highly transmissible but hardly virulent, because the survival rate is virtually 100 per cent? Or will it be more like rabies or tuberculosis, which continue to coexist with a host population seemingly forever? Unfortunately, although there have been more than 6,000 papers published on this question, no definitive answer is available.

It would seem a simple matter of applying Darwin's theory of natural selection to the virus's evolution. What will make virus survival and proliferation more likely—increased virulence of the disease in the host, or decreased virulence? The relevant theoretical relationships in those 6,000 academic papers are expressed in mathematical formulas, but we will describe the basic idea.

From the point of view of the host population, the objective is to make the reproduction number, R, as small as possible. For the virus, there is also a reproduction number R. In this case, R is the number of additional viruses that each virus can spawn and transmit to other hosts. The difference between the host R and the parasite's (that is, the virus's) R is that while the objective of the human population is to minimise R, the objective of the virus is to maximise R; i.e., to spread as quickly as possible. Like the host R, the virus's R is the product of how fast the virus spreads from one host to another (its transmissivity), and for how many days it can spread from that host; that is, the number of days for which the host is infectious.

For the purposes of this discussion, let us call the latter the duration. The central questions in most of the academic papers are: how long is the duration, and how is its length related to the transmissibility? The longer the duration, the more the virus would be transmitted to other hosts; its R would be higher.

Until the 1980s, the prevailing theory was the 'avirulence hypothesis'.[20] This hypothesis assumed that for a virus to be more transmissible, it would have to be less 'virulent'—that is, less lethal—because if it killed the host, that would shorten the duration of the time during which the virus could be transmitted. Therefore, like the common cold, the virus would become milder over time, even if more transmissible. The reason for this assumption was that the less lethal a virus is, the longer the average time for which the host lives, and therefore the longer the time the virus can spend living in the host and transmitting itself to other hosts.

Empirical studies, however—though difficult to perform because the variables are hard to define and measure—were not able to decisively confirm the avirulence hypothesis. In the early 1980s, Anderson and May and others presented another hypothesis,[21] known as the virulence-transmission trade-off. This hypothesis rests on the observation that if a virus has a higher transmission rate, it is likely to be more abundant in a host. Greater abundance means greater cost to the host, which means a higher mortality rate but also a lower daily rate of recovery if the patient does not die—that is, the patient is sick for longer. The higher mortality rate tends to reduce the virus's R because it can only live in the host and transmit itself for a shorter time. But the longer recovery time tends to *increase* the virus's R because it can live in the sick patient longer.

The virulence-transmission trade-off hypothesis arrives at an optimal transmissivity for the virus given that transmissivity increases mortality, but also increases recovery time for patients who do not die. It is a nice theory, but unfortunately attempts to verify it empirically have stumbled. The problem is twofold: first, it is difficult to gather data for the variables as defined in the model to verify it empirically; and second, other complicating factors can cause the relationship to be different from the result of the theoretical model. The result is that there is no reliable method as yet to predict with any certainty how the virus will evolve over time, and what its transmission rate and virulence will be. There are still hopes for the virulence-transmission trade-off hypothesis, but it has yet to be confirmed at a high level of confidence.

---

20. S. Alizon, A. Hurford, N. Mideo, and M. Van Baalen, 'Virulence Evolution and the Trade-Off Hypothesis: History, Current State of Affairs and the Future', *Journal of Evolutionary Biology* 22, no. 2 (2009): 245–259; Clayton E. Cressler, David V. McLeod, Carly Rozins, Josée van den Hoogen, and Troy Day, 'The Adaptive Evolution of Virulence: A Review of Theoretical Predictions and Empirical Tests', *Parasitology* 143, no. 7 (2016): 915–930; Miguel A. Acevedo, Forrest P. Dillemuth, Andrew J. Flick, Matthew J. Faldyn, and Bret D. Elderd, 'Virulence-Driven Trade-Offs in Disease Transmission: A Meta-analysis', *Evolution* 73, no. 4 (2019): 636–647.

21. Roy M. Anderson and Robert M. May, 'Coevolution of Hosts and Parasites', *Parasitology* 85, no. 2 (1982): 411–426.

Another phenomenon, however, leads to the conclusion that the virus will weaken over time. As many people in the population contract one variant of the virus or another, and as many people get vaccinated for the virus, their immunity to it and to future variants tends to increase.[22] This has been called 'hybrid immunity'—that is, immunity acquired from both prior infection and vaccination.[23] Therefore, there is a reasonable expectation that COVID-19, while it will be with us for a long time, will gradually become less and less of a problem over time.

Conclusion

The most salient—and dangerous—mathematical feature of the spread of disease is exponential growth. Exponential growth is especially problematic when the disease's transmissivity—its rate of spread, its R number—is large. If the rate of spread is not too great, and diligent test-and-trace methods are applied to find and isolate infectious disease carriers before they can spread the disease, the disease can be contained. But if the R number is so large that it overwhelms the capacity to test and trace, it can then spread exponentially, catastrophically exceeding hospital and medical care capacities. This was the case with the Omicron variant of COVID-19—though it was at least, for-tunately, less deadly than previous variants.

There may be little that can be done to contain a disease that is both highly trans-missive and highly virulent, except to ride it out until herd immunity. This is essentially what happened with the black plagues of the Middle Ages, though in those cases the problem was a lack of the medical knowledge needed to contain it. Nevertheless, for many countries of the world, insufficient preparation allowed COVID-19 to spread more than it needed to. With adequate preparation, it could have been contained through better test-and-trace methods and more isolation of the infectious. In advance of a likely future onset of another disease, mathematical modelling of varying hypo-thetical levels of transmissivity and virulence should be undertaken to determine what levels and types of preparation should be put in place to contain all but the most trans-missive, and thus uncontainable, of them. Cost-benefit analyses can be undertaken to determine what levels of defence against the spread of future diseases should be put in place to contain all but—to borrow a measure used to determine how much defence should be put in place against a flood or tsunami—the thousand-year disease. This anticipatory and preventive use of mathematical modelling may be even more essential than using it after a disease strikes.

22. William Hanage, 'After Omicron, This Pandemic Will Be Different', *The New York Times*, 19 January 2022, https://www.nytimes.com/2022/01/19/opinion/omicron-covid-surge.html.
23. Ivan Hung Fan-ngai, 'Beyond Hong Kong's COVID-19 Fifth Wave: Coping with the Coronavirus', *Asia Global Online*, 15 July 2022, https://www.asiaglobalonline.hku.hk/beyond-hong-kongs-covid-19-fifth-wave-coping-coronavirus?utm_source=Asia+Global+Institute&utm_campaign=783e7a6dbd-EMAIL_CAMPAIGN_2020_05_14_04_19_COPY_01&utm_medium=email&utm_term=0_c139173191-783e7a6dbd-381203146.

6

The Social Contract and Responses to COVID-19

Renu Singh

As the COVID-19 pandemic steamrolls through a third year, it has become increasingly evident that there will be several long- and short-term health, socio-economic, and political ramifications. This is not the first global or even global health crisis, and yet, with every new ordeal society learns to reassess, readjust, and redevelop as needed. On the one hand, SARS-CoV-2 had brought a number of age-old concerns and practices about sanitation, isolation, and public health more generally, back to the surface of public debate and political discourse. On the other, such concerns in the context of a much more globalised and interconnected world have posed new challenges, specifically about what the respective roles, responsibilities, and limitations of government and individuals in a given society should be. For example, both China and Italy have implemented some of the most stringent travel restrictions at different points in the pandemic—a policy echoed in the unprecedented introduction of border controls in the Schengen zone, which historically has allowed for free movement across the European Union starting in 2020. However, once implemented, Europe lifted such border controls much more quickly than China and several other countries that have maintained a zero-COVID policy—a policy also implemented for varying amounts of time and at varying levels of risk to public health. This shift towards increasingly stringent policies is also reflected in many of the COVID-19 public health measures across these contexts with the lockdowns, quarantines, and other policies put in place. Meanwhile, countries including the United States, Sweden, and the United Kingdom, while also reconsidering how stringent their public health and travel measures should be since the beginning of the pandemic, have fallen on the other side of the spectrum. In part, these differences reflect the public's reactions to these policies, with people holding different opinions about how much their governments should be involved in managing the risks of the pandemic and how much personal freedoms should be limited as a result.

All of these public health concerns allude to a theory as old as philosophy itself, describing an agreement—hypothetical or actual—among individuals about their rights and duties to each other and in the context of some form of government. This 'social contract' defines the moral and political obligations that the public and government have to themselves and each other, and in so doing provides the basic framework underlying how a society conducts itself. COVID-19 clearly illustrated the extent to which countries have very different social contracts based on their own contexts, histories, and public psyches. Faced with the same deadly threat of the coronavirus, countries have responded in very different ways over the last few years. Stringencies of policies and the relative prioritisation of health, trade, and economic policy by governments have varied. Likewise, what the public expects the role of their government to be in this crisis has also differed. Should governments mandate vaccines? How much of a priority is vaccine equity and how is it defined? For how long should mask mandates be in place or reinstated, if at all? Should there be quarantines? And if so, for how long and for whom? These questions are some of the most essential and controversial in the COVID-19 response and in defining the new norm in countries' social contracts going forward.

This chapter unpacks the idea of the social contract and applies it in the context of health policy and the world's response to the COVID-19 pandemic.

The Social Contract: An Introduction

The social contract provides a foundation of understanding upon which societies are built. This foundation of understanding requires that individuals have certain obligations to themselves and each other and where they voluntarily agree to either a tacit or explicit agreement based on their own self-interest and rationality. Social contract theory can trace its roots to Socrates's *Crito*, where he explains that he must remain imprisoned and face the death penalty in order to honour the very system of laws and norms in Athens that allowed for his existence and life. The laws and norms allowed for his parents and him to live the life they had led until the point in time of his imprisonment and execution, and in return, it was his obligation to uphold certain duties and responsibilities to the city and society of Athens.[1]

Social contract theory centres on the established expectation about what governments can and cannot do and what individual freedoms and responsibilities exist in any given society. The aim of the theory then, is to show why individuals in a given society endorse and comply with the formal and informal institutions (i.e., values, laws, etc.) in place, as with Socrates choosing to remain imprisoned and subjected to the other laws in Athens. However, there is no one theory for how this relationship between individuals and society should operate.

Modern social contract theory was developed by the British and French philosophers Thomas Hobbes, John Locke, and Jean-Jacques Rousseau. The basic premise

---

1.   Plato, *Crito*, Internet Classics Archive, accessed 13 September 2022, http://classics.mit.edu/Plato/crito. html; Internet Encyclopedia of Philosophy 'Social Contract Theory', accessed 13 September 2022, https:// iep.utm.edu/soc-cont.

behind each of their conceptions is that rational, free, equal-status individuals are in a State of Nature, and that the establishment of some type of a social contract via a government entity develops among these self-interested and rational individuals, forming a civil society that imposes rules and limitations to protect all. However, for Hobbes this State of Nature is comparable to a state of war, without morality and politics, where everyone is for themselves. As such, individuals choose to live under a sovereign with absolute authority in order to have a social contract that protects them.[2] Locke, on the other hand, views the State of Nature as a place where free, equal individuals do as they see fit to be their best selves while respecting the life, health, liberty, and possessions of others.[3] In this context, individuals accept a social contract in order to protect themselves against any transgressions by having a representative government. Finally, for Rousseau, the State of Nature also involves free individuals, but they succumb to dependencies, inequalities, and comparisons among themselves and need a social contract to break free from them and still be able to live together as a society.[4] The variation in these philosophers' ideas highlights how people can arrive at very different conclusions about what the social contract should look like and the problems it is meant to solve for society. These differences have implications for how individuals and societies address major governance issues, including health broadly but also emergencies like the COVID-19 pandemic.

The Social Contract and Health

Each theory of social contracts offers a justification for what a government provides the public and what the public is allowed to do. This can be applied to any sector in which the government is involved, and health is no exception. This balance of individual and societal needs, capacities, and responsibilities is central to both healthcare and public health policy. All healthcare systems have a social contract with the public emphasising the need to provide accessible, equitable, effective, and efficient care to whatever level they deem legitimate.[5] A classic tension also exists between growing demand for healthcare and public health services and declining economic means by which to do so.

As such, discourse on the role of government and individuals in healthcare and public health policy centres around questions of distributive justice, individuals' rights, and state and individuals' responsibilities. How accountable is the state for ensuring that conditions promote and even secure individual health? And to what extent are

---

2. Thomas Hobbes, *Leviathan* (Cambridge, MA: Hackett Publishing Company, 1994).
3. John Locke, *Locke: Two Treatises of Government*, ed. Peter Laslett (Cambridge: Cambridge University Press, 1988).
4. David Lay Williams, 'Book I', in *Rousseau's Social Contract: An Introduction* (Cambridge: Cambridge University Press, 2014), 26–63; Internet Encyclopedia of Philosophy, 'Social Contract Theory'.
5. Kumaran Senthil, Evan Russell, and Hannah Lantos, 'Preserving the Social Contract of Health Care—A Call to Action', *American Journal of Public Health* 105, no. 12 (December 2015): 2404, https://doi.org/10.2105/AJPH.2015.302898.

individuals, in turn, to be responsible for maintaining their own health and, further, to be held accountable for unhealthy behaviour—if at all?[6]

The development and reform of different welfare state systems is a testament to the fact that there is no single social contract around individual and community health. Countries approach it differently among themselves and also within their own contexts overtime. For example, the United Kingdom's National Health Service is one of the most socialised forms of medicine, providing free public healthcare to all permanent residents at the point of need, paid for by taxes. It was established to guarantee that everyone in the United Kingdom could seek healthcare when they need it, and yet it has also been criticised for being too all-encompassing and even intrusive as a 'nanny state', with too much influence on individuals' lives. In the context of these debates, the system has gone back and forth on how much spending and responsibility it has for the public's health.[7] At the other end of the spectrum, the United States does not provide universal coverage through the government, with Americans predominantly covered by private insurance through their workplace, and the right to healthcare being a less central tenet of the social contract. Publicly financed Medicare for the elderly, Medicaid for those with limited income and resources, and Tricare for military service members all exist, but private health insurance coverage is still predominant, with 67 percent of the population utilising this form.[8]

Of course, welfare states span several policy areas ranging from education, unemployment, and social security to healthcare, parental leave, and mortgage interest deductions. And policies, especially social security, unemployment, and mortgage interest deductions, show how all groups in society and not just those with low incomes, benefit from them. Thus, welfare policies and the welfare states that implement them reflect the social values and economic priorities of a country and the social contract that its government has with its people in light of such values and priorities.

The Social Contract and COVID-19

The COVID-19 pandemic has put each and every country's social contract on healthcare and public health to the test. A public health emergency in the form of a global pandemic immediately brought up questions of what public health measures should be in place and for how long, but also more fundamental questions of what the default state of health will be going forward and how much to prioritise prevention versus treatment.

---

6.   T. Patrick Hill, 'Health Care: A Social Contract in Transition', *Social Science & Medicine*, XIVth International Conference on the Social Sciences and Medicine, 43, no. 5 (1 September 1996): 783–789, https://doi.org/10.1016/0277-9536(96)00123-2.

7.   Nanny State Index, 'The Best and Worst Countries to Eat, Drink, Smoke & Vape in the EU', 2022, http://nannystateindex.org/.

8.   US Census Bureau, 'Health Insurance Coverage in the United States: 2020', Census.gov, accessed 26 May 2022, https://www.census.gov/library/publications/2021/demo/p60-274.html.

The very definition of what it means to be healthy has been questioned and changed since the first cases of COVID-19 appeared. When the pandemic started, a number of countries decided to prioritise a zero-COVID policy. All COVID-19 measures put in place by these governments, ranging from travel bans and quarantines to mask mandates and social distancing measures, aimed to bring the public back to a world where the coronavirus did not exist. Being healthy meant not getting COVID-19 and not having the virus in the community at all, ideally. Zero-COVID countries predominantly located in the Asia-Pacific were touted for their success in preventing COVID-19 cases and deaths before vaccinations were available and were thought of as representations of what the future would look like post–COVID-19.[9] However, as the virus became increasingly endemic around the world and vaccinations became more available, a new norm has been established—one of being healthy but 'living with COVID'. Countries still vary on where they stand on this idea of what being a healthy society means, and their social contracts have adjusted accordingly.[10]

One area has been the overall prioritisation of prevention versus treatment. As a public health issue, COVID-19 has underscored the importance of prevention in the form of better preparedness for the next virus and of public health measures (e.g., masks, social distancing, etc.) to address the current one. And yet, there has been much controversy and public discourse about what measures are truly necessary when also balancing the need for individual freedoms and for how long measures should be mandatory. The use of coercive policies in public health has been controversial. Consensus of where this balance lies has been especially difficult to reach as initial risk assessments began to change with the development and distribution of new vaccines and other treatment mechanisms.

Further, the discourse about the public health measures has been twofold. On the one hand, the focus has been on individual freedoms and whether or not the COVID-19 policies have been too coercive. On the other hand, there is also the issue of individual responsibility, centring on how much the interests of the collective should supersede that of the individual. This ties into the Rawlsian idea of impartiality being key to a social contract. The American moral and political philosopher John Rawls puts forward that establishing a fair and just society requires making decisions as if one were behind a 'Veil of Ignorance', where an individual is unaware of their particular hereditary, socio-economic, political, or other circumstances. In this 'Original Position', any rational individual should choose to distribute civil liberties and social and economic goods as widely as possible, having no bias from knowing the advantages or disadvantages of their own condition.[11] In the context of COVID-19, this would be the equivalent of any given individual making a decision on mask or vaccine mandates, the distribution of

9. Jay Patel and Devi Sridhar, 'We Should Learn from the Asia-Pacific Responses to COVID-19', *The Lancet Regional Health—Western Pacific* 5 (1 December 2020), https://doi.org/10.1016/j.lanwpc.2020.100062.

10. Darren Dodd, 'Living with Covid vs Zero Covid', *Financial Times*, 18 February 2022, https://www.ft.com/content/1c85e715-9a57-45af-8c47-ca652efef050.

11. Internet Encyclopedia of Philosophy, 'Social Contract Theory'.

vaccinations, social distancing measures, and other such policies without knowing their race, socio-economic status, nationality, medical history, and health status. However, even in an ideal world where individuals form opinions about the pandemic response through this approach, they will still hold differing opinions about the relative importance of health and economic outcomes for the government's policy decisions. Thus, both individuals and their societies could arrive at different conclusions about how the social contract should be formed in the pandemic.

Conclusion

In conclusion, the social contract is a fundamental institution in any society, demarcating what roles the government plays for the public, and what individual responsibilities and freedoms the public has to each other and for themselves. This theory has been a central tenet in every society that also adapts and adjustments overtime. While the social contract applies to all policy areas, this chapter focuses on its application to health, healthcare, and specifically COVID-19.

The roles and responsibilities of a government and the public to each other are reflected in healthcare policies answering questions ranging from what kind of welfare state exists, if any, to how much of a balance there is between public versus private expenditures on health and public health. There are a variety of welfare states and ratios of public-to-private expenditures on health, with countries like the United States on the more capitalist and economically liberal side of the spectrum, the United Kingdom on the other end with its system of more socialised medicine, and most other countries somewhere in between. At the core of the health policy debate in every country context is a divided perception of what the healthcare and public health systems represent—one centred on the idea that healthcare is about individuals' right to health and the other on how it is a government obligation to provide this as a public service. This divide and overall debate ultimately shape the social contract on this issue.

COVID-19 has been the most recent crisis to spark a reassessment of social contracts between governments, health systems, and the public worldwide. SARS-CoV-2 has brought forth an public health crisis that is unprecedented in living memory. Not since the 1918 flu has the world experienced such a dramatic loss of life due to a pandemic. As of July 2022, there were over 570 million COVID-19 cases and over 6.4 million deaths worldwide.[12] Thus, it certainly is not surprising that governments responded very differently to the threat posed by the novel coronavirus.

Without a clear playbook for how to deal with the virus, and with decisions needing to be made very quickly early in the pandemic, governments pursued varying approaches that were not always predictable based on pre-existing measures of health

---

12. Center for Systems Science and Engineering, 'COVID-19 Dashboard', Johns Hopkins University, accessed 13 September 2022, https://coronavirus.jhu.edu/map.html.

and overall state capacity.[13] However, as highlighted in some of the chapters of this book, a country's social contract generally, and in the sphere of health in particular, played an important role in influencing national level pandemic responses.

At the same time, the social contract in many countries has also been influenced by the disruptions emanating from the pandemic. After decades of experience and research indicating that coercive public health measures are largely counterproductive in efforts to mitigate disease, COVID-19 brought about a new norm. There has been a global shift towards greater acceptance of strict lockdowns, police-enforced social distancing and quarantines, tracking of movement for contract tracing purposes, and other coercive public health policies. The question then becomes, will these policies be effective enough to change perceptions and norms for the long term? Or are these policies merely a direct response to a particular public health and political problem that will peter out with time and with increasing pandemic fatigue, vaccine uptake, and biotechnological advances? Further, what will be the resulting, if any, amendments to the nature of healthcare? Will this have enduring effects on how people relate to their government in many countries as a consequence of the pandemic? It is too soon to know, but clearly a topic worth serious consideration in the future.

---

13. Matthew M. Kavanagh and Renu Singh, 'Democracy, Capacity, and Coercion in Pandemic Response: COVID-19 in Comparative Political Perspective', *Journal of Health Politics, Policy and Law* 45, no. 6 (December 2020): 997–1012.

7

The Economic and Social Consequences of the COVID-19 Pandemic

Michael Edesess and Christine Loh

From January 2020, the world experienced more than two years of severe global disruption brought on by the coronavirus SARS-CoV-2, which caused the pandemic disease COVID-19. The world shut down much of its day-to-day activities for a large part of this period, which led to a global recession. In fact, statistics could not capture the full extent of what happened to societies large and small during the pandemic. Not only lives were lost, an estimated 18 million died as a result of COVID-19 by the end of 2021,[1] but lifetime earnings were gone and many of those who became ill but recovered suffered a loss of earnings, which impacted their dependents. A large segment of people fell into poverty due to the pandemic in 2020 and the situation did not improve much in 2021 and even the first half of 2022. The associated stress and anguish carried incalculable but real costs too for individuals and societies.

The International Monetary Fund (IMF) described the pandemic in June 2020 as 'a crisis like no other', against the background of intensifying trade conflicts that began in 2018. The United States, under the Donald Trump administration, imposed punitive tariffs on a variety of products against multiple countries that affected global trade. Relations worsened especially between the United States and China, as the former complained about its huge trade deficit with the latter. By 2022, relations between these two largest economies in the world, together sharing nearly 45 per cent of global Gross Domestic Product (GDP), had become an all-out ideological and systems conflict. The Joseph Biden administration that succeeded the Trump administration characterised relations with China as 'a battle between the utility of democracies in the twenty-first century and autocracies'. The deteriorating relations between them affected how they saw each other's COVID-19 responses, as discussed in Chapter 9, when they could have cooperated to fight the disease. By February 2022, while COVID-19 had yet to recede in the world, a new phase of global disruptions burst forth with the war between Russia and Ukraine.

---

1. David Adam, 'COVID's True Death Toll: Much Higher Than Official Records', *Nature*, 10 March 2022, https://www.nature.com/articles/d41586-022-00708-0.

This chapter looks at the pandemic period in 2020–2021 and ends with observations about the state of the global economy in mid-2022 and the uncertain prospects for the future. The global economy had been ravaged by COVID-19—declared a pandemic on 11 March 2020 by the World Health Organization (WHO)—and its recovery is having to contend with war and its many spillover effects. According to a report issued in March 2022 based on a survey of business executives worldwide, their top concern had shifted from the pandemic, which had been identified as the top risk for the previous two years, to 'global instability and/or conflicts'.[2]

COVID-19 and Economic Contraction

The 'economy' is an abstraction, but it is not separate from society. It is through people and the aggregate of their activities that the economy is perceived and measured. An economic contraction is a decline in national output, which affects production, sales and consumption, employment, and personal income. The massive global economic contraction caused by COVID-19 in 2020 shut down industrial production, people stayed home, and everything closed, from offices to shops and restaurants, to schools and to places of worship. Clinics and hospitals worked overtime and were overwhelmed in many places for an extended period. Global GDP lost 3.6 per cent in 2020. While GDP had gone back into positive territory in 2021, the gains were relatively small when the losses in 2020 were considered.

Table 7.1 shows the changes in GDP of countries discussed in this book from the pre-pandemic year of 2019 and the first year of the pandemic in 2020, and the change in GDP between 2020 and 2021. In the first year, Vietnam and China, two developing economies that managed to suppress COVID-19 early on still managed positive growth. Other economies contracted although relatively slightly in the cases of South Korea and New Zealand, which acted relatively quickly and decisively. Some European economies experienced a massive GDP decline in 2020, and growth in 2021 did not make up for the loss in the previous year.

There were common themes during the pandemic even though governments of different countries reacted differently to COVID-19. Virtually all jurisdictions exerted some level of mandated social distancing and isolation of the infected, contact tracing, and travel restrictions to mitigate the spread of the disease, though those measures varied widely from place to place and over time. They all attempted to gain access to enough supplies of personal protective equipment (PPE) and medical equipment to protect healthcare workers and their populations. Governments also attempted to gain access to vaccines and to get their populations vaccinated, though there were

---

2. McKinsey, 'Economic Condition Outlook, March 2022', March 2022, https://www.mckinsey.com/~/media/mckinsey/business%20functions/strategy%20and%20corporate%20finance/our%20insights/economic%20conditions%20outlook%202022/march%202022/economic-conditions-outlook-march-2022.pdf.

Table 7.1: Change in GDP from (a) 2019 to 2020 and (b) 2020 to 2021

Countries	GDP Change between 2019 and 2020	GDP Change between 2020 and 2021
Vietnam	+2.9%	+3.78
China	+2.3%	+8.02
South Korea	−0.9%	+4.28
New Zealand	−1.9%	+5.06
Australia	−2.5%	+3.54
Sweden	−2.9%	+4.04
United States	−3.4%	+5.97
Germany	−4.6%	+3.05
Japan	−4.6%	+2.36
Canada	−5.2%	+5.69
Singapore	−5.4%	+6.03
Thailand	−6.1%	+0.96
France	−7.9%	+6.29
Italy	−8.9%	+5.77
United Kingdom	−9.4%	+6.76

Source: World Bank Data, https://data.worldbank.org/indicator/NY.GDP.MKTP.KD.ZG?locations=VN, and *Statistics Times*, https://statisticstimes.com/economy/projected-world-gdp-ranking.php.

inequalities in the availability and/or acceptance of vaccines across countries (see Chapters 2 and 4).

These common themes brought about similar economic and societal consequences in the domestic economies of the various countries and in the global economy. The heightened need for hospital beds and medical equipment, such as ventilators and PPE, as well as ambulances and refrigerated vehicles for transporting corpses, imposed severe stresses on hospitals, healthcare workers, and medical systems, especially in countries where measures to contain the disease were grossly insufficient to 'flatten the curve', i.e., to reduce the peak demand for these health-related goods and services to below their availability (see Chapter 5).

The shortages of PPE, especially face masks, which the general public around the world also sought to buy, was one of the items of panic buying and stockpiling in the early months of the pandemic. Toilet paper, hand sanitisers, and staple food products were swept up. Panic buying is an impulse and temporary reaction to anxiety and fear caused by an impending crisis. Even unneeded items were purchased because they were available in stores, leading to the emptying of shelves all over the world in 2020 and when new waves of COVID-19 emerged. Herd psychology was at play, propelling people to do what others were doing.

Government Support Schemes to Demobilise the Economy

The onslaught of COVID-19 was an enormous challenge to policy-makers and governments. China was the first country that had to deal with the new virus. By mid-March 2020, the world economy paused, and the challenge had become global. It was a new experience for all governments. COVID-19 presented a package of shocks; it was a health crisis, a social crisis, an economic crisis, and a political crisis all rolled into one on a global scale.

All governments stretched their budgets to relieve the financial pain of those who were affected by work stoppages and to stimulate their economies. Country after country put forward COVID-19 relief plans starting in February 2020. There were many types of relief from governments around the world—including handing out food, providing free facemasks, giving out cash, supporting companies to meet payroll, granting loan guarantees, extending mortgage and loan repayments, cutting taxes, and covering the costs of vaccination when they became available in 2021.

Political leaders around the world spoke of the funding needed to fight the consequences of the pandemic in terms comparable to fighting a war, except that it was not about mobilising resources and manpower for war but covering the cost of demobilising the economy so people could stay home. Agustin Carstens, the general manager of the Bank of International Settlement, an international financial institution owned by central banks to promote cooperation, noted that:

> The COVID-19 pandemic and the induced global lockdown are a truly historic event. Never before has the global economy been deliberately put into an induced coma. This is no normal recession, but one that results from explicit policy choices to avoid a large-scale public health disaster.[3]

The IMF noted that by October 2020, rich economies had provided on average 8.5 per cent of GDP in their relief packages in response to the pandemic. The United States, the world's leading economy, passed the Coronavirus Aid, Relief, and Economic Security Act (CARES) on 25 March 2020 after just a fortnight of negotiations amounting to a massive US$2.2 trillion, or 10 per cent of US GDP. CARES was a pay cheque protection programme for businesses, and also gave households money directly, and extended unemployment benefits. It was the largest fiscal support delivered to the economy ever. Germany, Italy, France, Spain, the United Kingdom, Japan, and South Korea devoted large portions of their pandemic packages to providing loan guarantees to help companies, which enabled employers to continue paying their employees at more or less full pay to large swaths of the workforce. In Germany for example, the loan guarantees amounted to more than 30 per cent of GDP, and the British government's loan guarantees amounted to around 15 per cent of the United Kingdom's GDP. Middle-income countries on average provided 4 per cent of GDP in their pandemic relief packages,

---

3.   Agustín Carstens, 'Countering Covid-19: The Nature of Central Banks' Policy Response', speech on 27 May 2020, https://www.bis.org/speeches/sp200527.htm.

while poor countries on average managed under 2 per cent of GDP.[4] With COVID-19 under control by April 2020, China was more restrained in doling out relief and aid. Nevertheless, its fiscal effort in 2020 still amounted to 5.4 per cent of GDP. In 2020, China loosened lending, funded infrastructure, transferred funds to local governments to aid their measures to fight the pandemic, cut taxes and fees, and provided some indirect payments to households.[5] Governments around the world provided further aid packages in 2021—too many to list here—after the initial ones, as the pandemic rolled on. Suffice to note that the pandemic has been very expensive for governments around the world.

The case of Hong Kong was noteworthy as an example of what a rich city did. Hong Kong was among the earliest to provide COVID-19-related relief. Its first round of relief was approved by the legislature on 21 February 2020 and by the end of 2021, four rounds of relief packages had been approved. The Hong Kong government cut taxes for low-salary earners, reduced profits tax, waived rates for millions of owners of domestic properties, provided all kinds of direct payment schemes to many sectors of business, and issued highly popular consumption vouchers to most residents to boost the economy. As the city was hit by the Omicron variant, the government issued two more rounds of relief between January and April 2022.[6]

Money did not come free of course. Hong Kong did not have to borrow because of the city's strong finances (see Chapter 11). Many economies had to borrow. The Organisation for Economic Cooperation and Development (OECD), a group of rich and higher-income economies, estimated that by the end of 2020, the total debt issuance by rich economies amounted to US$18 trillion with the United States accounting for about two-thirds, Japan for a tenth, and the rest divided among European countries.[7] Carstens explained the critical role played by the central banks of the rich economies that got things going and helped to shorten the economic contraction successfully:

> The actions of central banks . . . highlighted their central role in crisis management as they swiftly cut policy interest rates . . . In . . . urgent policy mobilisation, central banks' actions concentrated on large-scale purchases of government debt as well as credit support for firms and households. The latter encompassed funding for lending schemes, purchases of corporate debt, and support provisions for small- and medium-sized enterprises. This last set of measures is designed to travel the 'last mile'. The main objective is to prevent liquidity strains that could lead to bankruptcies of solvent firms and leave long-lasting scars on growth potential. These extraordinary actions were

---

4. IMF Fiscal Monitor October 2020, https://www.imf.org/en/Publications/FM/Issues/2020/09/30/october-2020-fiscal-monitor.
5. Yue Cao, Rebecca Nadin, Linda Calabrese, Olena Borodyna, and Beatrice Tanjangco, 'Pulse 1: Covid-19 and Economic Crisis—China's Recovery and International Response', *ODI Economic Pulse series*, 30 November 2020, https://odi.org/en/publications/economic-pulse-1-covid-19-and-economic-crisis-chinas-recovery-and-international-response.
6. Hong Kong Government, 'Anti-Epidemic Fund', accessed 13 September 2022, https://www.coronavirus.gov.hk/eng/anti-epidemic-fund.html.
7. OECD 2020, 'Sovereign Borrowing Outlook for OECD Countries 2020'.

designed precisely to flatten the mortality curve of businesses . . . Finally, let me say that the aggressive measures described, crossing the traditional boundaries between fiscal and monetary policies, are only feasible for central banks in advanced economies with high credibility stemming from a long track record of stability-oriented policies. This is strong medicine and should only be taken with extreme care.[8]

With two-thirds of the world's population living in middle- and low-income countries (excluding China) facing unprecedented economic damage from COVID-19, and lacking the monetary, fiscal, and administrative capacity to respond to the massive pandemic crisis, the role of the United Nations became vital to provide guidance and assistance, as well as to organise fundraising from the governments of richer countries and from philanthropic foundations. Chapter 2 details the role of the United Nations, the WHO, and other agencies in helping emerging economies. What was made available to low-income economies was far from sufficient and exacerbated global inequalities.

COVID-19 Exacerbated Inequalities

The experience of the pandemic depended on location, nationality, age, gender, and socio-economic status. Older people everywhere were more susceptible to catching COVID-19 and persons 65 or older had strikingly higher mortality rates compared to younger individuals, and men had a higher risk of death than women.[9] The poor suffered the most as a result of the pandemic. In 2021, the average incomes of people in the bottom 40 per cent of the global income distribution were 6.7 per cent lower than pre-pandemic projections, while those of people in the top 40 per cent were down 2.8 per cent. The reason for the difference was the higher-income earners recovered their income losses much faster than the poor earners. Between 2019 and 2021, the average income of the bottom 40 per cent fell by 2.2 per cent, while the average income of the top 40 per cent fell by only 0.5 per cent.[10] In the Asia-Pacific region, extreme poverty increased for the first time in 20 years.[11] A more graphic description was that 97 million more people were living on less than US$1.90 a day because of the pandemic, increasing the global poverty rate from 7.8 per cent to 9.1 per cent between 2019 and 2021. The next poorest group consisted of about 160 million people, living on less than US$5.50

8.   Carstens, 'Countering Covid-19'.
9.   N. David Yanez, Noel S. Weiss, Jacques-André Romand, and Miriam M. Treggiari, 'COVID-19 Mortality Risk for Older Men and Women', *BMC Public Health* 20 (2020), https://bmcpublichealth.biomedcentral.com/articles/10.1186/s12889-020-09826-8.
10. Carolina Sánchez-Páramo, Ruth Hill, Daniel Gerszon Mahler, Ambar Narayan, and Nishant Yonzan, 'COVID-19 Leaves a Legacy of Rising Poverty and Widening Inequality', *World Bank Blog*, 7 October 2021, https://blogs.worldbank.org/developmenttalk/covid-19-leaves-legacy-rising-poverty-and-widening-inequality.
11. Economic and Social Commission for Asia and the Pacific (ESCAP), Asian Development Bank (ADB), and United Nations Development Programme (UNEP), 'Building Forward Together: Towards and inclusive and Resilient Asia and the Pacific', March 2022, http://dx.doi.org/10.22617/TCS220113-2.

a day. The World Bank notes that inequality had also worsened within countries, as poorer households lost income and jobs at higher rates than richer households.[12]

In rich and middle-income economies, and in more developed parts of emerging economies, inequalities were exacerbated between those working in services, who were able to work at home and those working in sectors in which employees' physical presence is essential, especially in those sectors characterised by physical closeness of employees, such as in factories and meat-packing. This exposed those who needed to be present physically to a greater risk of catching the disease than those who could work from home. Workers in sectors that require physical contact with each other and with consumers, such as hospitality, restaurants, air travel, and tourism, were more likely to lose their jobs, temporarily or permanently. These were likely to be lower-paying jobs than those held by workers who could take advantage of e-meeting services, such as Zoom, whose common stock increased in price by more than 700 per cent between January and October 2020.

Education systems around the world faced unprecedented challenges due to the COVID-19 pandemic. The delivery of education massively shifted to distance-learning solutions in richer economies. Parents, who normally relied on schools to serve as day care and who needed to be physically present at work, and who still had work, were challenged to find ways to care for—and to occupy—their stay-at-home children. Online distance learning was far from ideal in educational terms for younger students. Schools and teachers had to learn how to teach online, which affected the quality of the experience. Distance learning also increased the marginalisation of the most vulnerable people, as only about half the world had access to the Internet and Internet stability differed from place to place. Students in poor economies missed many months of schooling and they had few means to catch up. The pandemic caused 1.6 billion students to be out of school during the peak period of infection in 2020.[13] Worse, predictions were that the likelihood of child labour would increase because of the need to supplement family income, and that more girls than boys would likely drop out altogether as schools re-opened.[14]

Privatising Risks While Socialising Gains

Government relief and aid packages all around the world were promulgated quickly to address the short-term COVID-19 impacts. The packages were massive in wealthy economies. There was no time to fine-tune them to focus on those who truly needed help. The huge government outlays to compensate the unemployed and to stimulate economies raised again an important concern that was last raised in a different form after the global financial crisis of 2007–2009. Then and in 2020, insufficient attention

---

12. Sánchez-Páramo et al., 'COVID-19 Leaves a Legacy'.
13. UNESCO, 'Education: From School Closure to Recovery', accessed 25 May 2022, https://en.unesco.org/covid19/educationresponse#durationschoolclosures.
14. ESCAP, ADB and UNEP, 'Building Forward Together'.

and funding to prepare for, or to prevent in advance a crisis that should have been foreseeable, resulted in the need for large government bailouts. In both cases, these bailouts tended to enhance the fortunes of the relatively well-off by driving up the value of stocks and other investments, while doing too little to alleviate the reduced circumstances of those who are not well-off, thus exacerbating inequalities, and privatising gains while socialising risks. This is particularly true in richer economies. Part of the assessment in the aftermath of the COVID-19 pandemic should address broader economic and philosophical questions: Is it possible that systemic changes to domestic and global institutions could alleviate these concerns? To what extent is it preferable for governments to invest heavily in preventive measures to avoid sudden, unpredictable, and possibly much larger expenditures later? These are questions not only for national institutions and governments, but also for global institutions like the IMF and the WHO, as discussed in Chapter 2.

Data showed that in April 2020, the savings rate in America increased from an average of 8 per cent in 2019 to 32.2 per cent in 2020—the highest figure ever recorded—and in Europe, it increased from 13.1 per cent in 2019 to 24.6 per cent in 2020.[15] What that meant was that in spite of the overall damages to the less wealthy, in some countries, such as the United States and Europe, government handouts were generous enough, together with mortgage payment suspensions, to enable many unemployed or stay-at-home people to save and either accumulate unspent money to fuel pent-up demand when restrictions eased, or to spend their time on internet-based activities such as online gaming and day-trading of shares of listed stocks. These activities, especially day-trading, tended to benefit the providers of the services, such as in the finance industry, who were wealthier. In the United States, the cheques households received under CARES and other rounds of stimulus payments enabled households to build up US$2.7 trillion in extra savings from the start of the pandemic to the end of 2021.[16] It helped to promote a rethinking of career paths, in some cases leading people to decide not to return to their original jobs, contributing to an employee pinch when the pandemic restrictions eased.

Regional Differences

Inflation began to spurt in 2022 as pandemic restrictions eased and activity revived in many economies. The pent-up demand and easy money from government COVID stimulus, together with supply-side constrictions due to disrupted supply chains, temporary work stoppages, and lockdowns in major Chinese cities in March–May 2022 all played a role. Among the main differences from country to country were that in some, most notably China, very severe measures to prevent the transmission of the

---

15. McKinsey Global Institute, 'Covid-19 Has Revived the Social Contract in Advanced Economies—For Now. What Will Stick Once the Crisis Abates?', 10 December 2020.
16. Rachel Louise Ensign and Orla McCaffrey, 'American Begin to Draw Down Pandemic-Era Savings', *The Wall Street Journal*, 6 July 2022.

virus were undertaken early, with noteworthy success, at least until the onset of the Omicron variant in 2022. In others, most notably the United States and the United Kingdom, relatively lax and late measures were applied to contain the spread in 2020. As a generalisation, the most stringent measures were undertaken in the Asia-Pacific region, including New Zealand and Australia. Countries in that region have suffered much lower numbers of hospitalisations and deaths per capita in 2020–2021 than the United States, the United Kingdom, and Europe. In the Asia-Pacific region, strong government restrictions and contact tracing were put in place to prevent hospitalisations and deaths. In the United States and the United Kingdom and some other countries, the emphasis was more on the trade-off and balance between preventing deaths and morbidities on the one hand and inflicting damage on the economy on the other. And yet paradoxically, in China particularly, as well as other countries that imposed strong measures to stamp out the virus in 2020–2021, normal economic growth returned quickly once the spread of the virus and its subsequent waves were contained.

Nevertheless, China's continuation with its zero-COVID policy after the onset of Omicron in March–May 2022 affected production there, which affected global supply chains, since China has a large manufacturing-export sector. In some quarters, this was seen as evidence that China's zero-COVID policy would be, and was, ultimately not as successful as first believed, leading to economic damage not only in China but in global markets. Some argued that China's policy prevented its population from building up herd immunity, whereas in other countries proximity to the virus tended to immunise populations in the long term. But with the development of effective vaccines that substituted for acquiring natural immunity from the virus itself (and for all vaccines, including those prevailing in China, the United States, and Europe, substantially lower rates of hospitalisations and deaths) this argument holds less force. The view from China was very different. China saw its COVID-19 policy as effective in curbing transmission at the fastest speed and at the lowest cost, and that it protected people's health while reducing its impact on the economy.

How China dealt with COVID-19 will be a topic of debate for years to come, not least because there were many unique aspects to the thinking of its leadership that were so different from other jurisdictions. The Chinese government went through enormous effort and great expense to contain COVID-19. As noted in Chapter 9, the highly transmissible Omicron outbreak in China in March 2022 led to restrictions and lockdowns in various places, including the major cities of Shenzhen, Shanghai, and Beijing. The Chinese formula for fighting COVID-19 involved mass testing and tracing on a huge scale and at great expense.[17] The justification was that this method and expense was considered much less than having to lock down the economy to save lives. By May 2022, the Chinese government announced large plans to bolster the economy, which were further expanded in the autumn. By mid-December 2022, COVID restrictions

---

17. Xu Wen, Cui Xiaotian, Dong Hui, Zhang Yukun, and Li Leyan, 'Five Things to Know about China's Plans for Regular Mass COVID Testing', *Caixin*, 3 June 2022.

eased substantially as the government realised the curbs were no longer working in face of the highly infectious Omicron and following public protests of what people saw as capricious restrictions by local authorities that weakened the economy and unreasonably affected their lives (see Chapter 9). Nevertheless, the full-year 2022 GDP for China was still expected to be around 3 per cent.

Rationality and Social Contracts

How one views society's response to COVID-19 could be explained by the work of the late Nobel prize-winning economist and political scientist, Elinor Ostrom. Ostrom theorised how people made decisions on following rules—the majority, referred to as 'norm users', were seen as willing participants to act for the collective good, but a minority of 'rational egoists' would only act if something was in their interest. Ostrom argued that 'rational egoists' would change their behaviour to avoid punishment because it would be in their interest to avoid punishment. In her view, those who acted in defiance of rules could negatively affect how willing participants behaved by influencing them to break rules. Thus, from a societal perspective, it would be important to punish the minority rule breakers to reinforce collective good norms.[18]

Using Ostrom's perspective, it could be said that the majority of Americans are 'rational egoists', while most of those in many Asian countries are 'norm users'. In the United States, the paramount value is individualism, while in many Asian societies, it is the well-being of the community. Thus, the implicit social contracts are different in the two regions. In Asia, it is considered a norm to act to support the community, and to obey and rely on the authorities. In the United States, authorities are not trusted, though this has not always been the case historically. It is, nevertheless, a norm to depend on oneself. This may partly account for the different actions in the two regions on the part of citizens and governments, and the different results. In the United States, masking, even during a pandemic, was scoffed at by a large percentage of the population, and in most places in the United States, one felt peculiar if one wore a mask; while in China and most of Asia, masking was accepted and performed by virtually all of the population, and one felt out of place if not wearing a mask.

These differences likely accounted for the differences in collective societal impacts of the pandemic. In the United States, divisions among the population increased. The approval of its president as well as institutions, legislators, media, and judiciary reached historic lows. Divisions increased not only in the United States but also in Europe and the United Kingdom over the issues of masking and vaccination. Some people were adamantly against getting vaccinated for a variety of reasons, including distrust of the vaccines. Even in Asia, social cohesion was tested when the Omicron variant hit in early 2022. There was heightened unease about restrictive government policies in

---

18. Elinor Ostrom, 'Collective Action and the Evolution of Social Norms', *Journal of Economic Perspectives* 14, no. 3 (Summer 2000): 137–158.

Japan[19] and South Korea.[20] With respect to Hong Kong, when the city was unable to contain the spread of Omicron in 2022, the public was angry that the authorities had lost the plot in COVID-19 management as many elderly people, who had declined to be vaccinated, died (see Chapter 11), moving Hong Kong from a location with one of the lowest daily COVID-19 death rates to the highest in the world. Rumblings of discontent even emerged in mainland China with the Shanghai lockdown in 2022. It remains to be seen what long-term impacts there might be on political trust in various jurisdictions.

As Chapter 1 pointed out, the Global Health Security Index (GHSI) in 2019 and 2021 on the preparedness of countries for a pandemic found that while no country was well prepared, the country that had the highest potential to be well prepared was the United States, and developing countries, including China, were ranked relatively lowly. And yet, it was the United States that floundered greatly. The authors of the GHSI acknowledged that beyond potential preparedness, political will to act was vital when a jurisdiction faced an infectious disease. The sociologist Ulrich Beck, coined the phrase 'organised irresponsibility', meaning a situation where 'individuals cumulatively contribute to risks without being held individually accountable'.[21] This perspective could be used to contrast the different actions taken by governments around the world. In Asia, the general public expectation was that the government must save lives, so the number of infections and deaths became the measure to judge policy effectiveness and also acceptance of tough measures that constrain personal freedoms. In the highly individualistic US 'rational egoist' culture, the notion of 'organised irresponsibility' may explain the public acceptance of a patchwork of lax official approaches that resulted in high infections and fatalities, as the majority of Americans saw lax approaches almost as a virtue.

The COVID-19 economic and social impacts were both short- and long-term. The long-term impacts will be debated for years. China's tough lockdown at the start crushed the virus in 2020, and there are insights and lessons to draw from that experience. A number of other economies also took fast action. This enabled the early revival of their economies. The closing of borders around the world limited cross-border transmissions and it took considerable time to resume; and for China and those countries that were successful in containing COVID-19 in 2020–2021, opening up represented considerable risk to their protected population. The United Kingdom and the United States had essentially re-opened their borders by April 2022 as they adopted 'living

19. Saya Soma and Yves Tiberghien, 'Japan Slams the Borders Shut on Omicron', *East Asia Forum*, 6 February 2022, https://www.eastasiaforum.org/2022/02/06/japan-slams-the-borders-shut-on-omicron.

20. Yoo-jung Lee and Yves Tiberghien, 'South Korea's Deepening Social Fractures amid COVID-19 Success', *East Asia Forum*, 28 October 2021, https://www.eastasiaforum.org/2021/10/28/south-koreas-deepening-social-fractures-amid-covid-19-success.

21. Cai Shouqiu provides a succinct summary of 'organised irresponsibility' in 'Rooting Out "Organized Irresponsibility"', 13 October 2020, *Caixin Online*, https://www.marketwatch.com/story/china-plagued-by-organized-irresponsibility-2010-10-13#:~:text=Ulrich%20Beck%2C%20a%20German%20sociologist,political%20hierarchy%20and%20organizational%20settings.

with COVID' policies. The contrast between them and China raised many commentaries that became politicised at a time of deepening ideological conflict, cast as between 'democracies and autocracies', which made it harder to reflect on the public health, economic, and social aspects of COVID-19. By the end of May 2022, the Chinese government announced a massive package of measures covering fiscal, financial, investment, and industrial policies to stimulate the economy, as other factors beyond the pandemic had emerged and China started to prepare for what might be a 'long COVID' global recession.

Long Economic COVID

Some patients who contracted COVID-19 found that deleterious effects continued for many months after its onset, leading to the coining of the term 'long COVID'. The pandemic itself, however, will also have lasting effects on the global economy as commerce continues to change in an era of resurgent nationalism, geopolitical tensions, and hyper-competition between groups of countries. These trends have raised questions about whether the post-COVID world might be less connected and less globalised. Even before the pandemic, complex forces had been pulling concurrently at both globalisation and deglobalisation. The forces are complex, and it is beyond this chapter to lay them all out. We focus on those aspects that the pandemic helped crystallise. Most obvious was the risk and danger of relying on global supply chains for PPE.

Globalisation of commerce had become the norm since the 1990s, as the widespread, blithe assumption that 'the world is flat' took hold, meaning the world was seen as a level playing field wherein all competitors, except for labour, have an equal opportunity. Flows of goods from lower-cost economies to consumers in higher-cost ones, and assembling parts in different countries, were so fluid that there was little concern about adopting 'just-in-time' supply chains that were highly economically efficient when all went well but not sufficiently resilient in case of supply shortages and bottlenecks along the chain. In 2020, there was a global severe shortage of PPE for a period of time as COVID-19 surged. The United States and many developed economies no longer had domestic suppliers for these goods. The competition for PPE was so intense that in one incident, the United States was accused of 'modern piracy' for diverting a shipment of masks intended for Germany,[22] and there was even competition for PPE between states and the federal government in America.[23] The call for reshoring of production, especially of PPE, drugs and other critical products intensified. Vaclav Smil noted:

22. Kim Willsher, Julian Borger, and Oliver Holmes, 'US Accused of "Modern Piracy" after Diversion of Masks Meant for Europe', *The Guardian*, 4 April 2020, https://www.theguardian.com/world/2020/apr/03/mask-wars-coronavirus-outbidding-demand.
23. Andrew Soergel, 'States Competing in "Global Jungle" for PPE', *US News*, 7 April 2020, https://www.usnews.com/news/best-states/articles/2020-04-07/states-compete-in-global-jungle-for-personal-protective-equipment-amid-coronavirus.

Questioning and criticising globalization has gone beyond narrowly ideological arguments, and the COVID-19 pandemic provided additional powerful arguments based on irrefutable concerns about the state's fundamental role in protecting the lives of its citizens. That role is hard to play when 70 percent of the world's rubber gloves are made in a single factory, and when similar or even higher shares of not just other pieces of personal protective equipment but also of principal drug components and common medications (antibiotics, antihypertensive drugs) come from a very small number of suppliers in China and India. Such dependence might fulfil an economist's dream of mass output at the lowest possible unit cost, but it makes for extremely irresponsible—if not criminal—governance when doctors and nurses have to face a pandemic without adequate PPE, when states dependent on foreign production engage in dismaying competition for limited supplies, and when patients around the world cannot renew their prescriptions because of the slowdowns or closures in Asian factories . . . the reshoring of manufacturing could be the wave of the future, both in North America and in Europe . . . we may have seen the peak of globalisation, and its ebb may last not just for years but for decades to come.[24]

The World Economic Forum, an annual gathering of senior business leaders and government officials, held in May 2022, noted that 'globalisation' was not fading but was continuing to evolve. The globalisation of services was increasing dramatically since the pandemic, while that for goods had stalled. COVID-19 led to the rise of services delivered online. This meant companies became comfortable with hiring people as employees and contractors to deliver services in different locations around the world and managing them remotely. However, the relocation of production of goods from high-income economies to low-wage economies had stalled even before the pandemic because firstly, what could be outsourced had been outsourced, and secondly, the tariffs imposed by the United States in 2018 under the Trump administration made cross-border commerce more challenging to plan, and especially challenging for Chinese exports. The pandemic focussed attention on the risk of extensive offshoring. This led to calls in rich economies to bring manufacturing jobs 'back home' to strengthen domestic economies. There were also calls for protecting workers' rights to enable wage-led growth rather than enabling the maximisation of corporate profits. The calls for reshoring manufacturing, and also improving wages for workers were often wrapped in anti-globalisation narratives.[25]

As far as PPE was concerned, the upsurge in talk about reshoring involved achieving 'supply chain resilience strategies' that could introduce buffers and redundancies into supply chains so that they could withstand stoppages and bottlenecks. Resilience and efficiency, however, are not close comrades. With added buffers and redundancies there are added costs and lowered efficiencies during the majority of times when those

24. Vaclav Smil, *How the World Really Works: A Scientist's Guide to Our Past, Present, and Future* (London: Viking), 133.

25. World Economic Forum, 'Davos 2021 – Preparing for Deglobalization', 26 January 2021, https://www.weforum.org/videos/davos-2021-preparing-for-deglobalization-english.

buffers and redundancies are not needed. Chapter 8 shows these issues are not easy to address and would require careful and skilful long-term policy-making.

It is worth digressing here to consider the trade rivalry between the United States and China. The Trump administration's tariffs imposed in 2018 averaged 19.3 per cent on US$335 billion of Chinese imports.[26] China reacted by imposing tariffs on US imports. Researchers studied how these tariffs affected trade flows in 2018–2019. Unsurprisingly, trade was depressed between the two countries—China's exports to the United States declined by 8.5 per cent and US exports to China fell by 26.3 per cent—but their punch-up did not depress overall global trade, which increased by 3 per cent. Researchers observed that:

> The US-China trade war raised concerns that the era of global trade growth would come to an end. Our results provide little support for this view, at least for the medium-run time horizon that is the focus of our analysis. Indeed, trade between the two largest economies, the US and China, declined significantly. However, we also find that trade among indirectly affected bystander countries, as well as trade between these countries and the US, increased substantially. As a result, global trade increased in the products targeted by the tariffs. Rather than merely reallocating global trade flows, the trade war appears to have created new trade opportunities for many countries.[27]

China had made it clear that it was ready to remove the tariffs as soon as the United States dropped its. The tariffs remained in place after a change of administration in 2021 in the United States. Despite inflation rising substantially by mid-2022, the Biden administration did not remove the Trump era tariffs imposed on Chinese exports.

The 'deglobalisation' narrative is tinged with nationalistic and competitive sentiments. While PPE was the reshoring posterchild with respect to the pandemic, more important still were products deemed critical to technology, especially computer chips, semiconductors, batteries, and advanced pharmaceuticals. New terms arose in 2021—'friend-shoring' and 'allies-shoring'—that reflected the notion that like-minded countries should cooperate to strengthen their economies and competitiveness against other rival systems. The leader of this coalition, the United States, was working with countries in Europe and together with Japan and South Korea as this book went to press. The intention is to 'unfriend China'.[28] These geopolitical factors make global cooperation much more challenging at a time when multi-lateral solutions are needed to not only regulate global trade but also deal with global crime, climate change, and, of course, fight pandemics. COVID-19 showed governments around the world took uncoordinated measures against a clear and present global threat to contain the transmission of a new infectious disease and to share vaccines.

26. Chad Brown, 'US China Trade Tariffs: An Up-to-Date Chart', 22 April 2022, https://www.piie.com/research/piie-charts/us-china-trade-war-tariffs-date-chart.

27. Pablo Fajgelbaum, Pinelopi K. Goldberg, Patrick J. Kennedy, Amit Khandelwal, and Daria Taglioni, 'The US-China Trade War and Global Relocations', National Bureau of Economic Research, Working Paper 29562, December 2021, https://www.nber.org/system/files/working_papers/w29562/w29562.pdf.

28. Mona Paulsen, 'Friend-Shoring', International Economic Law and Policy Blog, 21 April 2022, https://ielp.worldtradelaw.net/2022/04/friend-shoring.html.

The potential negative effects to international trade of 'friend-shoring' were made clear by the economist Raghuram G. Rajan, a former governor of the Reserve Bank of India. He noted that while diversifying production locations in the supply chain across countries to increase flexibility and resilience was appropriate, resurgent protectionism was not, and could pose a dangerous threat. Such a threat began with the tariffs introduced by the Trump administration and accelerated not only due to the supply chain difficulties during COVID-19 but also because of the war between Russia and Ukraine, and the imposition of sanctions on Russia by the United States and the European Union. Moreover, the 'friend-shoring' narrative by Western politicians was also due to their displeasure with China for its friendly relationship with Russia accompanied by Western dissatisfaction with both. Rajan pointed to another concern:

> friend-shoring will typically mean trading with countries that have similar values and institutions; and that, in practice, will mean transacting only with countries at similar levels of development. The benefits of a global supply chain stem precisely from the fact that it involves countries with very different income levels, allowing each to bring its comparative advantage to the production process . . . Friend-shoring would tend to eliminate this dynamic, thereby increasing production costs and consumer prices . . . friend-shoring would tend to exclude the poor countries that most need global trade in order to become richer and more democratic. It will increase the risks that these countries become failed states, fertile grounds to nurture and export terrorism. The tragedy of mass emigration will become more likely as chaotic violence increases.[29]

Inflation Uncertainty

As the world began to recover from the pandemic, concern about inflation, or more accurately, inflation uncertainty rose. Inflation was a major concern in the United States and elsewhere in the 1970s, which at one time exceeded 13 per cent in 1980. The United States Federal Reserve tightened the money supply in October 1979, which brought inflation under control at the cost of a severe, though short recession, in 1981–1982. Since then, inflation in the United States has been moderate, almost never exceeding 3 per cent annually since 1992 and dropping to historically low rates shortly before the pandemic. Although there was some warning of lurking inflation, especially when the Federal Reserve and other central banks adopted unconventional stimulative monetary policies after the 2007–2009 financial crisis in an attempt to spur economic activity, inflation did not in fact materialise. Low inflation appeared to be a persistent phenomenon in the global economy. The COVID-19 pandemic led to an economic slowdown and central banks acted to spur economies as noted above with massive aid packages. Research showed that in 2020–2021, the four major central banks in the world—the United States, Japan, Europe, and the United Kingdom—pumped in over US$11

---

29. Raghuram G. Rajan, 'Just Say No to Friend Shoring', *The Jordon Times*, 6 June 2022, https://www.jordantimes.com/opinion/raghuram-g-rajan/just-say-no-%E2%80%98friend-shoring%E2%80%99.

trillion to support their economies and the functioning of the global financial markets in response to the pandemic. This kind of monetary action is referred to as 'quantitative easing' and as Carstens warned, it is 'strong medicine'. It involves pumping money into their economies by buying assets, such as government bonds and asset-backed securities, which increases the value of those assets, and at the same time increases the size of the central banks' cumulative balance sheets.[30] When a central bank uses quantitative easing, it helps to lower the cost of borrowing thereby boosting spending and economic growth, which could lead to inflation. To control inflation, central banks have to play the challenging role of unwinding their asset purchases and at the same time increasing interest rates, ideally without disrupting economic growth.

Going into 2022, inflation surged as demand returned. Pent-up demand was strong as people could not spend during lockdowns, and demand was also fuelled by saving from generous government subsidies in rich economies, as explained earlier in this chapter. As demand surged, the war between Russia and Ukraine started on 24 February, and at the same time supply chains were affected by the renewed lockdowns in China as Omicron surged. The confluence of these factors affected the economies of individual countries and the global economy as a whole.

In the United States, inflation rose throughout 2021 from a low base to 7 per cent by December 2021 and averaged 4.7 per cent for the full year. Inflation was over 8 per cent from March and hit 9 per cent in June 2022. Critics complained the Federal Reserve had failed to fend off inflation resurgence.[31] Through 2021, the Federal Reserve had thought that inflation would improve gradually because it was a transitory problem—supply chain delays and worker shortages would self-correct. The fact that the Federal Reserve, arguably the most sophisticated central bank in the world, with its access to the widest possible array of data, was caught off guard by the return of inflation suggested that uncertainty about the level of inflation might prevail for the foreseeable future, complicating business and government planning and increasing the fear of hyper-inflation. The Federal Reserve changed tack in early May 2022 raising interest rates by 0.5 per cent and outlined a programme to reduce its asset holdings to fight inflation. In June, July and September 2022, it raised interest rates three times, each time by 0.75 per cent. raised

In the European Union, inflation averaged 5 per cent in 2021. By June 2022, it had exceeded 8.1 per cent. The European Union is made up of many economies—the average inflation rate does not reflect the diversity among the different economies. The European Central Bank retrenched from quantitative easing and raised interest rates in July 2022. Besides, Europe's energy supply has been disrupted and destabilized as a result of worsening relations with Russia. Reducing its dependence on Russian

---

30. The Atlantic Council, 'Global QE Tracker', accessed 13 September 2022, https://www.atlanticcouncil.org/global-qe-tracker.
31. John H. Cochrane, 'Why Hasn't the Fed Done More to Fight Inflation?', *Chicago Booth Review*, 27 April 2022, https://www.chicagobooth.edu/review/why-hasnt-fed-done-more-fight-inflation.

energy would take time and buying energy from elsewhere would impact global energy markets, the longer-term consequences of which are hard to predict.

Japan was in recession for much of 2021 and inflation remained in negative territory for the full year at −0.2 per cent. Indeed, Japan experienced deflation for nearly 30 years. By April 2022, inflation stood at 2.4 per cent and by September, it had climbed to 3 per cent, which was sharp for Japan, against an economic outlook clouded by the yet unknown length and consequences of the Russia-Ukraine war and its impact on energy and food prices—two major imports for Japan. China's inflation in 2021 was 0.9 per cent, but rose to 2.5 per cent in June 2022 amid rising energy prices, and logistic disruptions caused by the COVID-19 surge.

With so many factors at play, governments may be facing a period of inflation uncertainty, the economic consequences of which are difficult to predict but will surely not be conducive to economic stability. In short, the whiplash of economic activity caused by the COVID-19 pandemic, from economic lockdowns and slowdowns to a surge in pent-up demand coinciding with supply frictions, mixed with geopolitical conflicts and war, have increased uncertainty about inflation and about the global economy for some time to come.

Conclusion

The economic travails during the pandemic—the unemployment, the slowdowns in commerce, the burdens on essential workers—will be transient, but the long-term effects described above may be longer-lasting. The COVID-19 pandemic might eventually be seen as a global economic watershed. Paradoxically, a disastrous event, the onset of which was shared equally in virtually all countries of the world may wind up dividing countries, because of the realisation of the risks it posed—in spite of the obvious benefits—by their interdependency and tightly interlocking supply chains. The result is a general sense of worsening economic conditions. The Russia-Ukraine war and global decoupling attendant upon it are recent major contributors to that mood, but much of it began with awakened realisations about globalisation stemming from the pandemic. The net result could be more turbulent and unpredictable global economic conditions for years to come.

In the future, as noted above, an important question should be the subject of more searching inquiry than it has been in the past, both for national governments and for the global community. To what extent, and at what costs, should measures be adopted in times of relative calm to shore up national and global resilience against certain types of shocks that are predictable, but whose timing is unpredictable? At what point would the benefits of such measures exceed their costs? These events include pandemics and financial crises. Some countries, most notably the United States, apply massive resources and hedges in the form of defence budgets in an attempt to ensure resilience against war, but fail to do so to ensure resilience against pandemics and financial crises. Are there forms of economic analysis that can help to answer this question? This should be an important subject for further deliberation.

8

What Governments Should Do to Prevent Shortages of Medically Critical Products in Future Pandemics

Christopher S. Tang and ManMohan S. Sodhi

Introduction

This chapter uses the case of personal protective equipment (PPE) shortages in the United States as an example to motivate governments around the world to consider their strategies on how to manage the vulnerabilities in supply chains of medically critical items needed in a pandemic. The United States is the wealthiest economy globally, with a sophisticated healthcare system. The Global Health Security Index in 2019 and 2021 ranked it as having the best potential performance for pandemic preparedness (see Chapter 1). Even so, there were severe shortages of PPE and ventilators in the country in 2020 when COVID-19 emerged. Hence, the failure of the United States in this area provides sobering lessons for other jurisdictions. This chapter first highlights the PPE and ventilator shortages before examining the underlying causes and then making recommendations on measures to ensure supply chains of critical products can quickly respond to future pandemics and other major public health emergencies.

In 2020, the coronavirus SARS-CoV-2 put the entire world on notice with the COVID-19 pandemic, which continued into 2021 and 2022 with several waves and variants. In 2022, the Omicron variant rapidly drove a new phase of infections in many jurisdictions, including ones that had done well earlier to contain the virus. Over this period, COVID-19 created a worldwide health crisis not seen since the 1918 influenza pandemic. According to the World Bank, the world's real Gross Domestic Product (GDP) shrank by 3.4 per cent in 2020 relative to 2019, compared to a growth of 2.6 per cent in the previous year.[1] The US economy also shrank by 3.4 per cent year on year, while the Euro area and Japan experienced drops of 6.4 per cent and 4.6 per cent, respectively.

Economic consequences aside, COVID-19's toll on people was very high in many countries. By the end of July 2022, there had been over 572 million reported cases of infection. In May 2022, the United States has passed more than one million

---

1. World Bank, 'Global Economic Prospects', June 2022, https://www.worldbank.org/en/publication/global-economic-prospects.

COVID-related deaths, and the World Health Organization reported 15 million excess deaths worldwide over the two years from January 2020 to December 2021. Other estimates were even higher.[2] The sheer scale of the pandemic underscores the need for accelerated development and deployment of vaccines and drugs as preparation for future pandemics and access to medically critical products, such as PPE.[3]

The COVID-19 pandemic disrupted global supply chain operations from factories to ports, warehouses, and retail outlets. Severe shortages of PPE and ventilators in many countries revealed vulnerabilities in the supply chains of critical products at a time of acute need.[4] The severity of PPE shortages was a surprise, particularly in wealthy economies that supposedly had longstanding stockpiles and sound preparedness systems.

As demand for hospital care surged, frontline healthcare workers in many places had the same complaint—they were highly exposed but inadequately protected—and yet, they were the ones to help people survive contagion. The Lancet reported that healthcare workers were three times more likely than the general population to test positive for COVID-19.[5] PPE shortages are not just a worker's rights and an occupational health issue but a systemwide health challenge. Without proper protection, frontline healthcare workers are exposed to risks that make them more likely to become ill. Their falling ill leads to a decline in the number of healthcare professionals when the demand for care intensifies, thus reducing the quality of care and weakening the healthcare system.

Beyond healthcare workers, PPE shortages compromise mitigation measures, especially facemasks, which are crucial in reducing community transmission. Panic buying from the public everywhere in the world exacerbated the problem. COVID-19 has made it crystal clear that PPE availability is essential for responding to future pandemics effectively. Governments, hospitals, clinics, and corporations producing and selling PPE must rethink their supply chains. The public, too, has a role to play.

The above observations motivate us to structure this chapter as follows. We identify four underlying causes for PPE shortages based on the observed government response during the COVID-19 pandemic, and propose six recommendations for governments that involve all stakeholders to address these causes.

2. For excess deaths, see World Health Organization (WHO), '14.9 Million Excess Deaths Associated with the COVID-19 Pandemic in 2020 and 2021', 5 May 2022, https://www.who.int/news/item/05-05-2022-14.9-million-excess-deaths-were-associated-with-the-covid-19-pandemic-in-2020-and-2021. Others estimated deaths could have been as high as 18 million: David Adam, 'COVID's True Death Toll: Much Higher Than Official Records', Nature, 10 March 2022, https://www.nature.com/articles/d41586-022-00708-0.
3. We focus on medical PPE such as medical masks (surgical and N-95 masks), eye protection equipment (face shields and goggles), gloves, gowns, and coveralls, etc.
4. Based on a survey of 121 medical facilities in 2020, the WHO reported that fewer than 15 per cent of these facilities have access to the PPE they need (IFC (2021)).
5. Long H. Nguyen, David A. Drew, Mark S. Graham, Amit D. Joshi, Chan-Guo Guo, Wenjie Ma, et al., 'Risk of COVID-19 among Front-Line Health Care Workers and the General Community: A Prospective Cohort Study', Lancet Public Health, 31 July 2020, https://doi.org/10.1016/s2468-2667(20)30164-x.

Shortages of PPE during the Pandemic

COVID-19's high transmissibility and rapid spread resulted in many cases around the world requiring hospitalisation. Medical workers needed large quantities of PPE. Shortages stoked public fear and anxiety. The facemask shortage peaked in March 2020 in the United States, while news coverage of PPE shortages (facemasks, N-95 masks, medical gowns, etc.) and ventilators peaked the following month. Regardless of the media report peaks, PPE shortages were not resolved even by the late summer in the United States. In August 2020, 77 per cent of medical facilities in the United States had no supplies of one or more types of PPE. Earlier, from March to August 2020, two types of medically critical products were in severe shortage: facemasks and ventilators.

As COVID-associated hospitalisations skyrocketed in April 2020 and July 2020, the demand for PPE surged in the United States to protect healthcare providers. Prolonged shortages, especially of N-95 masks, have been linked to over 300 deaths and 60,000 infections among US healthcare workers by May 2020. The United States Centers for Disease Control (USCDC) initially recommended frequent hand washing and disinfecting surfaces as vital preventive measures. Then the USCDC further suggested facial covering and social distancing in early April. As different cities issued mandates requiring face coverings to slow the spread of COVID-19, demand for facemasks (mainly surgical masks) increased dramatically, leading to severe shortages.

Experts estimated a minimum need for an additional 45,000 invasive and 77,000 non-invasive ventilators in April 2020, considering the number of ventilators in stockpile or storage and the percentage of COVID-19 patients in intensive care units (ICUs) in need of invasive or non-invasive ventilators. On top of these shortages, over 2,000 ventilators in the US stockpile had either expired or were faulty and therefore unusable. Similarly, some states received unusable masks, gloves, ventilators, and other essential equipment from the national stockpile that had expired, rotted, or became otherwise non-functional. By the end of August, doctors and nurses were still reusing single-use N-95 masks and experiencing shortages of face shields and gloves.

Healthcare spending in the United States in 2019 was 17.7 per cent of GDP, by far the highest in the world. Wealthy countries like Germany, France, Japan, Sweden, and the United Kingdom spent between 10 and 12 per cent of GDP in 2019. China's spending that year was 5.4 per cent of GDP. Moreover, the country had warnings about a lack of preparedness. Despite the colossal healthcare budget and these prior warnings, Americans were shocked by PPE shortages for an extended period in 2020. Naturally, they raised questions about the United States' preparedness to respond to pandemics and other disasters. Indeed, the pandemic preparedness simulation in 2019, called the Crimson Contagion, had already noted shortages of PPE and ventilators, and highlighted other serious problems (see Chapter 9).

Four Causes for PPE Shortages

The COVID-19 pandemic showed that the supply chains for PPE and ventilators are highly vulnerable to disruption. While the media focused on complaints from health-care workers and the authorities' chaotic response to the shortages, the shortages were only *symptoms* of much deeper problems. We propose *four causes* to explain why the United States suffered from severe PPE and ventilator shortages—these issues should also be relevant to other jurisdictions.

Lack of long-term commitment

Whether geographically small or large, every country needs a long-term commitment to maintaining a stockpile of critical items. However, priorities and the level of commitment are often influenced by the day's politics. The United States' Strategic National Stockpile (SNS) was created as a warehouse of medical supplies, drugs, and vaccines.[6] It is overseen by the Department of Health and Human Services (DHHS) in coordination with the Department of Homeland Security. During the swine flu epidemic in 2009, the PPE distributed from the SNS—including some 85 million N-95 respirators—were not replaced. In 2011, then-President Barack Obama failed to get Congress to approve funds for replenishment. In 2012, Congress cut SNS funding by 10 per cent, and during the Ebola (2014–2015) and Zika (2015–2016) outbreaks, only half of the requested funding was supported by Congress. Individual states may also have built stockpiles. For instance, California amassed a considerable stockpile, including ventilators, under Governor Arnold Schwarzenegger in 2005. However, the stockpile was dismantled by Governor Jerry Brown in 2011 as a cost-cutting measure to reduce the state's budget deficit.

While managing the annual budget for preparedness to acquire PPE items is relatively simple, managing a stockpile of medical equipment for the long-term can be challenging because it requires significant investment in inventory management systems and personnel to ensure all items remain in good working condition. Even in the United States, the SNS inventory management system had not been updated for several years. Expired and faulty inventory was discovered only when urgently needed, suggesting that the SNS programme had not been consistently managed. Without knowing the exact number of functioning units in the stockpile, the authorities could not respond to disruptions in a time-efficient manner, thereby putting healthcare workers and the public at risk.

---

6.   The Strategic National Stockpile is a massive inventory-based approach for demand surges caused by public health emergencies. Suppose a community experiences a large-scale public health incident in which the disease or agent is unknown. In that case, the intent is to send a broad range of pharmaceuticals and medical supplies from strategically located warehouses throughout the United States in 50-ton containers to any state within 12 hours of the federal deployment decision.

Excessive reliance on overseas suppliers

The United States is the world's largest importer of facemasks, eye protection, and medical gloves, making it highly vulnerable to disruptions in the supply chains of PPE. Before the COVID-19 pandemic, PPE was considered a commodity that competes purely on price. Hence, it was cost-efficient for producers such as 3M, Dupont, and Honeywell to offshore (or outsource) the manufacturing of PPE to lower-cost countries, such as China, Malaysia, and Vietnam. Table 8.1 summarises the PPE trade flow among top importing and exporting countries as of 2019.

The global PPE market relies on global trade. However, the COVID-19 pandemic created a new wave of protectionism in 2020, with governments of twenty-four countries, including Germany and France, taking steps to ban or limit the export of PPE and medicines as cases surged in those countries.

Table 8.1: Top importing and exporting countries of PPE in 2019

PPE Products	Top Importing Countries	Top Exporting Countries
Masks (surgical and N95 masks)	US (34%), Japan (10%), Germany (8%), others (48%)	China (44%), Germany (7%), US (6%), Vietnam (5%), other (38%)
Eye protection (face shields and goggles)	US (29%), Canada (6%), Australia (6%), other (59%)	China (59%), US (6%), Germany (5%), other (30%)
Gowns and coveralls	US (37%), Germany (6%), France (6%), other (51%)	China (41%), France (9%), Vietnam (6%), other (44%)
Gloves	US (20%), Germany (20%), UK (6%), other (54%)	Malaysia (25%), Thailand (18%), China (18%), Germany (10%), other (29%)

Source: IFC Report, 2021.

Poor supply chain practices

The outsourcing of production overseas was not accompanied by proper risk management measures, even when the federal government was the purchaser. There was poor supply chain visibility of the supply sources. With severe shortages of PPE arising from the COVID-19 outbreak in 2020, the federal government eased regulations on vendor competition. It provided over US$1.8 billion to hundreds of unvetted contractors by the end of May. Federal agencies, states, local governments, and hospitals rushed to compete for supplies, and other countries were also looking to purchase more PPE—the result was the world's largest grey market in PPE and sky-high prices. Unethical and opportunistic suppliers cropped up to make a fortune, often without delivering quality products, if at all. Some imported products were found to be substandard. For example, the National Institute for Occupational Safety and Health found that 60 percent of sixty-seven different types of N-95 masks imported from China failed to provide adequate protection, offering as low as 24 per cent filtration instead of the required 95 per cent. Also, over 1,300 Chinese medical suppliers, including 217 N-95 mask manufacturers, used false addresses and non-working numbers in their registrations with the Food and Drug Administration (FDA). The problem was bad enough for the Chinese government to establish a new system of quality controls for exports of various medical supplies on 10 April 2020, including PPE products. The Chinese government was concerned that bad actors could negatively impact the whole PPE exporting industry.

The pandemic exposed how poorly various firms and the authorities had managed their supply chains. Many firms did not even know who their distant suppliers were. Based on a 2018 Deloitte survey,[7] some two-thirds of more than 500 procurement leaders from thirty-nine countries have limited or no visibility beyond tier-one suppliers. The FDA and hospital procurement systems also have virtually no supply chain visibility of their sources. The current FDA regulations require PPE manufacturers—for instance, 3M and Honeywell—to report only the locations of their factories rather than their domestic and overseas production capacity. Healthcare providers cannot manage their procurement risk without supply chain visibility. Providers cannot vet and track their suppliers to prevent adulteration and other quality issues without knowing their suppliers' identities. Consequently, time and resources will be wasted during a crisis such as during the COVID-19 pandemic.

Lack of capability for product design, development, and manufacturing

US President Ronald Reagan adopted supply-side economic policies in 1981, which called for tax cuts and deregulation of domestic markets. At the same time, China's 1978 economic reform created a perfect partnership: US corporations could offshore (and eventually outsource) their production to China by leveraging lower labour costs, and China could boost its economy by attracting outside investment. As China improved productivity, quality, and cost-efficiency, it became the 'factory of the world' for many goods. China became the largest producer of many items, including pharmaceutical ingredients (API) and PPE. While other low-cost producers have emerged, such as Malaysia and Vietnam, China remained the key exporter of PPE products. By contrast, decades of offshoring and outsourcing have hollowed out the manufacturing sector in the United States. By 2018, the share of manufacturing employment had dwindled to below 5 per cent of the US population. COVID-19 showed the difficulty of rapidly ramping up domestic production.

---

7.   Deloitte, 'Two in Three Procurement Leaders Have Limited or No Visibility Beyond Tier One of Their Supply Chain', 26 February 2018, https://www2.deloitte.com/uk/en/pages/press-releases/articles/procurement-leaders-have-limited-o-no-visibility.html. In the same vein, Choi et al. (2020) reported that, based on a survey conducted by Reslinic in late January and early February after the Covid-19 outbreak in China, 70 per cent of the 300 respondents said they were trying to identify which of their suppliers were in locked-down parts of the country.

During the pandemic, many US firms could not get PPE orders filled from their usual Chinese suppliers. This was because China had to first secure its supply of PPE after resuming manufacturing operations from its prolonged shutdown due to the COVID-19 outbreak and essentially locking down the country from 23 January 2020. In fact, with a new coronavirus first emerging in China in late 2019, China's demand for PPE increased. China not only restricted PPE exports but also imported a substantial portion of global PPE supplies in January and February 2020.

COVID-19 also showed how a pandemic can be an inflection point in the global political economy. As outbreaks emerged in different countries, various countries sought to corner the dwindling supplies. Besides China, other international producers of PPE, including Taiwan, Germany, France, and India, also restricted exports, contributing to much higher costs for those products worldwide. Even when Chinese factories could produce orders again as COVID-19 eased in China, shipping products to the United States and elsewhere was a significant challenge because global supply chains had essentially broken down. Governments worldwide closed borders and ports, imposed quarantine requirements on ocean freight personnel, and flights were greatly reduced.

Consider two examples of inadequate capability for producing PPE. When the supply from China looked uncertain, the apparent solution was domestic production and the following makeshift solutions:

Ventilators: In late March 2020, the United States government estimated that there would be severe shortages of both invasive and non-invasive ventilators. President Donald Trump used the *Defense Production Act* to ask US manufacturers to create consortia to produce ventilators quickly.[8] For example, automaker General Motors Company and Ventec Life Systems, a medical equipment maker, formed a partnership to build ventilators at a General Motors' plant in Kokomo, IN.[9] The consortium shipped 600 ventilators by mid-April and delivered 30,000 ventilators through the end of August to the DHHS. While such partnerships were needed at a critical time, the rushed project resulted in mechanical ventilators with basic features that could not fully support a patient's breathing, as there was little time to plan appropriately for design and production.

Facemask production: Considering the severe shortage of facemasks, the United States government asked two clothing companies, Hanes and Brooks Brothers, to retrofit their domestic factories to produce masks and gowns for medical professionals. Although basic facemasks are easy to make, a non-woven material from micro- and

---

8.   Federal Emergency Management Agency, 'Defense Production Act', accessed 14 September 2022, https://www.fema.gov/disasters/defense-production-act.

9.   At the same time, Michigan-based Creative Foam Corp. and Minneapolis-based Twin City Die Castings, both auto industry suppliers, repurposed their capacity to provide parts at high volume for the GM-Ventec endeavor. At first, the consortium planned to produce 30,000 of Ventec's flagship product with 700+ components for which it had identified most of the suppliers. The government balked at the $1 billion price tag. Hence, GM and Ventec switched to a more straightforward design with half the cost, but only the single ventilator function without oxygen-related features.

nano-polymer fibres using a conventional technology called melt blowing is needed for surgical[10] and N-95[11] masks to create filters to stop germs or minute particles from entering or exiting. The United States had limited capacity to make melt-blown fabric and could not quickly expand the production of melt-blown material domestically. The expensive equipment for making melt-blown fabric (approximately US$4 million each) was also in short supply. Due to worldwide shortages of surgical and N-95 masks, China suspended its exports of masks and melt-blown fabrics between late February and late March 2020, although exports had mostly resumed by April and export volume more than doubled compared to pre-pandemic levels. In March 2020, South Korea also temporarily banned the export of melt-blown material. The ban was lifted only in August when the in-country supply stabilised relative to domestic demand. Therefore, Hanes and Brooks Brothers could only manufacture basic masks, not the surgical or N-95 masks necessary to protect healthcare workers.

Thus, the lack of capability severely hampered the United States' response to the pandemic, especially regarding PPE shortages.

What Governments Can Do to Prepare Better for Future Pandemics

Government policy is essential to ensure adequate PPE and other medical supplies during emergencies. The example of the United States and the four root causes above contain lessons for stakeholders in other countries too. There is no single approach to secure the supply of PPE in both a time-efficient and cost-effective manner. Relying on stockpiling alone would be too costly and impractical. Focusing on domestic supply chains is not sustainable either, because of sharp demand swings. Developing capabilities takes commitment and a long-term coordinated plan. Therefore, any country needs to develop a 'proactive' plan that is based on a combination of the following strategies to prepare for future pandemics:

Develop an industrial policy

The shortages of PPE and ventilators should serve as catalysts to develop an industrial policy that can guide and focus on certain products and develop the requisite capabilities to deploy resources in time of need. During the decline of the automobile industry in the early 1980s, Labour Secretary Robert Reich argued that the United States should develop an industrial policy that focused on certain business segments to regain international competitiveness.

---

10. A proper surgical mask is usually made of three layers: an outer hydrophobic non-woven layer, a middle melt-blown layer, and an inner soft, absorbent non-woven layer. The outer layer is intended to repel water, blood and body fluids; the middle melt-blown layer is designed as the 'filter' to stop germs from entering or exiting the mask; and the inner layer is intended to absorb water, sweat and spit.

11. An N-95 mask is a respiratory protective device designed to achieve a very close facial fit and very efficient filtration of airborne particles. Unlike the surgical mask, the edges of the N-95 respirator are designed to form a 'seal' around the nose and mouth.

While not presenting a comprehensive industrial policy, President Joseph Biden has consulted with different departments for recommendations on strengthening the supply chains of vulnerable products.[12] The departments that took the lead for individual supply chains were the Department of Commerce on semiconductor manufacturing and advanced packaging; the Department of Energy on large capacity batteries; the Department of Defense on critical materials and minerals; and the DHHS, particularly its agency the FDA, on pharmaceuticals and APIs. The recommendations included steps to strengthen domestic manufacturing capacity for critical goods, recruit and train workers to make critical products, to invest in research and development that will reduce supply chain vulnerabilities, and work with US allies and partners to strengthen collective supply chain resilience. However, low-margin PPE was not included as a category. Low-margin PPE often suffers the worst shortages when demand surges in a major public health emergency. The only way to produce such low-cost, low-margin products profitably is to outsource production of these products to low-cost economies.

It is necessary to have an 'ecosystem' of designers, R&D centres, engineers, production engineers, and technicians to develop capabilities that can be deployed to create production capacity for critical products in times of need.[13] To do this, the government should engage the private sector and university research centres and provide the incentives necessary for the development and training of personnel with the requisite capabilities. Rather than just focusing on the products per se, different parts of the ecosystem should coordinate to improve the products and to develop manufacturing processes, as well as flexible capacity that could divert capacity to produce medical equipment to make ventilators and PPE when demand surges. Although there is domestic capacity for some types of PPE, for instance masks, the cost is substantially higher relative to imports, so either different production methods are needed, or the costs have to be effectively subsidised to keep a minimal capacity alive.[14]

Consider the case of iHealth Labs, the California-based subsidiary of Chinese manufacturer Andon Health that produced at-home COVID rapid test kits for the US government in 2022. Andon Health agreed to produce US$1.8 billion worth of test kits, which was five times its typical annual revenue.[15] Despite its small size, Andon Health was able to scale up due to its flexibility and capability to mobilise its regional supply chains in China.

12. The White House, 'Building Resilient Supply Chains, Revitalizing American Manufacturing, and Fostering Broad-Based Growth', June 2021, https://www.whitehouse.gov/wp-content/uploads/2021/06/100-day-supply-chain-review-report.pdf.
13. This notion of standby capability is also known as 'Industrial Commons' (Pisano and Shih 2009).
14. Joe Nocera, 'Why American Mask Makers Are Going out of Business', New York Times, 5 March 2022, https://www.nytimes.com/2022/03/05/business/dealbook/american-mask-makers.html.
15. Josh Nathan-Kazis, 'Why the U.S. Contracted with a Chinese Covid Test-Kit Maker You've Never Heard Of', Barron's, 3 March 2022, https://www.barrons.com/articles/covid-19-test-maker-ihealth-andon-health-51646318989.

By the same token, the US government will have to ensure there is a diversity of supply chains within the country that can be called up to meet a demand surge in a pandemic. For PPE production, America Makes (www.americamakes.us) is an Ohio-based non-profit organisation that 'supports the transformation of manufacturing in the United States through innovative, coordinated additive manufacturing and 3D Printing Technology Development and Transition, and Workforce and Educational Development'. Its members include government departments, private companies, and universities. For example, America Makes seeks to coordinate 3D printing capability with the FDA and the Veterans Health Administration to design a 3D printed mask approved by the FDA. Essentially, by coordinating different people with different expertise, America Makes enables the creation of approved PPE designs that can be manufactured with additive manufacturing capability within the country. In addition, America Makes has developed a knowledge-sharing platform (Digital Storefront) that shares the latest information with its members.[16] To a certain extent, America Makes is an ecosystem with standby capabilities that can be deployed to leverage 3D printing technology to develop and produce products when needed.

Education and job opportunities for students also need to be considered. For instance, after decades of offshoring and outsourcing manufacturing to benefit from lower costs, the United States need to significantly beef-up its overall industrial production capacities and capabilities. Many US students shy away from STEM (science, technology, engineering, and mathematics) as there had been fewer job opportunities in those areas. Currently, the United States produces around 500,000 STEM graduates per year, whereas China produced over 4.7 million since 2016. Not having enough STEM graduates results in not having enough talent for designing, developing, and producing equipment and technical products domestically. Unless there is a long-term commitment from the government, it will be challenging for the United States to re-establish these capabilities.

Long-term commitment is needed for manufacturing as well, especially for long-term manufacturing contracts, particularly when the demand is in the form of a highly uncertain surge. For example, 3.5 billion masks were needed annually during the pandemic, but demand will drop heavily during normal times. Also, while there was a panic to quickly produce ventilators in March 2020, there was an oversupply of ventilators at the end of August 2020 when less invasive treatments became more effective. In response to the ventilator oversupply, the US government cancelled the remainder of its contract with medical technology manufacturers.

---

16. The Storefront is 'an online platform where members can access member-exclusive information, project data, and intellectual capital assets, including project deliverables and artifacts along with their association to the Technology Roadmap'.

Encourage a 'hybrid' supply chain structure

During the first year of the pandemic, the annual demand for protective masks in the United States was 3.5 billion, or roughly 100 times more than the amount in the SNS. It is unrealistic and impractical to store billions of N-95 masks that expire after 3 to 5 years. Therefore, the government needs to develop standby capabilities with private sectors and universities and estimate the time needed to convert capability into actual production capacity. Given the urgency during times of crisis, this conversion time may be too long.

Therefore, it is necessary to develop a stop-gap solution to buy time while converting capability into capacity. Such a solution calls for a hybrid supply chain structure that supports domestic firms to sustain their global supply chains that serve the healthcare markets around the globe. At the same time, state governments should encourage firms to bring back at least some of their offshore manufacturing capacity, just like Texas and South Carolina are already doing.

Clearly, reshoring manufacturing for certain high-tech products requires the development of the previously aforementioned capabilities. Some firms, such as 3M and Honeywell, can certainly expand their supply chain operations for many PPE products in the United States. However, due to the sharp swings in the demand for these products, the US government may need to provide economic incentives, making it economically viable for a larger number of firms to expand domestic production. Using a combination of global and domestic supply chains, a company can cost-effectively produce products by leveraging its global supply chain operations in normal times and by shifting its operations to its domestic supply chain in a time-efficient manner when responding to a pandemic or some other public health emergency. Therefore, a 'hybrid' supply chain structure offers flexibility for the firm to operate its supply chain in a cost-effective or time-efficient manner.

Still, some challenges need to be considered:

Reverting to offshore purchasing before the next pandemic: With facemasks being imported to the extent of 90 percent or more before the pandemic, there was little capacity in the United States for making masks. The few small, focused manufacturers who had persisted did well during the pandemic in 2020–2022. However, the moment the pandemic is declared to be officially over, all indications are that hospitals will revert to their suppliers in China and elsewhere. To prevent these domestic manufacturers from going bankrupt, a possible solution is for the government to purchase masks made in the United States at the federal and state level or to support manufacturing costs.

Shifting PPE demand towards Asia: There are projections that Asia will increase demand for PPE over 2022–2025 as adoption increases in a continent with a population that is nearly eight times that of North America, currently the main source of demand for PPE. As such, there would be a greater impetus among global manufacturers at least to produce in the continent where they will experience demand rather than move facilities to North America. To counterbalance this trend, the US government—likely the federal government—will have to support a minimal level of domestic manufacturing capacity to enable them to be cost-competitive with Asian suppliers.

Supply chain raw material: Even if capacity is created domestically, there is a chance that raw materials or intermediate products will be imported. One example is non-woven fibre. When Hanes tried to manufacture N-95 facemasks in 2020, it discovered that the critical component of non-woven fibre had to be imported as there was no domestic capacity. Eventually, the company resorted to making essential masks rather than the preferred N-95 ones. To ensure sustainable production of N-95 masks domestically, a possible solution is for the government to provide R&D support to develop new materials and innovative production processes.

Actively manage stockpile inventory

Once the hybrid supply chain structure is established, the government can estimate the domestic production capacity of the domestic supply chain for producing critical products in times of need. Knowing this production capacity and the corresponding response time for production and distribution, the government can then determine the amount of inventory that the national stockpile needs to store. In addition to always maintaining the right inventory level, DHHS needs to conduct periodical audits, inspections, and rotations to ensure all stored units are usable.

By establishing standby capability, developing domestic supply chains, and keeping the right amount of PPE and medical equipment inventory, the authorities will be better equipped to respond to future pandemics. Additionally, the authorities can run stress tests and simulations to identify potential gaps throughout the entire ecosystem.

Encourage innovation

Currently, PPE such as surgical and N-95 masks are considered commodity products that compete on cost. As such, reshoring the production of PPE can be a risky venture when government purchases are based on the lowest cost. Consider the ill-fated investments in US facemask production. The severe shortages of N-95 masks in 2020 created investment opportunities for domestic production. When the number of monthly COVID-19-related deaths shot up in January 2021,[17] the orders for domestically made masks exploded. However, the orders for them vanished after China began exporting more masks at a much lower price. By September 2021, the American Mask Manufacturer's Association estimated that up to ten out of twenty-nine domestic mask manufacturers would go bankrupt. Domestic production cannot be sustained if the purchases continue to focus on procuring PPE at the lowest price because domestic

---

17. Whet Moser, 'The Deadliest Month Yet', *The Atlantic*, 2 February 2021, https://www.theatlantic.com/health/archive/2021/02/january-pandemic-deadliest-month/617898.

manufacturers are not cost-competitive due to higher wages and regulations. Therefore, to encourage domestic production, the procurement process must take the product's value (e.g., quality, full lifecycle cost, and environmental cost) into consideration. Doing so can create incentives for domestic companies to develop and produce innovative PPE products. For example, domestic firms can design PPE to fit different body and face shapes to increase comfort and protection. Designing *reusable* PPE made from biodegradable materials can reduce hazardous waste.[18]

Encourage individual responsibility

Preparing for future pandemics should be everyone's responsibility, not just the government's. Specifically, citizens can help curb the spread of future viruses by taking various precautionary measures (e. g., masking, social distancing, hand washing), enabling contract tracing, and participating in the requisite standards of testing and quarantining. Through participation, citizens can reduce the spread of the virus so that the demand for hospitalisation and PPE will not surge as quickly as it did during COVID-19. Public cooperation can buy time for developing more effective responses (e.g., adequate supply of the requisite materials) and for developing better treatments and vaccines. However, good and consistent communication from the authorities will be needed to galvanise the public at critical times.

The large-scale availability of at-home rapid test kits can make individual responsibility easier to bear as people would be able to test themselves at home and take steps to avoid spreading the virus.

Encourage the development of online platforms for response

In addition to developing the physical supply of PPE, online platforms can be considered when designing a coordinated response to identify and match supply sources and demand locations quickly. For instance, getusppe.org is an online platform to match the supply and demand of PPE in the United States. During the crisis, three young New Yorkers created Invisible Hands (invsiblehandsdeliver.org) to match volunteers with seniors and other at-risk groups in need of food and medication. In just two weeks of going online, the site attracted 7,300 volunteers who completed 600 deliveries in New York and New Jersey.

Once all these elements are implemented, we envision the United States and other countries can respond to a future pandemic. The national stockpile is the first line of defence. At the same time, the authorities should begin forecasting demand and check whether the backup capacity of the domestic supply chains can handle the predicted surge in demand. If not, the standby capabilities should be deployed, thereby

---

18. According to WHO (2018), it was estimated that disposed (medical) masks generate 1.6 million tons of plastic waste on a daily basis.

converting already developed capabilities into the capacity to produce the required amounts of critical products.

Conclusion

In recent years, there was insufficient realisation that the world had escaped narrowly from the SARS, MERS, Ebola, H1N1, and Zika epidemics.[19] On top of that, the likelihood of even more severe pandemics is increasing in the future with the growing world population, more encounters between humans and wildlife, and widespread human interactions.

It is, therefore, critical that governments combine different approaches to become more responsive and resilient when facing future pandemics. We have outlined six such approaches following the United States' experience with PPE shortages reflecting poor preparedness. No country can afford to be complacent about future pandemics that must be surely lurking around the corner.

---

19. Their reasons are simple: 'the presence of a large reservoir of SARS-CoV-like viruses in horseshoe bats, together with the culture of eating exotic mammals in southern China, is a time bomb.'

9

China and the United States

Mutually Incomprehensible Approach to Fighting COVID-19

Christine Loh

China and the United States, the two largest economies and most influential countries in the world, were polar opposites in how they fought COVID-19. This chapter discusses the beginning of the outbreaks in the two countries and subsequent waves, what they prioritised, the effectiveness of their interventions, and their considerations in 'opening up' and 'living with COVID'. Their different approaches illustrated their respective underlying conditions, politics, capabilities, cultures, and societies.

The assertion of their respective political will stemmed from a different sense of the 'social contract' in China and the United States. While there is no fixed or exact meaning of social contract, it broadly involves an implicit agreement by the people to follow policies and rules set by the government for the greater good of society. Chapter 6 provides a thorough discussion of the concept of the social contract. Furthermore, as explained in Chapter 1, trust matters a great deal too. The people are more likely to act in the interest of the whole because they trust their government to shape appropriate policies and rules, and/or they can rely on each other to abide by them. Chapter 1 provides details based on surveys about political trust in various countries, including China and the United States. In summary, political trust is high in China and low in the United States. While science and health advice were essential for political leaders in making decisions, COVID-19 showed the socio-economic, political, and cultural challenges that China and the United States faced.

China and the United States are physically large countries. China has a unitary political system, while the United States has a federal system. China has 1.4 billion people, and the United States has 330 million. The healthcare system is much more developed in the latter than in the former. It is beyond this chapter to drill down to what happened in specific localities of the two countries since there were many variations. This chapter stays at the national macro-level. Chapter 10 covers how neighbourhoods are organised in mainland China and the role they played in pandemic control, and Chapter 11 covers Greater China, which includes Hong Kong, Macao, and Taiwan. Reading the three chapters together provides a complete picture of the Chinese experience. Another distinguishing feature is the overall relationship between China and the United States when COVID-19 emerged. They were in the midst of a geopolitical contest with each other, which had a considerable impact on how they saw each other, including with respect to the pandemic. Their conflict is continuing and intensifying as COVID-19 continued into a third year and as this book went to press.

China's Response to COVID-19

China's response to COVID-19 could be seen in four phases:

1. Early uncertainties and missteps from December 2019 to 20 January 2020.
2. Interrupting transmission from 21 January to April 2020.
3. Normalising prevention from May 2020 to December 2021.
4. Olympics, Omicron, and opening up in 2022.

Legacy of SARS

The severe acute respiratory syndrome (SARS) epidemic in 2003 left a deep mark in China. It resulted in over 5,300 cases and over 540 attributable deaths, and the economy was affected. Worldwide, it affected 8,400 people and resulted in 916 attributable deaths. SARS was short-lived compared to COVID-19—only eight months separated the first reported case from the end of the epidemic. The legacy of COVID-19, by contrast, will be greatly felt for many years to come.

There was panic in January 2003 during the early period of the SARS outbreak in Guangdong. Rumours were rife about a strange disease, resulting in buying sprees of various folk medicine, drugs, and face masks. SARS spread to other parts of China— affecting Beijing particularly badly—and outside mainland China. Top leaders in Beijing were not properly briefed until mid-April 2003. However, once the leadership realised what was happening, China provided regular information and mobilised resources to act. SARS was contained quickly with the involvement of the World Health Organization (WHO).

SARS led to an overall assessment of the healthcare system in China. Investment in public health and the healthcare system had fallen behind, as the country prioritised economic growth. An important reform with respect to infectious disease management was the setting up of the automated Contagious Disease National Direct Reporting System (CDNDRS) in every hospital. This reporting system enables hospitals to report directly to the Chinese Centre for Disease Control and Prevention (CDC) to enable rapid response. It was also designed to minimise political interference. In 2003, the poor handling of SARS had much to do with the low awareness of the risk of infectious diseases among Guangdong provincial officials and Beijing officials, and what critics saw as the habitual downplaying or even concealing of 'bad news' from the highest authority in order to not cause panic and maintain stability. Since its creation, CDNDRS had been used and was thought to be a successful system. China's overall performance in infectious diseases has also improved. China dealt with H7N9, the avian flu that emerged in February 2013, in an exemplary manner. There were rumours that people could be infected from eating chicken but there was no widespread panic because the authorities took fast and effective countermeasures to keep people informed. H7N9 was lethal (fatality rate of 40 per cent) but not highly transmissible. China was widely praised for its new openness compared to SARS, and for its willingness to cooperate internationally.

Phase 1: Early uncertainties and missteps

COVID-19, a highly infectious fast-moving disease with a combination of unique characteristics (see Chapter 1), stumped the Chinese authorities in the early weeks of the outbreak. The contention centres around December 2019 to 19 January. There are many chronologies and viewpoints published by official sources, media organisations, and public health academics and other experts in specialist journals. Many books have also been written by political scientists, sociologists, journalists, and others with various interpretations, ranging from crude to thoughtful. There are essentially two contending narratives—one focuses on suppression and concealment, the other on reasonableness.

The first narrative targets the authorities for suppressing and hiding information. Frontline doctors in Wuhan started to see a rise in pneumonia-like cases during the flu season in November 2019. By early to mid-December, they could see some patients were not responding to flu medication.[1] They informed their immediate superiors, as they were supposed to do, who informed the local Wuhan health authorities. Doctors took fluid samples from patients and sent them to laboratories for analysis. Results showed the pathogen to be a SARS coronavirus, and the Wuhan health authorities were informed by 29 December. Frontline health professionals in Wuhan also shared what they were seeing with each other online. On 30 December, they got wind that it was a SARS coronavirus.[2] The leadership at Wuhan's hospitals should have activated the CDNDRS by then. Instead, the Wuhan health authorities sent out orders that hospital healthcare professionals were not to spread information about what they were seeing to avoid panic. The Wuhan Public Security Bureau was watching social media communication and issued a public report on 1 January 2020, that eight people had been summoned and reprehended for 'spreading rumours about the outbreak online'.[3] On the same day, the authorities closed the Huanan Seafood Wholesale Market in Wuhan

---

1. Retrospective research showed COVID-19 could have been circulating in mid-October to mid-November 2019 in China; Jonathan Pekar, Michael Worobey, Niema Moshiri, Konrad Scheffler, and Joel O. Wertheim, 'Timing the SARS-CoV-2 Index Case in Hubei Province', *Science* 137, no. 6540 (2021): 412–417.
2. Dr Ai Fen, head of the emergency department at the Wuhan Central Hospital, circulated the information on 30 December to other doctors when she found out that the pathogen was a SARS coronavirus.
3. The eight were all doctors who were sending social media messages to warn colleagues to take precautions against the virus. Dr Li Weiliang was one of them. Dr Li was 'summoned' and had to pledge in writing not to continue to spread rumours. He later became infected and died.

because some of the patients had been to the market and it was thought that the new coronavirus came from there, where many species of wildlife were sold.

Another questionable issue was over the slow release of genomic sequences by the Chinese authorities. Chinese laboratories were mapping the genetic sequence of the new pathogen. In one case, the laboratory at Fudan University in Shanghai received a sample on 3 January 2020 and had sequenced it by 5 January. The laboratory warned the Wuhan and Shanghai authorities, as well as the National Health Commission (NHC), China's ministry of health in Beijing, that it was from the same family as the bat virus that had spawned SARS. China only released the findings on 12 January after the Fudan sequence was uploaded online the day before.[4] Critics noted that an earlier release would allow for quicker development of a diagnostic test and antiviral treatments, and for others to get prepared.

The NHC sent two expert teams to Wuhan to investigate the outbreak—the first on 31 December and the second on 8 January. The experts sent to Wuhan thought the risk of human-to-human spread was low and that the situation was controllable, the consequence of which was the Wuhan city government proceeded with its annual political meetings on 6 January, followed by the provincial Hubei People's Congress meetings with over 600 delegates for five days starting from 11 January. Wuhan's annual Chinese New Year banquet with 40,000 families was also allowed to proceed on 18 January. It took a third team of experts to confirm that sustained human-to-human transmission was taking place the following day.

The reasonableness narrative focuses on the many unknowns in the early days of the outbreak in Wuhan. The authorities had to conduct detective work to rule out many suspects, such as known viral and bacterial pathogens from the clusters of similar pneumonia. COVID-19's many unique characteristics were unknown at the time, including its generally mild and self-limiting disease (as compared to 2003 SARS), long incubation period, asymptomatic spread, and high transmissibility.[5] The authorities' defence was that they acted as soon as cases were reported. On 30 December, the Wuhan health authorities issued an urgent notice to all local hospitals on the treatment of patients with pneumonia of unknown causes, and the NHC was informed. On 31 December, a first expert team was sent to Wuhan by the NHC to investigate. China informed the WHO about a new pneumonia on 3 January 2020. Chinese scientists confirmed the new coronavirus pathogen and its full genomic sequences were shared with the WHO

---

4.   Zhang Yongzhen led the Fudan team that sequenced the virus on 5 January. Zhang uploaded the genome to the US National Center for Biotechnology Information and notified the NHC, Wuhan Central Hospital that provided the sample, and the Shanghai health authorities that the virus was similar to SARS and that it spread by respiratory transmission, and he recommended the authorities take emergency measures to deal with the disease and to start developing antiviral treatments. For Zhang's own telling of what happened, see David Cyranoski, 'Zhang Yongzhen: Genome Sharer', *Nature*, 14 December 2020, https://www.nature.com/immersive/d41586-020-03435-6/index.html.

5.   Dr Gao Fu, head of the Chinese CDC, gave interviews that are available online about the early days of the detective work to explain China's perspective. See for example CCGT's interview with Gao about the early detective work, CGTN, 'Exclusive interview with Chinese CDC Director Gao Fu', accessed 14 September 2022, https://www.youtube.com/watch?v=q2PmAGvTCEQ.

on 12 January (see Chapter 2). The explanation for not publishing sequences earlier was that it was for the sake of accuracy. The general practice was to have at least two independent institutions do the sequencing before release.

President Xi Jinping was already informed about the outbreak in Wuhan by 7 January and had asked for it to be controlled. On 8 January, a second investigation team was sent to Wuhan to update the leadership. The issue of transmissibility and virulence was a vital piece of information to determine what needed to be done. Experts continued to advise the risk of human-to-human transmission was low. Ten days later, yet another team was sent, this time headed by China's famous respiratory doctor, Zhong Nanshan, as the leadership wanted greater clarity. By then, deaths were occurring—the first death from this new disease in China was announced on 10 January. Dr Zhong became famous during SARS when he spoke out against the authorities about the disease. Together with other experts, Dr Zhong conducted their assessment on 19 January and flew to Beijing immediately to brief leaders on 20 January that sustained human-to-human transmission was occurring. From Dr Zhong's various public statements, the discussion with leaders included policy priorities. The top leadership announced the same day that all levels of authority throughout the country 'should put people's lives and health first'. The NHC held a press conference at which Dr Zhong announced his findings and called on people not to travel to Wuhan. On 23 January, the lockdown in Wuhan and other cities in Hubei began. China declared the fight against the virus as an all-out 'people's war' and the whole country would be affected. The reasonableness narrative concludes that mistakes could happen in making battlefield calls in an unclear situation and China's overall action was not unreasonable despite mistakes by the local authorities in Wuhan and Hubei to suppress information. This narrative acknowledges suppression of information by the local authorities was wrong and the officials involved were subsequently held accountable and punished.

Structural, systemic, and habitual problems

Both the suppression-and-concealment and reasonableness narratives were quests for 'truth' although the vantage point of the viewer greatly affected perception. Those writing from a medical and health perspective tended to favour the reasonableness narrative, whereas those taking a political perspective tended to adopt the suppression-and-concealment narrative and were critical fundamentally of China's political system. Mainland Chinese analysts tended to explain the complexity of the Chinese political and public health systems, and pointed to specific problems that needed to be reformed.

The Chinese government itself explained the chain of events in a State Council paper published on 7 June 2020, starting with the local Wuhan CDC receiving information from a hospital about pneumonia cases of unknown cause on 27 December and informed hospitals under its supervision about it. The NHC was also informed and started to organise an expert team to conduct an on-site investigation in Wuhan on 31 December. The State Council paper does not cover earlier events. What it does show was the national government assumed authority over dealing with the disease from 20 January. Chinese analysts saw this step as necessary because of the fragmented and unclear nature of the Chinese political structure in the distribution of power between Beijing and the provinces and major cities.

COVID-19 exposed a number of China's governance challenges. Critics pointed to various longstanding failings of the Chinese system. Those in the medical profession saw the difficulty of getting urgent information quickly up and down the national CDC's layered structure in China (county, prefecture, provincial, national CDC, and then to the NHC) during the early days of the outbreak. Others pointed to the unequal relationship between health officials and the much more politically powerful provincial and municipal party secretaries, governors, and mayors. While the NHC and national CDC represent the national health authorities, they cannot easily interfere with local politicians. The local CDC officials and hospitals are answerable to the local leadership. It may be surmised that the CDNDRS was not activated because it got entangled with local political interference, as reporting needed the approval of the heads of hospitals who worked under the Wuhan health commission, which in turn took instructions from the Wuhan and Hubei leadership. During the days of the provincial political meetings, the Hubei health commission even stopped disclosing new infection cases.

Furthermore, officials could use unclear laws to shirk responsibility. For example, under the Law on Prevention and Treatment of Infectious Diseases, it is the NHC and the provincial health commissions that are responsible for issuing warnings of outbreaks and epidemics, whereas the Law on Emergency Response requires local governments to issue warnings. The contradiction encourages blame-shifting if something goes wrong. The mayor of Wuhan's defence was that while he knew about the outbreak, he claimed he was not authorised to disclose it.[6]

The mayor's acknowledgement that local leaders knew about the outbreak brings up another issue—the issuance and consideration of expert advice. Experts are often regarded as mere technicians with no independent agency, and information available to the experts is often tightly controlled by the authorities. A member of the first expert panel noted that at the beginning, the panel found no evidence of human-to-human transmission among close contacts put under quarantine, which to them suggested the virus had a low capability to spread among people.[7] Critics noted a tendency in China for experts to be conservative in their judgement of low-probability, high-impact situations, where a false judgement could lead to high political and/or social impacts.[8] A member of the second panel disclosed his panel was given false information in Wuhan

6.   Yang Zekun, 'Wuhan Mayor Says Will Resign If It Helps Control Outbreak', *China Daily*, 27 January 2020.
7.   Wang Xiaoyu, 'Q&A: Senior Health Expert Addresses Key Concerns Amid Outbreak', *China Daily*, 25 January 2020.
8.   Ye Qi, Coco Dijia Du, Tianle Liu, Xiaofan Zhao, and Changgui Dong, 'Experts' Conservative Judgment and Containment of Covid-19 in Early Outbreak', *Journal of Chinese Governance* 5, no. 2 (2020): 140–159, https://doi.org/10.1080/23812346.2020.1741249.

about whether doctors and nurses were infected.[9] The political leaders of Wuhan and Hubei did not want to disrupt their political meetings and Wuhan's annual banquet. It would have been difficult to proceed with those events had the expert teams sent to Wuhan on 31 December and 8 January concluded that human-to-human transmission was occurring. Critics saw such behaviour as the 'entanglement of political and economic interests' where the political and economic elites prioritised their interests over public health.[10] Nevertheless, even the national CDC showed a measure of understanding for the local authorities in Wuhan and Hubei that: 'They need to consider economic factors, and issues like family reunions over the Lunar New Year. So, what we [scientists] said was only part of their considerations.'[11]

Phase 2: Interrupting transmission

China's strength is in national mobilisation. China can act with speed, rigour, and effectiveness once decisions are taken at the top. The Chinese political and administrative systems can pull in the same direction although many details have to be worked out along the way that can be messy. It is what the public expects—the government is there to do big things that individuals cannot do, and the people are willing to submit to inconvenience and social control. Fighting an infectious disease is one such example. This is an important part of the ruling Chinese Communist Party's social contract with the Chinese people. Moreover, Chapter 10 explains how China's neighbourhoods are organised and the effectiveness of that system in mass mobilisation in times of need.

SARS provided a good example of China's mobilisation capabilities. It is worth listing the magnitude of that response in Beijing in 2003 to illustrate China's capacity to mobilise resources and the workforce despite many shortcomings in the health system then:

(1) Reducing person-to-person transmission through testing, isolation of SARS patients, tracing and quarantine of close contacts, and surveillance.

(2) Setting up more than 100 fever clinics in hospitals in Beijing, which played an important role in screening and triage.

(3) Building a new 1,000-bed SARS hospital in days in Beijing to deal with rising cases.

(4) Training large numbers of healthcare workers in the management of SARS patients, infection control and use of personal protective equipment (PPE).

(5) Sending large quantities of PPE and medical apparatuses to frontline healthcare workers.

---

9. Yu Liu and Richard B. Saltman, 'Policy Lessons from Early Reactions to the COVID-19 Virus in China', *American Journal of Public Health* 110, no. 8 (1 August 2020): 1145–1148; and Shen Kui, 'The Delayed Response in Wuhan Reveals Legal Holes', *The Regulatory Review*, 20 April 2020.

10. Li Zhang, *China and Global Capitalism* (Stanford, CA: Stanford University Press, 2021).

11. Jun Mai, 'Politics May Have Stalled Information in Wuhan Coronavirus Crisis, Scientist Says', *South China Morning Post*, 30 January 2020.

(6) Concentrating SARS patients in designated wards to help reduce transmission.
(7) Deploying thousands of local and military health workers for emergency management of the outbreak.
(8) Disseminating information to the public on the status of the epidemic and guidance on prevention.
(9) Dedicating substantial emergency funding to fight the disease nationally, including covering the medical costs of SARS patients by the state.

With respect to COVID-19 in 2020, the Chinese authorities essentially followed a similar path but on a much more substantial scale. From 23 January, the authorities imposed a variety of measures to cut transmission once national leaders decided the epicentre at Wuhan and Hubei had to be locked down. China's actions included:

(1) Suspending public transport with the closure of airports, railway stations, and highways to minimise transmission.
(2) Imposing travel bans throughout Hubei Province.
(3) Extending the Chinese New Year holiday nationwide to minimise transmission, as large numbers of people had already started their travel.
(4) Advising travellers who left Wuhan for the holidays to report their travel history and to self-quarantine for two weeks to prevent transmission; and postponing the re-opening of schools and factories nationwide to keep people at home.
(5) Centralising the allocation of PPE to give priority to the medical sector.
(6) Building 16 makeshift hospitals, called *fangcang* or cabin hospitals, over three weeks, starting in early February 2020, which provided 13,000 beds.

The *fangcang* is a type of field hospital mobilised by China at speed to tackle COVID-19. They were large-scale, low-cost, temporary facilities based in converted public venues, like stadiums and exhibition centres. They served to isolate the vast majority of patients with milder symptoms to minimise the spread to their families and colleagues. The *fangcang* provided medical care, disease monitoring, food, and social activities. Hospitals were reserved for those who needed serious medical care. The *fangcang* were decommissioned as COVID-19 subsided.[12]

China's anti-pandemic efforts also relied on mobilising medical personnel from across the country. Once an outbreak occurred in a certain place, medical professionals and supplies were quickly marshalled and dispatched there. Trained staff worked in shifts so that each sampling point could perform testing 24/7. Volunteer teams were also assembled to serve the community in need so that local residents could observe the quarantine rules to help prevent a large-scale outbreak.

---

12. Simiao Chen, Zongjiu Zhang, Juntao Yang, Jian Wang, Xiaohui Zhai, Till Bärnighausen, et al., 'Fangcang Shelter Hospitals: A Novel Concept for Responding to Public Health Emergencies', *The Lancet* 395, no. 10232 (2020): 1305–1314.

Moreover, mainland Chinese and Hong Kong experts began to provide a large number of research papers about the new disease through learned medical and scientific journals, such as *The Lancet, British Medical Journal, The New England Journal of Medicine,* and *Nature.* The earliest medical reports published in January 2020 described the symptoms of the new disease, warned that a high number of patients needed intensive care, noted fatality rates, and pointed out that human-to-human transmission had been occurring.[13]

The WHO described the totality of China's response as 'ambitious, agile and aggressive' in the history of disease containment. It included scaling up testing plus contract tracing, imposing temperature monitoring, requiring face masks, equipping healthcare workers with PPE, and massive scaling up of isolation and care capacities through deploying healthcare workers from other parts of the country to Wuhan. To cut transmission, an estimated 760 million people, half of China's population, were confined to their homes for an extended period.

As knowledge was gained about COVID-19, China was able to be more targeted in implementing its response with specific science and risk-based approaches that were less manpower heavy. Containment and mitigation measures were adjusted to different locations, contexts, settings, and circumstances. Messaging from Chinese leaders and the authorities was consistent about fighting the virus. Domestic transmission was controlled by March 2020, as cases dropped significantly. As China prepared for relaxation measures, Chinese digital companies developed a health passport embedded in China's popular mobile payment systems that could calculate the level of COVID-19 risk and assigned a colour code to define the user's permitted movements. From April 2020, China's focus switched to the containment of imported cases. All incoming travellers had to undergo a diagnostic test upon arrival and had to be quarantined for 14 days. China's success was symbolised by the end of the Wuhan lockdown on 8 April—the city put on a sound-and-light show and residents celebrated.

The Chinese public was highly critical of the government's handling of the early part of the outbreak in Wuhan, and the tough nationwide lockdown measures, but criticism eased as cases dropped and as many other parts of the world, including economies considered more advanced than China, such as the United States, failed to contain COVID-19 in 2020 and suffered high rates of hospitalisations and deaths.

Phase 3: Normalising prevention

As life resumed under the 'new COVID normal', China continued to face various outbreaks here and there—all were contained relatively quickly in 2020. On 7 May, the

---

13. Chaolin Huang, Yeming Wang, Xingwang Li, Lili Ren, Jianping Zhao, Yi Hu, et al., 'Clinical Features of Patients Infected with 2019 Novel Coronavirus in Wuhan, China', *The Lancet* 395, no. 10223 (2020): 497–506; and Jasper Fuk-Woo Chan, Shuofeng Yuan, Kin-Hang Kok, Kelvin Kai-Wang To, Hin Chu, Jin Yang, et al., 'A Familial Cluster of Pneumonia Associated with the 2019 Novel Coronavirus Indicating Person-to-Person Transmission', *The Lancet* 395, no. 10223 (2020): 514–523.

State Council published guidelines on the *Normalisation of Prevention and Control of the Covid-19 Epidemic*. The guidelines explained that the government would prioritise prevention, strengthen control in public places, expand diagnostic testing, leverage Big Data for health code development, do more research and development, and adjust risk levels and responses as needed. The authorities remained wary of resurgence, and cases could be imported. Chinese vaccines using inactivated-virus technology, similar to flu vaccines, were being developed and they became available in December 2020. Chapter 4 discusses the efficacies of the Chinese vaccines compared to other vaccines. China's aim was to achieve an 80 per cent vaccination rate by the end of 2021, so there was a mass vaccination drive. By the end of 2021, the vaccination had reached 85 per cent. China's cumulative case total for COVID-19 was about 100,000 with under 5,000 deaths at the time. The official view was that continuing with the zero-infection (zero-COVID) policy was right for China because of its very large population, and still inadequate national medical infrastructure, especially in the rural areas where 40 per cent of the population lives. A large outbreak could lead to the medical system breaking down with a huge number of fatalities. The appearance of the more virulent Delta variant in India in late 2020, followed by the highly transmissible Omicron variant in South Africa in late 2021 strengthened China's belief that its zero-COVID policy was correct, and it must be cautious in considering opening up. Chinese experts noted that countries that had relaxed their policies amid a drop in cases later suffered large numbers of infections. China continued to pounce on outbreaks here and there in 2021. They noted China's zero-COVID policy's approach to dealing with sporadic outbreaks was less costly than treating infected patients.[14] Chinese experts reframed the COVID-19 challenge by describing it as 'an era of epidemic normalisation', which meant China would have to coexist with the virus at some stage but that there should be a 'dynamic' aspect to China's policy that considered such factors as vaccination rates and better vaccines, the severity of variants, and how well COVID-19 was controlled around the world. The aim of any new policy should ensure normal socio-economic activities would not be disturbed too much, and that China could still prevent viral transmission effectively through testing and treating patients as quickly as possible—this would prove easier said than done in 2022 with the Omicron variant.

Phase 4: Olympics, Omicron, and opening up in 2022

Holding to the zero-COVID policy was important ahead of the Beijing Winter Olympics, scheduled for February 2022, when a large number of foreign athletes, officials, support staff, and journalists would arrive from many countries still with high numbers of COVID-19 cases. Those who tested positive upon arrival or during their stay were isolated. China's goal was to keep the games COVID safe and prevent

---

14. 'Top Infectious Disease Expert Defends China's "Zero Tolerance" Policy against Criticism It's Too Costly', *Caixin*, 2 November 2021.

transmission to its domestic population. A 'closed-loop system' was created for tens of thousands of people including medical staff and volunteers, who had to be shuttled through three competition zones up to 180 kilometres apart for 16 days and 109 events. A giant quarantine bubble had been created for the games, requiring meticulous planning, surveillance, management, and massive manpower. China pulled it off.

By mid-March 2022, the Omicron BA.2 subvariant had broken through in various parts of China, including the major cities of Shenzhen, Beijing, and Shanghai. COVID-19 restrictions were re-imposed to a greater or lesser extent. The Chinese formula remained mass testing, contact tracing, centralised quarantine, and lockdown if necessary. Shenzhen was locked down for a week in March, and Beijing for about four weeks in April–May; parts of Beijing had recurrent outbreaks into June. Most prominent was the two-month lockdown of Shanghai from mid-late March to the end of May. Initially, people were asked to stay home for a few days. Residents were not expecting a long lockdown and were psychologically unprepared for the extension and re-extension of the stay-home order, which exacerbated public anger as people did not know how long it would last. Residents also complained about many 'unreasonable' curbs, such as the erecting of fences to keep people within their residential compounds and evacuating people for disinfection of buildings. Other complaints included the poor conditions of quarantine centres, the shortage of food and medicine, and the lack of medical care for those with other illnesses. The Shanghai municipal government apologised for their COVID-19 unpreparedness and publicly thanked residents as restrictions eased on 1 June 2022. The battle was seen to be under a measure of control by late June.

The re-imposition of COVID-19 restrictions and lockdowns in China between March and May 2022 was not unreasonable. Research showed that having maintained a low infection rate in the general population through the pandemic, China had time to mass immunise its population, which had increased to 91.4 per cent by mid-April. However, the vaccine-induced immunity was insufficient to prevent outbreaks, and vaccine uptake in older adults remained lower than in other groups. From 1 March to 22 April, China saw more than 500,000 Omicron infections across the country with 93 per cent of them in Shanghai. Scientists estimated that in the absence of the Chinese formula noted above, there could have been a 'tsunami' of cases over a six-month period, resulting in over 112 million symptomatic cases, over 5 million hospital admissions, possibly 2.7 million intensive care admissions and 1.6 million deaths, with the main wave occurring between May and July 2022. Of the estimated fatalities, 77 per cent would have occurred in unvaccinated older individuals (see Chapter 5).[15] It was not surprising that when vice-premier Sun Chunlan visited Shanghai on 2 April 2022, she urged 'resolute' action to rein in COVID-19 despite the hardship caused to residents, and for the Chinese leadership to stay the course for the foreseeable future.

---

15. Jun Cai, Xiaowei Deng, Juan Yang, Kaiyuan Sun, Hengcong Liu, Zhiyuan Chen, et al., 'Modeling Transmission of SARS-CoV-2 Omicron in China', *Nature Medicine* 28 (10 May 2022): 1468–1475.

The complaints about the over-zealousness of officials and the bungling of aspects of the Shanghai lockdown led the NHC to issue orders in June 2022 that local authorities should not take unnecessary measures to restrict people's movements and business operations. Nevertheless, Chinese leaders felt they needed to stick to the winning formula of mass testing and tracing plus quarantine because there could be further mutations and China's overall healthcare conditions could not cope with massive numbers of cases. They felt China's overall numbers justified their approach—from the start of the COVID-19 outbreak in 2020, China had 2.42 million cases and 14,600 deaths, still very low compared to other countries, such as the United States and the United Kingdom. The argument in the summer of 2022 was over whether it was the right policy for China to continue regular mass testing all over cities, as the cost and effort would be enormous. Testing booths and centres mushroomed. Shanghai reportedly had one testing station for every 1,000 to 3,000 residents by the end of May 2022, and 15,000 stations in June. Estimates showed it could cost CNY60 billion for all cities with more than one million residents to build and maintain an adequate number of testing centres in 2022, and another CNY350 billion would be needed to conduct tests every 48 hours from May to December 2022.[16] The Chinese government justified the expense on the basis that it would be less costly than lockdowns. Experts were concerned about whether public support would wane, as pandemic fatigue set in, and whether the vast sums needed for testing could be better spent on protecting vulnerable groups who should be vaccinated, especially the non-vaccinated elderly, where China had not done well enough. While the overall vaccination rate was over 91 per cent by June 2022, the rate for people over 60 was around 83 per cent, and less than 50 per cent of those over 80 had received two shots. Like in other jurisdictions, many elderly people remained worried about whether vaccines would harm them and their efficacy (see Chapter 11 on vaccine hesitancy). At the end of June, China relaxed quarantine requirements for close contacts and inbound travellers, but did not change its zero-COVID policy—an indication that the leadership was trying to find the right combination of measures to keep the virus in check while avoiding shutdowns of its economy. By the end of July 2022, it could be seen that COVID control measures became somewhat less stringent, which in the words of Sun was for 'precision', not relaxation. COVID-19 cases continued to appear here and there. At a news briefing on 13 October 2022, when China's total COVID deaths was around 26,600, Liang Wannian of the NHC, explained why China's zero-COVID policy could not be done away with yet:

> Although the fatality rate . . . of Omicron is lower than that of the original strain and other variants, it can still lead to large numbers of infections due to its fast and stealthy transmission and ability to evade immunity. As a result, the absolute number of deaths across a certain population would still be quite large, and the disease's population-mortality risk remains higher than that of influenza . . . If we relax our virus-control

16. Xu Wen Cui Xiaotian, Dong Hui, Zhang Yukun and Li Leyan, 'Five Things to Know about China's Plans for Regular Mass COVID Testing', *Caixin*, 3 June 2022.

measures, there is bound to be a spike in new infections, and even many serious cases and deaths. We cannot stand to see such a severe consequence.[17]

Yet, the Chinese government started to adjust its COVID strategies on 11 November 2022 with new rules. On 27 November, the government announced that it was embarking on a campaign to vaccinate the elderly, and on 7 December 2022 it relaxed restrictions substantially when COVID cases were rising. The leadership had multiple reasons to pivot: the control methods were no longer working with the highly infectious Omicron with R0 as high as 22[18] and the authorities had to respond to protests for the economically damaging restrictions, as well as the poorly executed lockdowns in various localities. Mike Ryan, a WHO director, explained that it was not the lifting of restrictions that caused cases to increase; Omicron had been spreading because the control measures in themselves were no longer stopping the disease. He believed that: 'China decided strategically that was not the best option anymore . . . so the challenge that China and other countries still have is: are the people that need to be vaccinated, adequately vaccinated, with the right vaccines and the right number of doses and when was the last time those people had the vaccines.[19]

The leadership pivoted after consulting experts that relaxation and lowering fatalities could go together. While some modelling studies suggested that the lifting of strict restrictions could infect between 160 million and 280 million people—resulting in some 1.3 million to 2.1 million deaths, Dr Zhong Nanshan noted that Omicron had a fatality rate of about 0.1 per cent, about the same as ordinary seasonal influenza and that the current Omicron could be described as a 'novel coronavirus cold.[20] All experts agreed that the risk was highest among unvaccinated older adults, but that it was possible to minimise severe disease and deaths if the authorities went all out to ramp up vaccination and boosters for the elderly. The WHO and experts recommended that China should intensify vaccination—experts thought a three-dose regimen for older people could reduce fatalities by over 60 per cent. Loosening restrictions was seen as a means to incentivise people to get a third dose. Further studies showed a fourth shot would also be helpful. Other essential measures included using antiviral therapies to block viral spread, which required stockpiling drugs, as well as train more medical staff and increase the number of hospital beds. One study showed that China could reduce deaths by 89 per cent by treating those with COVID symptoms with antiviral drugs,

17. Wang Xiaoyu, 'Experts: Dynamic Zero-COVID Policy Still Key', *China Daily*, Hong Kong edition, 14 October 2022.

18. An R0 of 22 meant one infected person could infect 22 persons (see Chapter 5 on R0). Zhou Xiaoming, 'COVID Rules Reflect Ground Realities', *China Daily*, Hong Kong edition, 23 December 2022.

19. Emma Farge, 'China's COVID Spike Not Due to Lifting of Restrictions, WHO Director Say', *Reuters*, 15 December 2022.

20. 'New Edition of China's COVID-19 Control Protocols to Be Released Soon: Zhong Nanshan', *Global Times*, 15 December 2022. It was also reported that an unverified document suggested 248 million people in China were infected by COVID between 1 and 20 December, see Josephine Ma, 'Beijing's Covid Wave May Have Peaked but China's Tsunami of Cases Is Months from Easing: Experts', *South China Morning Post*, 24 December 2022.

including ones manufactured by western pharmaceutical companies, something China was reluctant to do in 2021. Moreover, experts advised managing China's reopening in 2023 using a well-coordinated approach so as not to over-burden the health system was a top priority.[21]

United States' Response to COVID-19

The United States had the highest cumulative total of COVID-19 cases and deaths in the world at the end of 2021—50 million and 800,000 respectively, which by 1 June 2022, had risen to over 83 million and over a million deaths, despite having the world's highest concentration of science and technical knowledge. Its experience could be conveniently viewed through three phases that represented the approaches of two successive administrations, and a third phase of 'living with COVID' in 2022.

1. The Donald Trump Era—January 2020 to December 2021
2. The Biden Administration—January 2021 to December 2021
3. Living with the virus—from January 2022

Phase 1 was dominated by Donald Trump and the decisions made by his administration in 2020, when there were many surprising missteps. There are many scholarly and popular publications on this period. The White House chief of staff admitted on 25 October 2020 that 'we're not going to contain the pandemic . . . because it is a contagious virus' and that the administration would focus on 'vaccines, therapeutics and other mitigations'.[22] Phase 2, starting in 2021, may be seen as a time for remedial action by the administration of Joseph Biden, but even with greater effort, it was hard to assert control. Beyond the personalities of the two presidents and their appointed officials, there was the longstanding neglect of identified weaknesses in US pandemic preparedness. Moreover, the underlying US culture of resisting restrictions, even in the face of contagion, was also a confounding factor in dealing with COVID-19. Phase 3 deals with how the Biden administration coped with 'living with COVID' as the Omicron variant and subvariants emerged, followed by the easing of pandemic restrictions in end-March 2022. Pandemic fatigue had set in, despite the fact that health experts called for caution.

21. 'China Epidemiologist Urges Faster COVID-19 Vaccination among Vulnerable Groups', *Xinhua*, 12 December, 2022; 'China Launches Second COVID-19 Booster Shot', *Xinhua*, 14 December 2022; Smriti Mallapaty, 'Can China Avoid a Wave of Deaths if It Lifts Strict Zero-Covid Policy?', *Nature* 612 (8 December 2022): 203; Kathy Leung, Gabriel M. Leung, and Joseph T. Wu, 'Modelling the Adjustment of COVID-19 Response and Exit from Dynamic Zero-COVID in China', *medRxiv*, 14 December 2022, https://doi.org/10.1101/2022.12.14.22283460.
22. Devan Cole, 'White House Chief of Staff: We Are Not Going to Control the Pandemic', *CNN*, 25 October 2020.

A warning: Crimson Contagion

'Crimson Contagion', the simulation exercise in 2019, showed many deficiencies in US pandemic preparedness. The exercise involved various federal, state, local, private, and public institutions. It was based on an outbreak of a novel influenza spreading from returning visitors to China that ended up infecting over 100 million Americans, hospitalising millions of patients, and resulting in over 500,000 deaths. The exercise showed that the authorities had limited capacity to respond, and that states would experience multiple challenges in obtaining resources from the federal government due to a lack of standardised, well-understood, and properly executed resource request processes. The assessment report also pointed to federal agencies lacking the resources and capacities to respond and predicted they would have problems in coordination.[23]

Similar problems had been foreseen even earlier. In 2005, the White House published a national pandemic strategy, after which various government departments issued recommendations and guidelines to lay out priorities, and articulate the roles and functions of federal, state, and local authorities. Critics were concerned about the uneven capabilities and capacities of state and local agencies to respond. As many agencies and private sector health institutions had to act swiftly in an emergency, the ability of federal agencies to coordinate had also been questioned. The United States was considered to have coped reasonably well with the H1N1 pandemic of 2009–2010, referred to as the swine flu, that originated in Mexico.[24] A closer examination of subsequent reviews flagged a warning that the country's public health capacity could have been overwhelmed had the outbreak been more widespread or more severe. Reports noted that decades of chronic underfunding meant that many core systems were not prepared for epidemic and pandemic emergencies. To strengthen preparedness, experts made a range of recommendations that included:

1. Ensuring public health departments had enough resources to provide on-the-ground responses, and for hospitals and clinics to increase surge capacities.
2. Improving communication and coordination among federal, state, local authorities, and the private sector in preparedness.
3. Investing in pandemic planning and stockpiling antiviral medications, vaccinations, and PPE, including replenishing stocks.
4. Enhancing research and development abilities to rapidly develop a vaccine and ensuring inoculation capability in a short period of time.

---

23. David E. Sanger, Eric Lipton, Eileen Sullivan, and Michael Crowley, 'Coronavirus Outbreak: A Cascade of Warnings, Heard but Unheeded', *New York Times*, 19 March 2020.
24. By the time it waned in August 2010, virtually all countries had reported confirmed cases. In 12 months, H1N1 was estimated to have caused 60.8 million illnesses, over 270,000 hospitalisation and over 12,400 deaths in the United States, and an estimated 151,700 to 575,400 deaths globally. Statistics from the US Centers for Disease Control and Prevention (USCDC), '2009 H1N1 Pandemic (H1N1pdm09 virus)', accessed 14 September 2022, https://www.cdc.gov/flu/pandemic-resources/2009-h1n1-pandemic.html.

5. Improving strategies to limit the spread of disease, ensuring people have sick leave benefits, and that communities were prepared to limit public gatherings and close schools as necessary.

6. Ensuring all those who needed care during an emergency could be cared for, as that would help to limit the spread of a contagious disease to others, and that the institutions that provided care were compensated.

The problems were well-document by numerous reports of the Government Accountability Office between 2009 and 2013 expressing concern about the level of pandemic preparedness,[25] and other inspection reports in 2014 and 2016 noted the urgent need for improvements.[26] The *Crimson Contagion* laid bare US vulnerabilities on the eve of the COVID-19 outbreak.

Phase 1: The Donald Trump era

The United States Centers for Disease Control and Prevention (USCDC) is answerable to the Department of Health and Human Services, which is headed by a politically appointed secretary. The USCDC came to know that there was a pneumonia of unknown cause in Wuhan on 31 December 2019, and it circulated the information in an internal document. By 2 January, senior national security and White House officials were alerted, and there was concern about the outbreak spreading. The USCDC issued a health advisory on 7 January to local health departments and healthcare providers about the outbreak in China and requested US healthcare providers to ask patients with severe respiratory illness about their travel history and notify the USCDC where relevant. By 20 January, when China announced human-to-human transmission was occurring, the USCDC activated its Emergency Operation Center to 'support public health partners' to respond domestically. The first confirmed case in the United States, announced on 20 January, was a man who had visited Wuhan. He felt ill and went to a doctor on 19 January after hearing of the USCDC's health advisory. In a 28 January intelligence briefing, Donald Trump was advised that the new virus could be the biggest security threat of his presidency.[27] Meanwhile, US officials stationed in China were planning to evacuate their citizens from Wuhan, and the first group of about 200 evacuees landed at an air base in California on 29 January for observation and screening.[28] Shortly thereafter, the State Department authorised the departure of all its China-based employees.

25. GAO published critical reports to the US Congress about pandemic preparedness in 2009, https://www.gao.gov/products/gao-09-334; in 2011, https://www.gao.gov/assets/gao-11-632.pdf; and in 2013, https://www.gao.gov/assets/gao-18-362.pdf.

26. Department of Homeland Security Office of the Inspector General reports in 2014, https://www.oig.dhs.gov/reports/2014-08/dhs-has-not-effectively-managed-pandemic-personal-protective-equipment-and, and in 2016, https://www.oig.dhs.gov/sites/default/files/assets/2017/OIG-17-02-Oct16.pdf.

27. Jamir Gangel, Jeremy Herb, and Elizabeth Stuart, 'Play It Down: Trump Admits to Concealing the True Threat of Coronavirus in New Woodward Book', *CNN*, 9 September 2020.

28. A subsequent review showed not all the staff sent to the airbase had infection control training, protective gear

Even though senior officials were concerned about the virus, their public communication was low-key. Dr Anthony Fauci, head of the National Institute of Allergy and Infectious Diseases, and the head of the USCDC, described the risk to Americans as 'low'. They did not want to cause panic. The news media reported many other health professionals saying the seasonal flu posed a greater threat than this new disease. On 30 January 2020, the first case of person-to-person transmission was reported in the United States of a person who had not been to China but had been in touch with someone who had. The United States announced a public health emergency on 31 January, a day after the WHO declared a Public Health Emergency of International Concern (PHEIC; see Chapter 2). This was a clear signal for countries to prepare for outbreaks. Dr Fauci and the USCDC head continued to say that the risk to the United States was low through February, when what was unfolding in China was severe. Their tone only changed in March 2020.

The most important step in the early days should have been containment through ramping up testing and tracing so that the authorities could identify where and how the disease was spreading and use the information to guide intervention measures (see Chapter 1). Critics faulted the USCDC and the Food and Drug Administration (FDA) for a series of decisions that delayed testing.[29] The United States could have used an available diagnostic test developed in Germany that the WHO was recommending and used it to make testing kits. Although unlikely, it could also have used China's. The United States wanted to develop its own more complex test that would supposedly be more precise. Most unfortunate, its testing kits turned out to be defective.[30] Critics also found fault in restricting testing to only individuals with a known travel history and who sought medical care for specific symptoms, and for confining the use of its test to a limited group of laboratories. Taken together, very little testing was in fact done and precious time was lost in tracking the spread of the virus at the early stage. Dr Fauci described the US roll out of testing as 'a failing' of the system. He noted 'the idea of anyone getting (a COVID-19 test), the way people in other countries are doing it— we're not set up for it'.[31]

For some infections, testing and tracing should go together at the early stage of an outbreak. Contact tracing should start when someone tested positive. A tracer should interview this person to identify contacts, such as family members and co-workers. Tracers should inform the contacts so they could quarantine themselves and get tested.

was not worn to avoid 'bad optics', and there was no overall plan for infection prevention; see Dan Diamond, 'US Handling of American Evacuees from Wuhan Increased Coronavirus Risks, Watchdog Finds', 29 January 2021, *Washington Post*, https://web.archive.org/web/20210207054532/https://www.washingtonpost.com/health/2021/01/28/wuhan-americans-evacuation.

29. Cary Coglianese, 'Obligation Alleviation during the Covid-19 Crisis', *The Regulatory Review*, 20 April 2020; and Jaimie Ding, 'Why Are Rapid Antigen Tests Tough to Find?', *Los Angeles Times*, 10 January 2022.

30. US Department of Health and Human Services, 'Summary of the Findings of the Immediate Office of the General Counsel's Investigation Regarding CDC's Production of Covid-19 Test Kits', 19 June 2020, https://www.documentcloud.org/documents/6953861-6-19-20-Summary-of-the-Findings-of-the-Immediate.html.

31. Elizabeth Chuck, '"It's a Failing. Let's Admit It", Fauci Says of Coronavirus Testing', *NBC News*, 12 March 2020.

The purpose of testing, tracing, and isolation is to break the chain of transmission. In some parts of the United States, more than 50 per cent of the people who tested positive provided no details of contacts when asked; and where contacts were provided, a high portion could not be reached. Insufficient resources and lack of technology support made tracing virtually impossible. Even where there was funding, it was hard to hire enough contact tracers and marshal them efficiently. Public resistance to disclosing information was also a problem.[32]

From 2 February 2020, the Trump administration restricted non-citizens other than the immediate family of citizens and permanent residents from entering the United States if they had been to China within the previous fortnight.[33] It restricted travel further as the WHO declared COVID-19 had become a pandemic, and President Trump declared the COVID-19 outbreak a national emergency on 13 March. There were deeply divided views within the White House and among experts on what to do and how to implement measures. On 16 March, the White House finally issued guidelines calling on the public to limit travel and avoid social gatherings of more than ten people for the next 15 days—later extended until 30 April 2020.

The White House's guidelines did help. However, critics saw them as too little, too late. By then the United States had seen not only the aggressive Chinese response with lockdowns and how Asian economies were dealing with COVID-19, but also the devastating situation in Italy (see Chapter 12). The political priority and messaging, however, was to promote a return to normality as soon as possible. Restricting activities was felt to be anathema to the *raison d'être* of the country. The social contract between the rulers and the people in the United States is based on as few restrictions on individual freedom as possible. States started to abandon or reduce mitigation measures towards the end of April 2020 so that their economies could bounce back. By year-end, cases surpassed 20 million with nearly 350,000 deaths.

The Trump factor and choice

Americans did not hear a unified and consistent message from their government. Trump's messages from January to early March 2020 were that the virus was 'under control', the United States was 'in very good shape', his administration was 'doing a great job', and that the 'risk to the American people remains very low'.[34] The president was a frequent commentator on his unique understanding of the science, risks, and cures.

---

32. Dyani Lewis, 'Why Many Countries Failed at Covid Contact-Tracing—But Some Got It Right', *Nature*, 14 December 2020, https://www.nature.com/articles/d41586-020-03518-4.

33. Estimates showed 40,000 residents had returned to the United States from China after the ban took effect, and in the month before the travel restrictions, about 300,000 people had travelled to the United States from China; Steve Eder, Henry Fountain, Michael H. Keller, Muyi Xiao, and Alexandra Stevenson, '430,000 People Have Traveled from China to U.S. Since Coronavirus Surfaced', *New York Times*, 15 April 2020.

34. According to contemporaneous interviews with Trump, he was regularly briefed and knew that the virus was dangerous, airborne, and highly contagious. He played it down publicly because he did not want to cause panic. Bob Woodward, *Rage* (New York: Simon and Schuster, 2020).

His messaging started to change in four ways from mid-March after the WHO declared COVID-19 a pandemic. First, he described himself as 'a wartime president' to fight the virus; second, he started to attack China by calling the virus 'Chinese' and attacking the WHO for incompetence; third, he switched to a success narrative of the US response— 'We've made every decision correctly' even as infections and fatalities climbed; and finally, criticisms were 'enemy statements'.[35]

By June 2020, pandemic restrictions had become politically and socially divisive as the United States hit two million confirmed cases and new infections rose in 20 states. COVID-19 became increasingly partisan in the run-up to the presidential election, as could be seen from the disagreements over wearing facemasks. When Trump decided he would not wear one, it became a political statement. His harshest critics accused him of 'pandemicide' for proceeding with large rallies that enabled the spreading of the virus among his mostly unmasked supporters.[36] In 2021, the wearing of facemasks continued to be controversial in the United States with court cases striking down facemask mandates.

The Trump administration's choice was to leave response strategies to the pandemic to the states. Critics alleged it was because Trump did not want to be held responsible for failure, and by passing the responsibility to the states, there would always be others to blame. The United States had a patchwork of strategies on imposing mitigation measures such as face masking in public, limiting gatherings, issuing stay-at-home orders, restricting out-of-state travel, and closing schools and day-care centres. The federal government chose not to centralise and coordinate the purchase of PPE and medical equipment, which led to states bidding against each other for scarce supplies in the global marketplace when the federal government was also bidding. One view was that the perpetual struggle over relative power and autonomy between federal, state, and municipal authorities was inevitable and that the fragmentation of authority, policy-making, and implementation was a part of America's experience in its constitutional history.[37] Another view put the blame on the president for not choosing to lead a coordinated national response to fight COVID-19, as could be done under the constitution and laws. Those who held this view argued that early, decisive national coordination for containment, mitigation, and procurement and distribution of PPE and equipment supplies could have reduced the state and local governments' disadvantages early in the

---

35. There are numerous 'fact checks' relating to Donald Trump's many statements related to COVID-19 by media organisations. An early check was Justin Fishel, Elizabeth Thomas, and Lauren Lantry, 'Fact Check: Trump's Coronavirus Response Plagued with Misstatements', *ABC News*, 16 March 2020. For another study in which Donald Trump was considered a major driver of misinformation, see Sarah Evanega, Mark Lynas, Jordan Adams, and Karinne Smolenyak, 'Corona Misinformation: Quantifying Sources and Themes in the COVID-19 "Infodemic"', https://allianceforscience.cornell.edu/wp-content/uploads/2020/09/Evanega-et-al-Coronavirus-misinformationFINAL.pdf.

36. Laurie Garett, 'Trump Is Guilty of Pandemicide', *Foreign Policy*, 18 February 2021, https://foreignpolicy.com/2021/02/18/trump-is-guilty-of-pandemicide.

37. Greg Goelzhauser and David M. Konisky, 'The State of American Federalism 2019–2020: Polarized and Punitive Intergovernmental Relations', *Publius: The Journal of Federalism* 50, no. 3 (2020): 311–343.

pandemic, which could have saved lives and boosted the economy.[38] Chapter 8 provides an in-depth discussion of the shortage of PPE in the United States. Perhaps the US federal system is bound to produce many variations, which in itself is not necessarily a problem if the leadership was there to bring society together during the pandemic and forge consensus and coordination.

Phase 2: The Biden administration

Trump lost the November 2020 election to Biden, who was sworn in as president in January 2021. Biden's early focus was to continue to ramp up vaccination, as they had become available by the end of the previous year. Chapter 4 discusses vaccines; suffice to acknowledge here that the United States has an advanced industrial and technological base for vaccine development, and this was its undoubted strength. Developing vaccines as quickly as possible was seen as the silver bullet to defeating COVID-19. Once available, the challenge was to get people vaccinated to reduce their risk of infections and severe COVID-19. In the early days of the outbreak in the United States, there was a moment when the Trump administration thought that herd immunity could be achieved through doing very little so that the people would be infected and thereby become immune. The United Kingdom had thought of adopting such an approach at one time and it was Sweden's approach in 2020 (see Chapter 12).

The Trump administration's major contribution to fighting COVID-19 was *Operation Warp Speed*, announced on 15 May 2020. This was a public-private sector partnership to get vaccine companies to work at speed and scale. The United States funded it by applying a part of its COVID-19 stimulus package and using funds shifted from other projects. By October, contracts had been awarded to support the development and production of six vaccines, with obligations of about US$10 billion. Under the programme, vaccine companies could build production plants to make millions of doses even before they were proven to be effective. Pfizer, a German vaccine developer not part of the partnership, received a US$1.9 billion advance purchase agreement in July. The US funding not only removed the financial risk for these companies to develop vaccines before they were authorised by the FDA or shown to be effective, but also gave the companies immunity to lawsuits if something unintentionally adverse arises from the use of their vaccines.[39] The two most successful vaccines produced by Pfizer and BioNTech, and Moderna, tried a new messenger RNA (mRNA) technology to trigger an immune response inside the body.

---

38. Beverly A. Cigler, 'Fighting Covid-19 in the United States with Federalism and Other Constitutional and Statutory Authority', *Publius: The Journal of Federalism* 51, no. 4 (2021): 673–692.
39. Under existing law, the US government invoked the Public Readiness and Emergency Preparedness Act (2005) that empowers the Secretary for Health and Human Services to give legal protection to companies making or distributing vaccines and treatments unless there is wilful misconduct. Time limits do apply to the protection of the pharmaceutical companies under the Act.

An early decision of the Biden administration was to reverse the Trump administration's decision that states were responsible for getting people vaccinated, which led to a slow roll out. Federal agencies were enlisted to set up large-scale vaccination sites, and the military assisted. Between March and June 2021, cases declined steeply as the vaccination rate rose. President Biden and his administration felt victory was at hand by early July 2021. The USCDC ended indoor masking for vaccinated people. Anticipating lower demand, laboratories that made test kits reduced production. Some states scaled back on reporting COVID-19 data. Despite consistent messaging and more effort, the vaccination rate remained stuck at around 60 per cent due to vaccination resistance. The Biden administration admitted that it did not see the Delta and Omicron variants coming.[40] The Delta variant was able to re-infect people who had previously been infected and caused more severe disease in unvaccinated people than previous strains did. Healthcare workers and hospitals were under strain once again as cases rose. In 2021 there were 470 million COVID deaths, more than had occurred in 2020 under the Trump administration. The USCDC recommended on 29 November 2021, that everyone 18 and older should get a third 'booster' dose of vaccination and broadened the age range for vaccination to include children 5 years and older. By the end of 2021, the United States had many concurrent variations in dealing with COVID-19 adopted by states, cities, counties, school districts, universities, and workplaces. In general, the low-vaccination communities had lax restrictions, while high-vaccination ones tended to have more stringent measures.

Phase 3: Living with the virus

In January 2022, the Omicron BA.1.1 subvariant was the dominant strain in the United States. By early February, infections had topped 76 million, and deaths shot over 900,000. Yet, a line of argument had taken root by March that while permissive policies in some states did not stop COVID-19, their overall results were not much worse than those states that had many restrictions, such as masking and forced vaccination. The narrative was that it was better to 'live with COVID' and be free of restrictions, especially as the level of community immunity was thought to be sufficiently high with 66 per cent of all Americans having received two vaccines and 29 per cent having had a booster dose. It was also thought that a high proportion of the unvaccinated had some infection-related protection. Hence, some three-quarters of the population was estimated to have some level of immunity, and people were considered less likely to need hospitalisation even if cases surge in yet another wave. Moreover, antiviral therapies could help, although Congress axed US$15 billion of COVID-related funding in March 2022 that included spending on providing therapies, as well as bolstering testing capacity. By May 2022, confirmed US deaths from COVID-19 had surged passed a million.

---

40. Noah Bierman, '"We Didn't See Omicron Coming," Harris Says', *Los Angeles Times*, 18 December 2021.

Various federal guidelines on such measures as masking in public places had expired and were replaced by a county assessment system based on local case counts and hospitalisation. Local authorities were to make their own rules at a time of high pandemic fatigue. Essentially, the United States was 'living with COVID'. In June and July 2022, the Omicron subvariants BA.4 and BA.5 were prevalent. COVID-19 cases were about five times higher than they were in the summer of 2021, reporting about 100,000 new cases each day and further spikes were considered possible as few restrictions were in place anywhere. However, hospitalisation rates were far lower than in the first two years of the pandemic and therefore thought to be manageable. By the end of July 2022, there were still substantial numbers of cases resulting in workers being out sick, including healthcare workers. On 19 September, Biden said the pandemic was essentially 'over' for the United States.[41] At the time, there were still about 400 deaths per day in the United States.[42]

Observations

The greatest criticism of China was its failure before 20 January 2020 to come clean on the emergence of a new disease. Information was suppressed by officials in Wuhan and Hubei until they were caught out and the central authorities mobilised to contain the new virus. In today's world of instant communication, it is impossible to hide information for long. The news of the appearance of an atypical pneumonia was already circulating on 30 December 2019, on ProMED, a global online forum that public health specialists look at (see Chapter 2).[43] China cannot easily dismiss the view that its political system could not be trusted despite many positive reforms and advances. When push came to shove, information about the new coronavirus was suppressed somewhere along the chains of responsibility. The greatest criticisms of the United States were negligence and failure of leadership, as the White House and the Trump administration ignored and downplayed available information about the new disease and failed to take action to contain the virus that led to a loss of control resulting in high infection and fatalities.

Mutually incomprehensible approaches

The Chinese Communist Party is the ruling party in China on an ongoing basis. It must continue to deliver strong governing performance to justify its continuing leadership. In other words, its legitimacy comes from performance. In facing a new infectious disease, the leadership used the number of cases and fatalities to judge its own performance.

---

41. 60 Minutes, *CBS*, 18 September 2022, https://www.cbsnews.com/news/president-joe-biden-60-minutes-interview-transcript-2022-09-18/.
42. Jacob Stern, 'Hundreds of Americans Will Die from Covid Today', *The Atlantic*, 16 September 2022.
43. ProMED, or Program for Monitoring Emerging Diseases of International Society for Infectious Diseases, is a non-profit scientists' organisation.

The Chinese people supported these key performance indicators in the government's COVID-19 approach. There was an alignment in how the authorities and the people saw their social contract with each other.

Chinese leaders were advised by experts that China's strategy ought to focus on containment at the epicentre in Wuhan and Hubei. There was no proven treatments or vaccine for a new coronavirus in January 2020. China decided on the toughest approach to suppress the virus through a lockdown to cut human-to-human transmission for an extended period; and used strong mitigation measures elsewhere in the country. Chinese experts considered this strategy was the key to China's success. Chinese leaders decided to accept the enormous pain this would cause to the people and the economy. The political risk was high—losing the fight would hurt the credibility of the leadership and the Chinese Communist Party. The Chinese government's approach was only possible because the Chinese people had a very high level of political trust in the national government. From the people's perspective and despite much complaint and suffering, it was precisely at such times that leaders had to make tough decisions.

The enormity and courage of China's choice in 2020 could be seen from the WHO Beijing resident representative's description of the Wuhan lockdown—that it was 'unprecedented in public health history' and mass quarantine 'was new to history'. That view should be seen within the context of prevailing views. For example, a WHO publication in March 2019 did not recommend quarantine because 'there was no obvious rationale for this measure, and there would be considerable difficulties in implementing it'.[44] Another report published six months later by the Center for Health Security at Johns Hopkins University noted quarantine was likely not effective in controlling highly transmissible respiratory pathogens like influenza and highlighted the 'difficulty of implementing such measures on a large scale'.[45]

There was a measure of gloating among US and other Western commentators starting in February 2020 that the virus could be China's 'Chernobyl Moment' and that the Chinese leadership might collapse. By March 2020, China's methods were crushing the virus. Containment measures through extensive testing, tracing, and isolating cases, as well as stopping non-essential activities, helped to cut transmission. The result of the extended lockdown in Wuhan and Hubei was remarkable—it set a new historical example in infectious disease control. The level of trust that the Chinese had in their government rose to 90 per cent in 2020. US experts did not miss the effectiveness of the

44. WHO, 'Non-Pharmaceutical Public Health Measures for Mitigation the Risk and Impact of Epidemics and Pandemics Influenza', Global Influenza Programme, 19 September 2019, https://apps.who.int/iris/bitstream/handle/10665/329438/9789241516839-eng.pdf, 16.
45. Johns Hopkins Center for Public Health, 'Preparedness for a High-Impact Respiratory Pathogen Pandemic', September 2019, https://www.centerforhealthsecurity.org/our-work/pubs_archive/pubs-pdfs/2019/190918-GMPBreport-respiratorypathogen.pdf, 57.

Chinese approach,[46] but it was probably unworkable in the United States as Americans' trust in their government was no more than 40 per cent.[47]

The US experience could not be more different than China's. As a two-party system with regular elections for the legislature and the presidency, a change of leadership presents a fresh start. The legitimacy of the US political system comes from elections, and if performance was found wanting, the people could elect different leaders with different policies at the next election. Despite elections, political trust in the United States is low, as discussed in Chapter 1. Beyond the issue of political trust, there were too many arguments within the White House on what to do in 2020. There were arguments about the cost of mitigation to keep COVID-19 in check, and there were strong views that the cost outweighed the benefits. What was agreed was for the US government to support the speedy development of vaccines to bring about herd immunity. This justified the enormous funding for vaccine development. It set a record in the speed of their development and approval for use in about a year. Although vital in the fight against COVID-19, vaccines were not the quick one-time 'silver bullet' that had been hoped for due to vaccination resistance by a not insignificant portion of the population, and boosters were also needed as effectiveness waned after several months. The lesson here is that the availability of vaccines did not mean other forms of protection were no longer needed.

As China's efforts were bearing fruit, the United States had 40,000 COVID-19 deaths by mid-April 2020. Trump said deaths could be 50,000 to 60,000, then revised it to 60,000 to 70,000 before further adjusting it to 100,000 deaths the following month. In early May, the White House projected 100,000 to 240,000 deaths if good mitigation measures could be implemented.[48] Infections and fatalities continued to rise through 2020. The United States had lost its way, as containment failed in the early days and mitigation measures were patchy. Beyond what critics called 'the Trump factor', the many disconnects and vulnerabilities of the US healthcare system, as shown by the *Crimson Contagion* simulation in 2019, proved accurate with the onslaught of COVID-19. This was not just the inattention and neglect of one administration or a particular congressional term of office, as the problem could be traced back many years.

Indeed, a change of administration in January 2021 and greater attention to dealing with the virus could not overcome many years of budget cuts that led to a myriad of weaknesses in the healthcare system, especially as dealing with COVID-19 became a highly charged partisan issue in the country. For example, Republican-led states fought the Biden administration for overstepping its authority with a plan to require most US

46. Harvey V. Fineberg, 'The Weeks to Crush the Curve', *New England Journal of Medicine* 382, no. 17 (23 April 2020), https://doi.org/10.1056/nejme2007263.

47. According to the Edelman Global Trust Barometer Report, the rate of public trust in the Chinese government was 84 per cent in 2018, 86 per cent in 2019, and 90 per cent in 2020. Over the same period, Americans' trust in their government ranged from 37 per cent to 40 per cent.

48. Patrick Smith, 'Trump Warns Coronavirus Death Toll Could Reach 100,000', *NBC News*, 4 May 2020, https://www.nbcnews.com/politics/politics-news/trump-warns-coronavirus-death-toll-could-reach-100-000-n1199161.

workers to be vaccinated or regularly tested. In a January 2022 ruling, the Supreme Court allowed the mandate for health workers but blocked the vaccinate-or-test mandate for other workers on the basis that it was for the states, not the federal government, to decide. It is beyond the ambit of this chapter to discuss these legal issues. Suffice to note that it is very much a part of US political culture to use the courts to settle issues that are seen as affecting the division of power between the federal and state governments.

The US political leadership was always greatly concerned about the health of the economy. Opening up the economy in 2020–2021 and 'living with COVID' in 2022 were the dominant narratives alongside 'freedom of choice' in limiting restrictive mitigation measures. In the United States, it was seen as acceptable to open up at the expense of a higher number of infections and deaths. The Chinese leadership put health and lives first, the consequence of which was to stay with a long period of stringent measures. Yet, despite the initial shock of the harsh lockdown, China's economy started to improve in May 2020. In 2020, China's GDP grew 2.3 per cent and 8.1 per cent the following year, while that of the United States was at –3.5 per cent in 2020 and 5.7 per cent the following year (see Chapters 7 and 11). The US political establishment is unlikely to ever concede that China did a valiant job that produced positive results in 2020 and 2021. Likewise, it is difficult for the Chinese leadership to understand why Americans could accept such a high death rate from COVID-19.

Readiness to live with the virus: Different calculus

For governments, deciding on when to end pandemic measures or when to reinstate them during a new wave involves a complex balancing of health, economic and social concerns. Cases and deaths tend to decline during periods when stringent measures are in place but rebound when those measures are lifted. In March 2022, a group of prominent US public health experts suggested 60,225 as the number of acceptable yearly deaths from COVID-19 and other respiratory illnesses combined for the United States, which worked out to be one death per 2 million Americans, or 165 per day nationwide. This would be like an extremely severe season of the flu. At that rate, US hospitals could still cope.[49] Critics were concerned that death from COVID-19 was being normalised in the United States. In April 2022, the USCDC decided the decision to loosen or tighten restrictions would be made at the local country level depending on the capacity of its hospitals to handle a new influx of patients. The Chinese too had to grapple with how to proceed. The explosion of Omicron cases in the spring of 2022 that resulted in lockdowns confirmed China was unready to 'live with COVID'. By the summer of 2022 in the United States, the issue was whether facemasks should be re-imposed as

---

49. Dolores Albarracín, Trevor Bedford, Thomas Bollyky, Luciana Borio, Rick A. Bright, Lisa M. Brosseau, et al., 'Getting to and Sustaining the Next Normal: A Roadmap for Living with Covid', March 2022, https://www.rockefellerfoundation.org/wp-content/uploads/2022/03/Getting-to-and-Sustaining-the-Next-Normal-A-Roadmap-for-Living-with-Covid-Report-Final.pdf.

infections rose (albeit relatively mild) but there was also a concern that it might be hard to enforce due to public resistance. Americans were enjoying being free from COVID restrictions. The American political establishment saw China's situation as being stuck in the mud. The Chinese government had to pivot to 'live with COVID' by December 2022, realising that its control methods were no longer working against Omicron and that vaccinating vulnerable groups became a matter of the highest priority, together with promoting booster shots, and importing pharmaceuticals produced by Western companies that had proven to be effective. As China faced a tsunami of Omicron cases at the end of the year, new COVID cases trended up in the United States alongside a spike in other infections, and the worst influenza season in two decades, further straining American healthcare capacity.

In the midst of the US-China conflict

The Trump administration marked the time of a visible and widening split in Sino-American relations. COVID-19 arrived as conflicts in trade and technology were already in full swing. An early spat arose from Trump calling the virus the 'Chinese' virus and the 'Kung flu'. On 24 March 2020, a bipartisan resolution was passed to condemn China's handling of the virus outbreak. In April 2020, several class-action suits were filed against China, seeking trillions of dollars over the outbreak in the United States, including one by the state of Missouri and another by Mississippi. It was perhaps too hard to accept that the carnage was caused by the fault of their own government. On 30 April 2020, Trump said he had reasons to believe COVID-19 originated from a virology laboratory in Wuhan. Since then, the issue of the origin of COVID-19 became an issue of not just scientific exploration but political contention between the two countries and will likely continue into the future (see Chapter 1).

A new narrative developed as the United States and Europe began to 'live with COVID' by easing restrictions during the first quarter of 2022. This narrative emphasised that China's success with its zero-COVID policy could not be sustained because tough mitigation would be increasingly costly while also having reduced effectiveness in face of the highly transmissible Omicron, and that China's refusal to abandon its policy was due to systemic obstinacy. China was annoyed that the head of the WHO, Tedros Adhanom Ghebreyesus, said on 10 May 2022, that 'we don't think that it is sustainable, considering the behaviour of the virus now and what we anticipate in the future' and that a 'shift in approach would be very important', as the Chinese leadership was dealing with the outbreak in Shanghai. One line of criticism was that the Chinese leadership could not easily adjust its policy because it had invested so much in its zero-COVID policy that it had become political and a part of the ideological competition between the lackadaisical West versus the more cautious Chinese approach,[50] while another line of criticism was the Chinese political system was too autocratic and rigid to change

50. Jeremy Goldkorn, 'China's Covid-19 Spike and a Clash of Civilization', *SupChina*, 1 April 2022.

even when it was in its own best interest to do so.[51] Critics of China saw the 'living with COVID' versus the cautious Chinese approach in black-and-white terms rather than considering whether they were appropriate under the circumstances. Furthermore, critics saw China as posing a threat to the world because there would be more and more outbreaks, resulting in more and more lockdowns that would lead to unhappy citizens, greater economic gyrations, and frequent disruptions to global supply chains that would harm not only the Chinese economy but the rest of the world too.[52] When there were isolated grumbles in September and October, and explicit protests in November 2022, it was seen as confirmation that the authoritarian system face a major crisis. These perspectives were variations of the 'Chernobyl Moment'. As this book went to press, the situation was grave—Omicron swept across China very quickly. The leadership's pivot to managing COVID relaxation and prioritising vaccination among the elderly and providing enough antiviral therapies for its people, including imported ones, once again tested the Chinese Communist Party's ability to mobilise resources, gain the cooperation of the Chinese public, as well as whether it could manage China's reopening in a way that minimised fatalities and economic damage.[53] The chaotic scenes that Americans witnessed in 2020 in the United States in clinics, hospitals, and mortuaries with their first COVID wave was happening in China.

Negative views about China might have also been affected by the overall negativity in the West, particularly the United States, about China and its political system. Naturally, Chinese officials saw things differently. A line of defence was out-of-control COVID-19 in China would not serve anyone's economic interest and would hinder supply chains. The Omicron outbreak in 2022 did not lead to China closing down the country and its economy—the government believed that while officials were not blameless, China had learnt to target closures to limit socio-economic impacts. China's main defence lies in numbers. If the Chinese people had died from COVID-19 at the same rate as Americans between January 2020 and May 2022, China's COVID-19 fatalities would be more than 4.2 million. China's COVID-19 fatalities at the end of May were 14,600, and in early October were under 26,600 compared to over a million in the United States. According to Ma Xiaowei, the director of the NHC, 'China's anti-epidemic experience shows that having 1.4 billion people holding the line of defence is the greatest contribution to international anti-pandemic efforts'.[54] Along this line of thinking, China has 18.3 per cent of global population and contributed 0.16 of COVID cases and 0.08 per cent of related deaths worldwide. This meant COVID's incidence

51. Huang Yanzhong, 'The Collateral Damage in China's Covid Was: Are Beijing's Harsh Measures Undermining Its Old on Power?', *Foreign Affairs*, 17 May 2022.

52. Ian Bremmer and Cliff Kupchan, 'Risk 1: No Zero Covid', Eurasia Group, 3 January 2022, https://www. eurasiagroup.net/live-post/top-risks-2022-1-no-zero-covid.

53. Kathy Leung, Gabriel M. Leung, and Joseph T. Wu, 'Modelling the Adjustment of COVID-19 Response and Exit from Dynamic Zero-COVID in China', *medRxiv*, 14 December 2022, https://doi.org/10.1101/20 22.12.14.22283460.

54. Jack Lau, 'China Sticks to Strict Plan: Health Minister Says Swift Response Means Time Needed to Contain Outbreaks Has Been Cut from a Month to Two Weeks', *South China Morning Post*, 3 December 2021.

rate in Mainland China was only 1/483rd of the United States', and its mortality rate was 1/785th of that of the US. From this perspective, the Chinese leadership saw no reason for critics to cast doubt on its zero-COVID strategy.[55] As for disruptions to global supply chains, China's total imports and exports for 2021 exceeded US$6 trillion for the first time, and it could be argued that China played a role in keeping supplies up and prices down. Nevertheless, the Chinese economy had slowed down in 2022, and it was a cause of public discontent. More concerning still was losing the grip on Omicron and having to face rising fatalities. China paid the price of having failed to prioritise vaccinating the elderly and promoting booster shots, plus the earlier refusal to import Western-produced vaccines and antiviral drugs when the Chinese COVID-control methods no longer worked to stop the spread of Omicron. The Chinese government had to pivot when it realised that it had to.

Beyond conflict to cooperation

The Delta and Omicron variants provided two important signals for the world. First, new variants could indeed evade the protection of vaccines, and second, not only should social restrictions continue to some extent depending on circumstances—a particular tough message for Americans—but as long as people across the world remained unvaccinated, new strains of the virus would continue to develop, and the increased transmissibility and immune escape of the latest variants will mean that herd immunity through vaccination alone is likely impossible. Hence, there could be more ups and downs in infection rates until the pandemic truly receded.

Cooperation between China and the United States will help end COVID-19 and prepare for future pandemics. Over the decades, the two countries had in fact worked together positively. The two countries have many areas where cooperation would be helpful instead of finger-pointing at each other. Chapter 13 provides a record of their previous cooperation and makes observations about the areas in which they could cooperate.

---

55. Wang Xaioui, 'Experts: Dynamic Zero-COVID Policy Still Key', *China Daily*, Hong Kong edition, 14 October 2022.

10

Pandemic Control in China's Gated Communities

Hualing Fu*

Introduction

A key global strategy to contain the coronavirus disease 2019 known as COVID-19 has been the implementation of social distancing measures (SDMs), in particular Stay-at-Home (SaH) orders. Given the epidemiological consensus at the time that social distancing significantly reduces transmission and that the ability of a country to contain the spread of infections depends on the degree to which SaH orders and other SDMs are enforced and complied with, few countries, if any, have not imposed lockdowns of sorts to some degree, in particular a range of SaH orders, placing a significant part of their population, if not all, under quarantine for various durations.[1] To a large degree, the success or failure of these measures has depended on citizens' willingness to change their behaviours to comply with SaH orders.

The existing literature indicates a range of factors, both subjective and objective, to explain compliance. Subjective factors include substantive support for the measures, trust in the government, political values, and obligations to obey regulations, broadly defined to include the impact of deterrence and the sense of fairness.[2] Some studies show that civic and moral education, and the appeal to altruism or a sense of solidarity, have some short-term positive impact on compliance with SDMs; an invocation of a degree of fear is also found to have more explanatory power in motivating behaviour

---

*   The author would like to thank Calvin Ho, Eric Ip, Christine Loh, Shitong Qiao, and the reviewers for their insightful comments on the earlier version of this chapter and Chloe Tang and Kinson Cheung for their research assistance.

1.   Minah Park, Alex R. Cook, Jue Tao Lim, Yinxiaohe Sun, and Borame L. Dickens, 'A Systematic Review of COVID-19 Epidemiology Based on Current Evidence', *Journal of Clinical Medicine* 9, no. 4 (2020): 967; Stella Talic, Holly Wild, Ashika Maharaj, Zanfina Ademi, Wei Xu, Evropi Theodoratou, et al., 'Effectiveness of Public Health Measures in Reducing the Incidence of Covid-19, SARS-Cov-2 Transmission, and Covid-19 Mortality: Systematic Review Ad Meta-analysis', *BMJ* (2021): 375.
2.   Chris P. Reiders Folmer, Megan A. Brownlee, Adam D. Fine, Emmeke B. Kooistra, Malouke E. Kuiper, Elke H. Olthuis, et al., 'Social Distancing in America: Understanding Long-Term Adherence to Covid-19 Mitigation Recommendations', *PloS one* 16, no. 9 (2021), https://doi.org/10.1371/journal.pone.0257945.

change.[3] Others have pointed out that one's political views (Democrat or Republican in the American context) have some predictive power on whether or not one will adhere to SDMs.[4]

Compliance with SaH orders can hardly be achieved without coordinated action, effective enforcement, and adequate material and psychological support on the part of the government. In the United States, while people generally felt compelled to obey the law, supported the principle of social distancing, and were concerned with the consequences of non-compliance, 'only a minority of Americans indicate that they always follow social distancing measures'.[5] In Italy, public authorities struggled to deal with significant non-compliance with SaH rules.[6] Sheth and Wright reported significant violations of the SaH order in California, concluding that relying on risk aversion or altruism would not achieve compliance.[7] Even in Canada, where compliance was high across all provinces, there was still a substantial proportion of norm-breakers.[8]

In order to secure adequate compliance, objective factors also need to be factored in, including people's capacity to follow SaH orders, opportunities to violate the measures, costs and benefits of adherence, and social norms in terms of adherence, i.e., whether others around are also in compliance. A key factor is the practical capacity to adhere to SDMs—people do not follow rules that are hard, if not impossible, to follow. Effective implementation of SaH orders demands support for residents in isolation and monitoring to enforce the orders.

This chapter examines the unique role that grassroots residential social organisations in China have played in supporting and enforcing pandemic control measures. In explaining China's performance in containing the pandemic before the sudden reverse of the restrictive policy in November 2022 after a nationwide protest COVID restrictions,[9] commentators have attributed this to the Chinese Communist Party's

3. Craig A. Harper, Liam P. Satchell, Dean Fido, and Robert D. Latzman, 'Functional Fear Predicts Public Health Compliance in the COVID-19 Pandemic', *International Journal of Mental Health and Addiction* 19, no. 5 (2021): 1875–1888; Janice Y. C. Lau and Shui-Shan Lee, 'Legal Provisions for Enforcing Social Distancing to Guard against COVID-19: The Case of Hong Kong', *Journal of Law and the Biosciences* 8, no. 1 (2021): 1–14.

4. Marcus O. Painter and Tian Qiu, 'Political Beliefs affect Compliance with Government Mandates', *Journal of Economic Behavior and Organisation* 185 (2021): 688–701.

5. Reiders Folmer et al., 'Social Distancing in America'.

6. Briscese Guglielmo, Nicola Lacetera, Mario Macis, and Mirco Tonin, 'Compliance with COVID-19 Social-Distancing Measures in Italy: The Role of Expectations and Duration', National Bureau of Economic Research, IZA Discussion Papers no. 13092 (2020).

7. K. Sheth and G. C. Wright, 'The Usual Suspects: Does Risk Tolerance, Altruism, and Health Predict the Response to COVID-19?', *Review of Economics of the Household* 18 (2020): 1041–1052.

8. For the Canadian case, see Jean-Francois Daoust, Éric Bélanger, Ruth Dassonneville, Erick Lachapelle, and Richard Nadeau, 'Is the Unequal COVID–19 Burden in Canada Due to Unequal Levels of Citizen Discipline across Provinces?', *Canadian Public Policy* 48, no. 1 (2022): 124–143.

9. China had been successful in reaching its zero COVID-19 goal. For example, prior to the outbreak of the Omicron variant, 'China has reported only 0.05% of the total number of global cases despite making up 19% of the world's population'; Jin-Ling Tang and Kamran Abbasi, 'What Can the World Learn from China's Response to Covid-19?', *BMJ* 375 (2021), https://www.bmj.com/content/375/bmj.n2806. For reports on China's anti-COVID restrictions protests in November 2022, see, for example, Helen Davidson, 'Covid Restrictions Lifted on Guangzhou and Chongqing after China Protests', https://www.theguardian.com/world/2022/

decisive move to lock down cities at a high social and economic cost and to the capacity both to mobilise human and material resources to build hospitals to isolate those infected with the virus, and to send medics and support to the most infected cities to treat patients. Another feature that has characterised the Chinese strategy and is receiving increasing attention is the broad societal participation and the ability of residential communities to enforce SDMs and, in particular, SaH orders, enabling residents to respond to the pandemic and to comply with pandemic control measures with resources and confidence.[10] In what was dubbed by the Party as the people's war against the COVID-19 pandemic, Chinese urban communities showcased the effectiveness of the unique governance style in inducing compliance under certain political conditions. What makes Chinese urbanites more willing to participate in pandemic control enforcement and more compliant with SaH orders? And when will the willingness to comply and participate be withdrawn?

Emergencies and Authoritarian Advantage

Chinese urban communities are part of the overall political system and need to be situated in that larger political context.[11] China's political system, with its democratic centralism, coupled with its ability to shape public opinion and exert discipline and control, is well-equipped to manage novel crises.[12] Chinese commentators have

---

nov/30/us-and-canada-urge-china-not-to-harm-zero-covid-protesters-amid-calls-for-crackdown.

10. For a growing body of literature, see, for example, Qiulan Chen, Lance Rodewald, Shengjie Lai, and George F. Gao, 'Rapid and Sustained Containment of Covid-19 Is Achievable and Worthwhile: Implications for Pandemic Response', BMJ 375 (2021), https://www.bmj.com/content/bmj/375/BMJ-2021-066169.full.pdf; Jinghua Gao and Pengfei Zhang, 'China's Public Health Policies in Response to COVID-19: From an "Authoritarian" Perspective', Frontiers in Public Health, 15 December 2021, https://doi.org/10.3389/fpubh.2021.756677; Jue Jiang, 'A Question of Human Rights or Human Left?—The "People's War against COVID-19" under the "Gridded Management" System in China', Journal of Contemporary China 31 (2022): 491–504; Feng Xu and Qian Liu, 'China: Community Policing, High-Tech Surveillance, and Authoritarian Durability', in COVID-19 in Asia: Law and Policy Context, ed. Victor V. Ramraj (Oxford: Oxford University Press, 2021), 27–42; Xiaolin He, Ping Jiang, Qiong Wu, Xiaobin Lai, and Yan Liang, 'Governmental Inter-Sectoral Strategies to Prevent and Control COVID-19 in a Megacity: A Policy Brief from Shanghai, China', Frontiers in Public Health (2022), https://doi.org/10.3389/fpubh.2022.764847; and Guobin Yang, The Wuhan Lockdown (New York: Columbia University Press, 2022).

11. Article 21 of the PRC Constitution explicitly mentions these organisations ('neighbourhood organisations') in the context of public health. It states: 'To protect the people's health, the state shall develop medical and health care, develop modern medicine and traditional Chinese medicine, encourage and support the running of various medical and health facilities by rural collective economic organizations, state enterprises, public institutions and neighbourhood organizations, and promote public health activities.'

12. Jacques deLisle and Shen Kui, 'Lessons from China's Response to COVID-19: Shortcomings, Successes, and Prospects for Reform in China's Regulatory State' University of Pennsylvania Asian Law Review 16, no. 66 (2020): 66. Jonathan Schwartz, 'Compensating for the "Authoritarian Advantage" in Crisis Response: A Comparative Case Study of SARS Pandemic Responses in China and Taiwan', Journal of Chinese Political Science 17, no. 3 (2012): 313–331; and Victor C. Shih, 'China's Leninist Response to COVID-19: From Information Repression to Total Mobilization', in Coronavirus Politics: The Comparative Politics and Policy of COVID-19, ed. Scott C. Greer, Elizabeth J. King, Elize Massard da Fonseca, and Andre Peralta-Santos (Ann Arbor: University of Michigan Press, 2021).

confidently and, nearly universally, pointed to that systemic advantage over liberal democracies. As Gao and Zhang put it:

> Because collectivist societies are supposed to cooperate more for the benefit of the majority, individual interests need to be sacrificed when necessary. Democracies, on the other hand, advocate for individual freedom, and governments must implement policies within the limits of what is legally permissible. Such institutional constraints inevitably cause numerous inconveniences in responding swiftly to disasters and crises.[13]

Regime type seems to have mattered less in shaping states' initial responses during the crisis as the pandemic has created a global authoritarian movement that witnessed a sudden surge of executive power and steady weakening of democratic accountability.[14] The traditional liberal states have scrambled to impose some emergency measures suitable to their respective constitutional traditions and made a turn in their governance towards authoritarianism.[15] In managing the pandemic, the differences between democracies and statist/authoritarian states have diminished. As Fukuyama points out:

> In the end, I don't believe that we will be able to reach broad conclusions about whether dictatorships or democracies are better able to survive a pandemic. What matters in the end is not regime type, but whether citizens trust their leaders, and whether those leaders preside over a competent and effective state.[16]

Yet, as liberal democracies learn to act uncomfortably and often awkwardly in authoritarian ways, they encounter formidable political, legal, and social resistance.[17] The legislature may refuse to endorse pandemic control legislative initiatives or act to dilute the expansion of executive power that may be needed to implement effective control. Similarly, the judiciary, holding the executive legally accountable, may review and invalidate some of the executive excesses. More importantly, citizens, frustrated by continuous lockdowns and SaH orders, may rebel through non-compliance and open protest, as has been widely observed in democracies.[18]

---

13. Gao and Zhang, 'China's Public Health Policies in Response to COVID-19'.
14. Richard Horton, 'Offline: Is Democracy Good for Your Health?', *The Lancet* 398, no. 10316 (2021): 2060; David Gilbert, 'These 30 Regimes Are Using Coronavirus to Repress Their Citizens', *Vice*, 9 April 2020, https://www.vice.com/en_us/article/dygbxk/these-30-regimes-are-using-coronavirus-to-repress-their-citizens.
15. Stephen Thomas and Eric C. Ip, 'COVID-19 Emergency Measure and the Impending Authoritarian Pandemic', *Journal of Law and the Biosciences* 7, no. 1 (2020): 1–33.
16. Francis Fukuyama, 'The Thing That Determines a Country's Resistance to the Coronavirus', *The Atlantic*, 30 March 2020, https://www.theatlantic.com/ideas/archive/2020/03/thing-determines-how-well-countries-respond-coronavirus/609025; and Ilan Alon, Mathew Farrell, and Shaomin Li, 'Regime Type and COVID-19 Response', *FIIB Business Review* 9, no. 3 (2020): 152–160. For a general survey of state capacities, see Ramraj, *COVID-19 in Asia: Law and Policy Context*.
17. Sarah Engler, Palmo Brunner, Romane Loviat, Tarik Abou-Chadi, Lucas Leemann, and Andreas Glaser, 'Democracy in Times of the Pandemic: Explaining the Variation of COVID-19 Policies across European Democracies', *West European Politics* 44, no. 5–6 (2021): 1077–1102.
18. See, for example, Maciej Kowalewski, 'Street Protests in Times of COVID-19: Adjusting Tactics and Marching "as Usual"', *Social Movement Studies* 20, no. 6 (2021) 758–765; and T. Plümper, E. Neumayer, and K. G. Pfaff,

How to explain the different responses among different regimes to the pandemic control emergency measures? For liberal democracies in general, the gap between the normal and the exceptional was sharp, and the restrictions on rights and freedoms during the pandemic made real differences, both epistemologically and empirically. Under pandemic control measures, public gatherings were banned, rallies and processions were barred, and freedom of mobility was curtailed. These restrictive measures, which may be commonly accepted and even taken for granted under authoritarianism, may produce shocks, be met with resistance and are, in any event, hard to implement in democracies.

The Chinese political system is well-equipped to manage novel crises. The authoritarian advantage is referred to as democratic centralism, in which a constitutionally entrenched Communist Party monopolises political power to exercise 'absolute leadership'. There are no effective checks and balances, and the decision-making process is, in McCubbins' terms, 'decisive' or even 'tyrannical'.[19] Under democratic centralism, China's pandemic control efforts are defined as 'centralization, coercive intervention, and state paternalism'.[20] The decision to impose a total lockdown on first Wuhan, a city of over 11 million people, then Hubei, a province of 65 million people, and finally on most of the other provinces was a decisive moment in China's war against the virus,[21] a move that received initial disbelief, shock, and suspicion in the international community, but later became a standard preventive measure that was widely adopted.[22] The lockdown illustrated the decisiveness and swiftness of the system in sharp contrast with some of the democratic gridlocks that have been commonly observed. By the time Shanghai was totally locked down in 2022, what the Party-state is capable of achieving its policy objectives regardless of the costs was laid bare.[23] After all, this is the same Party that implemented the One Child Policy and other massive projects unprecedented in human history. Political systems with concentrated political power may be able to act decisively while others with more fragmented political powers—subjecting decisions to multiple veto points and excessive checks and balances—may succumb to gridlock and political paralysis in the process.[24]

'The Strategy of Protest against Covid-19 Containment Policies in Germany', *Social Science Quarterly* 102 (2021): 2236–2250.

19. Mathew D. McCubbins, 'Gridlock', in *The Encyclopedia of Democratic Thought*, ed. Barry Clarke and Joe Foweraker (Abingdon: Routledge, 2000), 325. See also Gary W. Cox and Mathew D. McCubbins, 'The Institutional Determinants of Economic Policy Outcomes', in *Presidents, Parliaments, and Policy*, ed. Stephan Haggard and Mathew D. McCubbins (Cambridge: Cambridge University Press, 2001), 21–63.

20. Gao and Zhang, 'China's Public Health Policies in Response to COVID-19'.

21. Eddie Yu, 'An Analysis of China's Strategy in Combating the Coronavirus Pandemic with the 3H Framework', *Public Administration and Policy: An Asia-Pacific Journal* 24, no. 1 (2021): 76–91.

22. Keith Bradsher, 'As China Fights the Coronavirus, Some Say It Has Gone Too Far', *New York Times*, 20 February 2020, https://www.nytimes.com/2020/02/20/business/economy/china-economy-quarantine.html.

23. See, for example, Bloomberg, 'China Lockdowns Cost at Least $46 Billion a Month, Academic Says', https://www.bloomberg.com/news/articles/2022-03-29/china-lockdowns-cost-at-least-46-billion-a-month-academic-says?leadSource=uverify%20wall.

24. McCubbins, 'Gridlock', and Alon, Farrell, and Li, 'Regime Type and COVID-19 Response'.

In addition, the Party-led system can mobilise national resources to launch a sustained political campaign, setting aside legal rules and marginalising legal institutions in accomplishing its goals,[25] leading to human rights abuses.[26] This whole national system, which has often been referred to when China demonstrates its ability to coordinate national resources to train athletes,[27] has a long history and goes far beyond sports. Facing a crisis or a challenging task of national significance with limited resources, the Party is razor-sharp in its focus. It can mobilise all available resources to achieve its goal. In the process, it does not tolerate doubts, distractions, or disobedience and is ready to silence and crush, if needed, any sign of resistance.[28] This type of multi-functional government with the power of total mobilisation is commonly regarded as a Chinese political advantage.[29] The capacity to mobilise resources, evidenced in the record-breaking speed in building specialised hospitals; manufacturing and supplying medical supplies, especially protective equipment, in large quantities; drafting 42,600 medical doctors and experts to affected areas at short notice;[30] and the seamless coordination, vertical and horizontal, of operations, is regarded as a strength that can barely be matched in any liberal democracy.[31]

The Chinese political and constitutional design demonstrates fewer differences between normal operations and crisis management. One may even argue that part of the Chinese system has already normalised and routinised exceptional or emergency measures, so it is ready to encounter crises with a high degree of preparedness. Examples abound. Political rules of the Party have de facto legal effect in normal times or during a crisis, as Article 1 of the Chinese Constitution declares that 'Leadership by the Communist Party of China is the defining feature of socialism with Chinese characteristics'. There are few if any veto points in the decision-making process; the Party controls the press and imposes censorship of news; it routinely punishes rumours through criminal law and police power; prohibits demonstration and protest at all times; the routine police monitoring and control of population movement and residence is a feature of China's urban management, and the mass surveillance does not spark significant privacy concerns from the society; and Chinese courts encourage and subtly enforce the settlement of disputes expediently through mediation. What is regarded as

---

25. Patricia M. Thornton, 'Of Constitutions, Campaigns and Commissions: A Century of Democratic Centralism under the CCP', *The China Quarterly* 248 (2021): 52–72.

26. Jue Jiang, 'A Question of Human Rights or Human Left? – The "People's War against COVID-19" under the "Gridded Management" System in China', *Journal of Contemporary China* 31, no. 136 (2022): 491–504.

27. Fan Wei, Fan Hong, and Lu Zhouxiang, 'Chinese State Sports Policy: Pre- and Post-Beijing 2008', *The International Journal of the History of Sport* 27, no. 14–15 (2010): 2380–2402.

28. Cox and McCubbins, 'The Institutional Determinants of Economic Policy Outcomes'.

29. '杀猫、封路、强制隔离，中国式抗疫是如何形成的？', *Initium Media*, 4 March 2020, https://theinitium.com/article/20200309-mainland-coronavirus-mergency-management/.

30. Hao Jin, Ligong Lu, Junwei Liu, and Min Cui, 'COVID-19 Emergencies around the Globe: China's Experience in Controlling COVID-19 and Lessons Learned', *International Journal for Quality in Health Care* 33, no. 1 (2021): 1–5; Yu, 'An Analysis of China's Strategy', see note 19.

31. He et al., 'Governmental Inter-Sectoral Strategies'; Jingjing Yan and Dahei Zhao, 'Administrative Mechanism of Joint Participation and Cooperation in the Early Stages of the COVID-19 Outbreak in Wuhan', *Risk Management and Healthcare Policy* 13 (2020): 723–731.

normalcy in China could be possible only under emergency measures elsewhere. Due to the lack of a clear distinction in the conceptual framework and institutional choices between normalcy and emergency, China can move into crisis management mode with far less resistance.

Authoritarian advantages notwithstanding, the political design and the power to mobilise *per se* cannot fully explain the Chinese ability to enforce the SaH order and SDMs. The world is not short of authoritarian leaders who can act decisively and expediently or political systems that do not admit any checks and balances or external accountability. States that are able to pull in national resources to achieve certain political goals or manage a crisis also abound. This is the 'despotic power', in Mann's terms, to assert control *over* society, which explains Chinese decisiveness and resourcefulness.[32] China's operation depended, however, on more than despotism and autocratic decision-making. When China launched a people's war against the pandemic, the battleground was shifted to residential communities at the grassroots level, and the despotic power had to penetrate the social fabric and become what Mann referred to as the 'infrastructural power' *through* society that is manifested through the routine.[33] The pre-crisis neighbourhood organisations, as they were mobilised by the Party-state to combat the pandemic, coupled with a high level of political trust in the government and the resulting voluntary compliance, proved to be the most crucial aspect of the Chinese ability to trace, monitor, and control, which in turn further legitimised, solidified, and reinforced the operating system.

Shequ, *Xiaoqu*, and Gated Communities

The Chinese residential community (*shequ*) is the place where SaH orders and other measures are enforced. It is the site where the Party-state displays its infrastructural power. A Chinese community is composed of three elements on a long spectrum that includes government offices, parastate and civil society organisations, and commercial firms, which together formed the backbone of the people's war against the pandemic.[34]

---

32. Michael Mann, 'The Autonomous Power of the State: Its Origins, Mechanisms and Results', *European Journal of Sociology/Archives européennes de sociologie* 25, no. 2 (1984): 185–213, 185; 'Infrastructural Power Revisited', *Studies in Comparative International Development* 43, no. 355 (2008), https://doi.org/10.1007/s12116-008-9027-7; and 'The Sources of Social Power Revisited: A Response to Criticism', in *An Anatomy of Power: The Social Theory of Michael Mann*, ed. John A. Hall and Ralph Schroeder (Cambridge: Cambridge University Press, 2005), 343–396.

33. Mann, 'Sources of Social Power Revisited'. For an application of Mann's conceptualisation of power on China, see Michael W. Dowdle, 'Infrastructural Power and Its Possibilities for the Constitutional Evolution of Authoritarian Political Systems: Lessons from China', in *Authoritarian Constitutionalism*, ed. Helena Alviar Garcia and Gunter Frankenberg (Cheltenham: Edward Elgar, 2019), 76–94.

34. Beibei Tang, 'Grid Governance in China's Urban Middle-Class Neighborhoods', *The China Quarterly* 241 (2020): 43–61. For studies of Chinese urban communities, see Martin King Whyte and William L. Parish, *Urban Life in Contemporary China* (Chicago: University of Chicago Press, 1984); Benjamin L. Read, *Roots of the State: Neighborhood Organisation and Social Networks in Beijing and Taipei* (Stanford, CA: Stanford University Press, 2012); and Luigi Tomba, *The Government Next Door: Neighborhood Politics in Urban China* (Ithaca, NY: Cornell University Press, 2014).

The government includes the Street Office (SO), the lowest level of Party-state power in urban China. Within the SO jurisdiction, there is a neighbourhood police station called a *paichusuo* (PCS) in charge of population management and public order. Under the SO, there is a parastate organisation called the Residential Committee (RC), a semi-autonomous organisation elected by and composed of local residents to manage neighbourhood affairs. Each RC is composed of a number of small communities (*xiaoqu*), often in the form of a gated community with walls to mark its boundaries and protect it from outsiders. The RC may set up a service station at a *xiaoqu* to maintain contact with residents in the jurisdiction. Under Chinese law, residents in a *xiaoqu* are entitled to form a homeowners' association (HoA) through an election among the homeowners. An HoA is a self-regulatory body formed to protect the rights and interests of homeowners. Each *xiaoqu* may engage a Property Management Company (PMC) to manage the residential buildings and provide services for the residents. A *shequ* is often a high-density ecosystem with complicated hierarchical and horizontal relations in which the Party-state, society, and market interact with each other to maximise their respective interests.

The *shequ* is a unique political design. At its core, as Read noted, is 'a dense network of standardized cells, with state-defined boundaries, covering all or virtually all of the urban geography'. The structure and designs are inherited from long historical practice and in significant ways, 'grow out of a more regimented vision of how society is to be ordered'.[35] Underlining this unique infrastructure is the Chinese *hukou* system, which registers persons by household and assigns each individual, at birth, to a community. The Party has upgraded the system into a panopticon to allow the state, through the neighbourhood police, to monitor and control the entire population.[36] The neighbourhood community exists first and foremost for government control over urban societies.

Significantly, control is extended through a parastate organisation, the RC, and a network of social groups, whose leaders, often endorsed, and from time to time chosen, by the residents, work for and with government officials on a wide range of matters concerning the community. Beyond extending government control to the fabric of the communities, the RC and the social groups also represent local interests in their interaction and bargaining with the local state. Policing, public health, and poverty alleviation are concerns of both the government and the community. The dialogical, 'socialised',[37] or 'associative'[38] process in which both contention and accommodation take place,[39] and through which the state integrates residents into state projects and residents make their claims, not only allows the state to calibrate its control but also solidifies and strengthens the social fabric. Through formal and informal links, the

35. Read, *Roots of the State*, 3.
36. Michael R. Dutton, *Policing and Punishment in China: From Patriarchy to 'the People'* (Cambridge: Cambridge University Press, 1992).
37. Sophia Woodman, 'Local Politics, Local Citizenship? Socialized Governance in Contemporary China', *The China Quarterly* 226 (2016): 342–362.
38. Read, *Roots of the State*, 4.
39. Tomba, *The Government Next Door*, 165.

community structure engenders dynamic state–society synchronisation and mutual support. Under this structure, citizens' 'belonging, participation and entitlement, and state obligation' all gravitate towards the residential communities, and the neighbourhood becomes the site of political action in China's urban governance.[40]

Shequ is a hodgepodge of organisations with different identities, interests, and priorities, which interact hierarchically and horizontally. The RC is legally an autonomous organisation, the PMC is a commercial entity serving the interests of residents who pay them, and the HoA jealously guards the interests of the Chinese middle classes. The SO is the lowest organ in the Party-state system and is staffed by low-ranking bureaucrats whose duties are to coordinate the bread-and-butter affairs of the urban communities. When the COVID-19 pandemic hit, the Party started to intervene directly in community management, connecting the SO, RC, PMC, and HoA into a network to form a defensible space against the virus.

Since the outbreak of COVID-19, local people's congresses and city governments in most provinces have enacted local legislation and rules to require *shequ* organisations, especially the PMC and HoA, to follow the leadership of the SO and RC and to take active steps to implement pandemic control measures, in particular in posting information flyers, disinfecting public areas, taking the temperature of visitors, monitoring residents who returned from other regions, enforcing social distancing rules, and so on, all contingent on evolving circumstances.[41] The *xiaoqu*—the little gated community—formed the basic unit in China's people's war on the pandemic; and China's massive SaH order was enforced under the leadership of the SO and RC, with the active participation of the PMC and *xiaoqu* residents, all supported and reinforced by the police in the PCS. Through this particular organisational structure, national pandemic control policies were announced and sent to residents, individuals were isolated, monitored and supported, and those who test positive were sent to designated places for quarantine. A well-led, resourceful, and well-organised community structure with disciplined participation is a necessity to make the SaH order practical and enforceable. However China's pandemic control strategy is perceived and assessed, the gated communities are an essential part of it.

The Street Office and the Residential Committee

Let us examine these community structures in more detail. The SO and the RC are the two key institutions in Chinese urban communities. The SO and the RC were institutionalised in Chinese cities in 1954 according to the particular social and political

---

40. Woodman, 'Local Politics', 343.
41. '广州市人大常委会表决通过《关于依法全力做好新冠肺炎疫情防控工作的决定》', The People's Government of Guangzhou Municipality, 12 February 2020, https://www.gz.gov.cn/xw/gzyw/content/post_5660731.html; '关于疫情防控期间进一步加强住宅小区物业管理的通知', Tieling Housing and Urban-Rural Development Bureau, 2 July 2020, http://60.18.233.39:8082/eportal/ui?pageId=115383&articleKey=895319&columnId=277495.

environment at the time. They played an important role in mobilising politically isolated social groups into a unified leadership, extending administrative control, and offering a more systematic way of political recruitment.[42] An SO is established as a sub-agency of a district or city government to take charge of an area referred to as an administrative street. To avoid any possible 'fragmentation of power', an SO was restricted to a minimum level in terms of resources and responsibilities.[43]

Despite the drastic social and economic changes that have taken place in Chinese cities, the role of the SO remains largely unchanged in that, as the most basic level of government, its principal function is to enhance the governance capacity at the basic level, framed as to work with stakeholders to build streets that are 'civilised', 'vibrant', 'convenient', and 'peaceful', with its work clearly identified as 'local', 'social', and 'mass-oriented'. In concrete terms, the SO should respond to complaints to the city government from local residents and address their concerns; in addition, SO officials should appear on the frontline in coordinating works and services from different government departments and solve whatever problems may arise in the locality.[44] The SO is front and centre in the Party's effort to build a responsive state.

The RC is a 'basic level' parastate organisation that was established directly by the Constitution and is governed by national law. The RC is designed as a 'self-management, self-education and self-service entity' and is tasked with community public affairs, such as policing, poverty alleviation, and dispute resolution. It also has a legal duty to promote the implementation of laws and policies, and to reflect the views and complaints of residents to the government. As a self-regulatory body, its members are elected either by all eligible residents and households, or by representatives from small groups within an RC. An RC receives supervision, guidance and, above all, financial support from the SO. It is commonly observed that members of an RC maintain 'affective connections' with officials and at the same time build 'personal relations' with residents in the community,[45] in which 'an active, proximate, and responsive state' is interacting and coping with 'disagreement, contentions, and resistance' from the communities.[46]

Property management companies and homeowners' associations

The traditional neighbourhood system has gone through a period of renewal with the privatisation and commodification of residential housing, forming the typical Chinese

42. Janet Salaff, 'The Urban Commune in Communist China', *The China Quarterly* 29 (1967): 82–110; 'Urban Residential Committees in the Wake of the Cultural Revolution', in *The City in Communist China*, ed. John Wilson Lewis (Redwood City, CA: Stanford University Press, 1971), 289.
43. Franz H. Schurmann, *Ideology and Organisation in Communist China* (Berkeley: University of California Press, 1968), 379.
44. 北京市人民代表大会常务委员会，'北京市街道办事处条例'，http://www.bjtzh.gov.cn/tzzfxxgk/c109720/202101/1332302.shtml.
45. Schurmann, *Ideology and Organisation*, 346; Read, *Roots of the State*, 4.
46. Read, *Roots of the State*, 4.

gated residential communities. With the rise of the Chinese middle class and the availability and popularity of privately owned condominiums, Chinese cities have witnessed a fundamental shift towards clear demarcation, assertion, and protection of property rights. With this broad background, PMCs emerged to manage residential communities in high-density, high-rise residential buildings.[47]

The PMC, as a commercial entity, operates on a contract basis with the residents in a community to offer management services on a fee-for-service basis. The PMC is well-resourced, commercially organised, and embedded in the community to offer routine services. It is a formidable player in China's urban community with a staggering influence on people's livelihoods. Take Hangzhou, for example, where over 700 PMCs manage over 4,000 *xiaoqu* and buildings in the city and where over 50,000 employees of those PMCs were on the frontline in enforcing SDMs. Another notable example is Vanke Property Development, a single company that has 2,663 residential projects and 639 business projects. Its more than 50,000 employees participated in the services of over 5 million households during the pandemic.[48]

Side-by-side with the PMC is another prominent organisation—the HoA, a companion entity that has grown together with the PMC. Both are products of China's bourgeoning residential housing market. As it happens, disputes over property rights and management issues abound, and the PMC, as a matter of routine, often gets into disputes with residents. The PMC is often controlled or owned by the developers that built the housing projects and occupies an advantageous position vis-à-vis the often disorganised residents. In response, aggrieved residents use the HoA platform to protect their rights in legal and political ways.[49]

Ownership of private property in urban condominiums creates a common identity and shared interest for the owners, who, united under a common cause, demand the protection of their legal rights, efficient management of their property, and good governance of the neighbourhood. The government clearly recognises property rights and has created procedures to form HoAs under the guidance of the SO and the RC, and with the limited participation of the developers. While the government grants the right to organise the HoA through a democratic process, a rare situation in the Chinese political system, and to seek legal and political protection of rights in a collective and organised manner, these rights are strictly limited to their implementation in the immediate neighbourhood.[50]

Riding on the tide of social management innovation, the government has become more interventionist in pre-empting disputes between the two entities. Clearer rules have been made, and the SO and RC are more proactive in establishing co-governance

47. Shitong Qiao, 'The Authoritarian Commons: Divergent Paths of Neighborhood Democratization in Three Chinese Megacities', *American Journal of Comparative Law* (forthcoming, 2023).

48. '新华社经济分析报告：强化物业管理构建社区疫情防控"安全线"', 19 February 2020, https://www.sohu.com/a/374168882_214444.

49. Ngai Ming Yip, Rongui Huang, and Xiaoyi Sun, 'Homeowners' Activism and the Rule of Law in Urban China', *China Journal of Social Work* 7, no. 2 (2014): 175–188.

50. Qiao, 'The Authoritarian Commons'.

involving all stakeholders and are more ready to take political action to root out net-working, public protests or other 'radical actions' on the part of some of the HoAs.[51] In the urban management setting, the HoA is regarded as a potential spoiler of the established arrangement, whereas the PMC and the developers behind them are able to build and maintain a close alliance with the government, which is interested in little more than maintaining stability.[52]

Beyond giving the SO and RC more resources and mandates to manage urban communities and, in particular, to improve relations between the PMC and HoA to maintain local stability, the other step that has been taken is the building of the Party at the community level and the invocation of Party mechanisms. While the RC does not have any legal or administrative authority over the PMC, just as the SO does not have any direct authority over the RC, the political mechanism of the Party serves as the golden thread to tie all the loose pieces together. While the local government, the PMC, and the HoA may have their unique interests and concerns, the political interest of the Party transcends all. Each autonomous unit has a Party cell, which can be used to exercise political leadership over Party members in the PMC and Party members in the whole community.[53]

When the pandemic broke out, the government immediately tapped into the resources and organisational capacity of PMCs in China and folded them into the pandemic control mechanisms. PMCs, being a permanent presence in the gated com-munity, had no choice but to participate. While accusations that PMCs may have shed their responsibilities from time to time, they worked hand-in-glove with the govern-ment and the residents and by and large performed extra, out-of-contract tasks at their own expense for pandemic control purposes. Indeed, they have been treated as if they were a government entity in performing a wide range of pandemic control responsibili-ties such as checking the identities and conditions of vehicles and individuals entering or leaving a community, disinfecting public places, enforcing SDMs, arranging food deliveries to households, and any other tasks that needed to be done. In order to rec-ognise PMCs' contributions, some well-off cities provided them with subsidies for the additional costs that PMCs may have incurred.[54]

The institution that is conspicuous by its absence from the entire pandemic control campaign is the HoA, which has gained much popularity in its fight for property rights since its inception. As many studies have shown, the government is hostile to the for-mation of any independent organisations, including HoAs, and has taken steps to limit

---

51. Ngai-ming Yip and Yihong Jiang, 'Homeowners United: The Attempt to Create Lateral Networks of Homeowners' Association in Urban China', *The Journal of Contemporary China* 20, no. 72 (2011): 735–750; Ying Xia and Bing Guan, 'The Politics of Citizenship Formation: Homeowners' Collective Action in Urban Beijing', *Chinese Journal of political Science* 19, no. 4 (2014): 405–419.
52. Qiao, 'The Authoritarian Commons'.
53. 钟发亮、刘磊: '城镇化进程中创新社区党建工作', 广州大学学报（社会科学版）（2018）（17: 10）: 66–73。
54. '新华社经济分析报告: 强化物业管理构建社区疫情防控"安全线"', 19 February 2020, https://www.sohu.com/a/374168882_214444.

their growth.[55] According to some statistics, about 20–30 per cent of eligible residential communities have created HoAs, and a very small percentage of the established HoAs (5–10%) operate actively. The difficulty of collective action has prevented them from expanding as the legislation allows.

Despite their high profile, HoAs have not been able to grow into a formidable force to reckon with and have played a marginal role, if any, as institutions in enforcing pandemic control rules in their own *xiaoqu*. In the best-case scenarios where an HoA has played an active role, it was its members who volunteered their services in their personal capacities, using their social and political capitals to serve their communities.[56] Two main reasons may explain the marginalisation of HoAs. First, pandemic control measures are regarded as a highly politicised activity, and SO and RC leaders are hands-on in directing and organising enforcement and coordinating support. The heavy presence of officials, including those civil servants or Party members who are seconded to the communities—to be discussed below—crowded the HoA out, except for its members' voluntary participation under government leadership. The democratic procedure in the decision-making of the HoA is such that participation in pandemic control work would require the authorisation of the Owners' Committee with the support of half of the owners of the units, which may have rendered it impossible for an HoA to use its resources to support the pandemic control work, given the isolation and social distancing requirements. The historical image of the HoA as a representative organ of homeowners standing against the PMC on economic matters and against the local government on political matters has not helped either.

The neighbourhood police

The neighbourhood police station, the PCS, is at the heart of the system in maintaining public order in general but has only played a supplementary role in pandemic control enforcement. Their presence is mainly to ensure compliance, take action when voluntary compliance and persuasion of community leaders have failed, and punish delinquents when required.[57]

The principal duty of the PCS is to maintain order within its jurisdiction, including maintaining and updating a population/household database, organising community crime control, monitoring suspicious populations, and carrying out other matters related to law and order within a defined territory. Policing in the neighbourhood is preventive, aiming to pre-empt potential disorder. In that sense, the police, through

---

55. Qiao, 'The Authoritarian Commons'.
56. One report from Shanghai, where the HoAs were better developed than those elsewhere and developed a cooperative relationship with the government, said the level of volunteerism of the HoA members reached 80 per cent (Qiao, 'The Authoritarian Commons').
57. Kai Lin, Shan Shen, Ivan Y. Sun, and Yuning Wu, 'Policing Pandemic in China: Investigating the Roles of Organizational Adjustment, Procedural Justice, and Police Trustworthiness on Public Compliance', *Police Practice and Research* (2022), https://doi.org/10.1080/15614263.2022.2127717.

their deep-rooted, proactive policing, make the community and the people visible and legible to the state, thus enhancing the state's capacity to know, monitor, and control.

Chinese police forces, compared to their Western counterparts, are small in size and have less visibility. One of the key features of the Chinese policing system is the embedding of policing and maintenance of order in the communities where the police serve. This mass-line policing, as it is known, promotes the concept of co-governance and shared responsibility, where the police receive public input and support while at the same time enhancing the self-policing capacity of the communities. The strength of the Chinese police lies in the development of a mode of policing by people who know the community and have routine interactions with residents on non-policing matters, rather than by strangers who remain at arm's length from the communities. It is both 'bottom up' and 'inside out',[58] making police work subtler, less confrontational, and often more effective.[59]

In China, some efforts have been made, especially in the 1980s, to create what was called dynamic policing—highly visible and quick to respond and adapt to the changing social and economic environment. With the arrival of migrant workers en masse in the mid-1990s and the increase in social mobility, traditional community control and policing styles were placed under great stress and, from time to time, were criticised for being too static and ill-equipped to control a dynamic society in great social and economic transition. Instead of embedding policing in community work to enhance self-policing capacity, police were asked to withdraw from the community and to launch swift and effective responses to crimes; instead of visiting households and chatting in the neighbourhood, police were forced to put their limited resources on the streets so as to become visible through routine patrols. There was a clear shift from maintaining order to enforcing the law and from preventive community work to rapid response to crime scenes and emergency calls. Doubts were even cast on the viability of the PCS as an institution, and suggestions were made to uproot the police from the community so as to professionalise the service. This was a paradigmatic shift in strategic thinking about policing, crime, and punishment in China.[60]

By the late 1990s and early 2000s, China was facing new challenges. While the periodic crackdowns on crime had achieved an impact in terms of incapacitating and deterrence, suppressing the crime rate to a comparatively low level, social conflict and protest had increased at speed and to a degree that exceeded the capacity of the existing institutions. Petitions to Party authorities and public protests were perceived to be spiralling out of control and posed a threat to the political order. Not surprisingly, the vast majority of conflicts came from local communities and could have been prevented, resolved, or otherwise stopped at the level where they arose in the first place. Institutions were required to go back to the basics to halt the further escalation of social

58. Kam C. Wong, *Police Reform in China* (Abingdon: Routledge, 2017).
59. Lena Y. Zhong, *Communities, Crime and Social Capital in Contemporary China* (Cullompton: Willan, 2009).
60. Fu Hualing, 'Patrol Police: A Recent Development in the People's Republic of China', *Police Studies* 13 (1990): 111.

conflict—courts were forced to settle cases through mediation so that matters would truly end when the case files closed, and police were ordered to go back to the communities where the root causes of China's social problems were located.

At that particular juncture, community policing (*shequ jingwu*) became fashionable and was systematically promoted within the police in partnership with other relevant authorities. Some coastal cities piloted it in the late 1990s, and by the early 2000s, community policing was rolled out nationwide.[61] A contentious issue was why China resorted to US policing for inspiration in developing community policing rather than reflecting on its own experiences from the not-so-distant past and whether there were any meaningful differences between the neighbourhood policing that the PCS had developed and the newly imported community police.[62] Nevertheless, the police did return to the communities, and when they did so, they encountered residential communities that had been transformed beyond recognition, with high-rise residential towers dotting the city landscape and where strangers of different social and economic backgrounds came together to rebuild their communities, now referred to as 'little communities'.

The new community police in China addressed the security concerns of the *xiaoqu*, and the resulting policing measures, in turn, reinforced the *xiaoqu* identity and a shared sense of community. The Ministry of Public Security, together with the Ministry of Civil Affairs, which has jurisdiction over community development, jointly issued instructions to establish community policing in China.[63]

Part of the reform was, in fact, to return to the old-style neighbourhood policing with which the Chinese police were familiar. Under community policing orders, local police are required to participate in the RC activities and coordinate the management of local affairs;[64] in particular, they are required to give guidance and offer supervision on community mediation, monitor the rehabilitation of offenders on probation, and carry out neighbourhood patrols.[65] The main thrust of the police reform, especially since 2003, has been to enhance local and community capacity and, within the police, to 'sink' the workforce and resources all the way down to support the PCS and reengage the community. A heavy presence of the police on the streets was no longer a priority; instead, the urgent work was to equip *shequ* organisations to develop their self-policing capacity, with the understanding and expectation that disputes mostly arose at a low level and should be solved, if not pre-empted, at this low level. Not directly related to the pandemic, the police in 2020 launched a nationwide campaign of one million

61. Yuning Wu, Shanhe Jiang, and Eric Lambert, 'Citizen Support for Community Policing in China', *Policing: An International Journal of Police Strategy & Management* 34, no. 2 (2011): 285–303.

62. Lena Y. Zhong, 'Community Policing in China: Old Wine in New Bottles', *Police Practice and Research: An International Journal* 10, no. 2 (2009): 157–169.

63. Wu et al., 'Citizen Support', 288.

64. Ibid., 288.

65. Steven F. Messner, Lening Zhang, Sheldon X. Zhang, and Colin P. Gruner, 'Neighborhood Crime Control in a Changing China: Tiao-Jie, Bang-Jiao, and Neighborhood Watches', *Journal of Research in Crime and Delinquency* 54, no. 4 (2017): 544–577.

police officers entering households,[66] in which the police were required proactively to engage communities to improve police–society relations.

There is a new element to modern community policing, which China learnt from US criminology. In maintaining order in the new neighbourhoods with a high population density in high-rise towers, the police encouraged the creation of a 'defensible space' to control crime and disorder through physical design.[67] The new design resulted in a gated community with restricted membership, limited access, and extensive monitoring. It is a community with a strong sense of insiders versus outsiders and one that treats outsiders as strangers with great suspicion, if not outright hostility. In its ideal form, retired residents are organised to serve as floor monitors, building monitors and block monitors. All the security measures are also maintained and reinforced by paid private security working closely with the PMCs, supported by the PCS and enhanced by surveillance technologies such as high-definition cameras and face-recognition tools. Thus, the small communities are all fortified against criminals or 'bad elements' in society. When COVID-19 broke out and the government demanded isolation, Chinese communities were immediately mobilised and prepared for it.

Grids and grid monitors

Perceiving a declining governance capacity at the grassroots level and the potential of technology-enhanced social management, the Party created a grid system in 2013 to upgrade and renew *shequ* management so as to entrench the stability (*weiwen*) of the mechanism that had been initiated a decade earlier.[68] The new grid system was mapped onto the existing *shequ* structure, injecting more resources into the communities and enhancing the monitoring capacity of the state.[69]

Under the grid system, each RC is further divided into several zones, or 'grids', clearly demarcated and identified, with specific allocations of responsibility. In a pilot district for grid reform in Beijing, for example, the 17 SOs and 205 RCs were further divided into 589 grids in 2010, and each was allocated a person living within the grid as a grid monitor. The grid system was finalised in Beijing in 2014, and by 2017, Beijing had been able to integrate urban administration, policing, and social services within the grid system. The grid was introduced as an urban governance reform and designed as a system of total control: where there is a community, there are grids; where there is a

---

66. Liu Yang, '全国公安机关深入开展"百万警进千万家"活动 热情服务群众 守护一方平安', *People's Daily*, 1 July 2021, http://www.gov.cn/xinwen/2021-01/07/content_5577609.htm.

67. Oscar Newman, *Creating Defensible Space* (Darby, PA: Diane Publishing, 1966).

68. Dali L. Yang, 'China's Troubled Quest for Order: Leadership, Organisation and Contradictions of the Stability Maintenance Regime', *Journal of Contemporary China* 26, no. 103 (2017): 35–53; and Jonathan Benney, 'Weiwen at the Grassroots: China's Stability Maintenance Apparatus as a Means of Conflict Resolution', *Journal of Contemporary China* 25, no. 99 (2016): 389–405.

69. Tang, 'Grid Governance in China's Urban Middle-Class Neighborhoods'; Jiang, 'A Question of Human Rights'.

grid, there is someone in charge; and when there is someone in charge, that person is held accountable—a visible return of a technology-enhanced *baojia* system.

The grid system serves two functions: one is to solidify control, and the other is to address specific concerns of residents and enhance services. Distinct from the traditional RC mechanisms that rely on face-to-face contact between community leaders and residents, the grid offers a digital platform that contains comprehensive personal and community data. Indeed, a key duty of a grid monitor is the responsibility to collect and update the data to facilitate control and service. The dataset would create a transparent *shequ*, exposing individuals and communities to the state. The creation of the digital grid would be transformative, shifting the control of the old style that is 'traditional, reactive, qualitative and diverse' to a new style that will be 'modern, proactive, quantitative and systematic'.[70] The grid is a sophisticated tool to maximise control by identifying events promptly, allocating responsibilities swiftly and offering solutions effectively. In essence, the grid governance system refocuses on pre-emptive control at the grassroots level. It aims to streamline and rationalise management responsibilities at different levels of government and to enhance multi-institutional coordination of police, social services, and other government departments—which had previously operated in isolation—into a single control network. The grid makes rapid and targeted actions possible.[71]

The second function is to improve public services and, in so doing, enhance government accountability. Once a request for service is made on the online platform, it triggers an upward information flow that demands swift and effective action from those with responsibility. The grid system, while not making the government's responsibilities transparent and comprehensible to residents, does create a mechanism to hold officials accountable to the rhetoric of the Party. At the heart of the system is the grid monitor, who feeds information to the government for action.

Each grid generally has one monitor, who may be assisted by a few other grid workers. They are supported by SO officials, RC members, and also by PCS police. The backgrounds of grid monitors vary. When the grid was created, local governments recruited a large number of full-time grid monitors to work in the communities. For example, in one district in Changde city, Hunan province, in 2014, the district government contracted a technology company to build a grid information platform for the district. It created 577 grids out of 92 *shequ*, with an average of 350 to 500 households per grid.[72] It then recruited over 500 grid monitors, who were said to be young and well-educated. There is a clear trend to professionalise grid monitors, as evidenced by the use of uniforms, recruitment of recent university graduates, and training before deployment. Grid monitors see themselves as the chiefs of staff of their respective grids, giving answers to residents and at the same time monitoring behaviour, entering data,

70. Tang, 'Grid Governance in China's Urban Middle-Class Neighborhoods'.
71. Ibid., 44.
72. http://theory.people.com.cn/n/2014/1127/c40531-26105462.html.

solving disputes, and reporting suspicious individuals to the police, all similar functions to those that RC members used to and continue to play.[73] Many grid workers are indeed recruited from residents in the grids working part-time or full-time.[74]

It is difficult to estimate how many grid workers there are in China. *Legal Daily* reported that four and a half million grid workers went into a 'state of war' in China after the COVID-19 outbreak.[75] Reports from the grassroots level are more informative. In one street in Luohu, Shenzhen, there are 81 grids, covering a total of 100,000 people. Another community with 15,000 people is divided into nine grids with six grid monitors.[76]

Grid monitors, like other community leaders and volunteers, play an indispensable role in the pandemic control operation. They serve multiple functions. First, they are the police within the gated community, checking and verifying the movement of residents, and especially isolating those who have returned from high-risk areas, persuading and forcing residents to comply with social distancing rules, stopping outsiders from entering their communities, deciding who can leave the community and for how long, and from time to time physically restraining or even assaulting residents who are trying to sneak out. Grid monitors and other gird workers may not be government officials, but they enjoy government powers.

Second, they serve as social workers and medics. They provide public health information and remind residents to take preventive measures; they answer questions from residents, offer comfort and therapies as best as they can, and in any event, maintain near-constant communications; they facilitate COVID-19 testing as the government requires; liaise with hospitals and quarantine facilities on behalf of residents who need quarantine at designated places; and they persuade senior citizens to get vaccinated.[77] Finally, they are service providers for residents under the SaH order, doing the tedious work of receiving food and other daily necessities ordered by residents and organising and coordinating deliveries and pick-ups.

'Sinking' and volunteering

The Party did not leave the *shequ* alone, of course, to enforce the SaH order. Effective enforcement of the regulations on the Chinese scale requires direct state support and also state supervision. China's President Xi Jinping called on 10 February 2020 for the construction of a people's frontline and demanded government officials and

73. Sa Ze，'那个掌管小区综合治理"神经末梢"的人', *China Digital Times*, 24 July 2021, https://chinadigital-times.net/chinese/668681.html.
74. '有一种力量，叫"中国网格员"', *China Digital Times*, 3 October 2021, https://chinadigitaltimes.net/chinese/663429.html.
75. Liu Ziyang, '450万网格员筑牢疫情社区防控"第一道防线"', *Xinhua*, 10 March 2020, http://www.xinhua-net.com/legal/2020-03/10/c_1210507945.htm.
76. Sa Ze，'那个掌管小区综合治理"神经末梢"的人'.
77. Wu Lumu，'重庆渝北：网格化管理"十到位"筑牢防疫 最后一公里', *China Economic Net*, 7 February 2020, http://www.ce.cn/xwzx/gnsz/gdxw/202002/07/t20200207_34231032.shtml.

Party members 'sink' (*xiaochen*) to the *shequ* during the lockdown.[78] In Wuhan, by 27 February 2020, close to half a million civil servants, employees in public institutes, and Party members were sent to communities to enforce the lockdown.[79] When Xi'an imposed its lockdown in late 2021, it sent 64,000 cadres to monitor and serve the 13 million people in the city.[80] There was a certain specificity as to who went where and a degree of stability in the temporary assignments. In a Wuhan example, eight Party members from a District Bureau of Justice, divided into two groups, were sent to assist the 9th and 10th grids of a community with a total of 760 households.[81] But there was no clear division of labour among these cadres, which led to complaints from those who had to perform whatever tasks were presented to them, including getting to know the communities by memorising the names and addresses of the residents, helping to check and verify the travel histories of residents, taking temperatures, or simply purchasing and delivering goods for residents.

The 'sinking' process is decisive, and even war-like and military in style. Mobilising cadres and marching them to specific grids requires rigid organisation and careful coordination. Life as a 'sinking' official was tough and risky, but working on the frontlines was a political mission of the highest order and a test of one's political loyalty. In addition to civil servants assigned by administrative decisions, the Party has also mobilised its members in other public sectors to serve in the *xiaoqu*. For example, school teachers are not civil servants and are not normally required to work at *xiaoqu* even if they are available. But teachers who are Party members were still called upon, as Party members, to 'volunteer' at a *xiaoqu*. Like civil servants, these Party members were assigned to a specific *xiaoqu* to join the pandemic control teams. The sheer size of the population under SaH orders necessitates societal support beyond those in the public sectors, and there were isolated calls by city governments for non-government organisations (NGOs) to also participate in serving the communities. When a new wave of the pandemic hit Xi'an at the end of 2021, the provincial government made an uncharacteristic appeal to social organisations, largely those under government control, requesting them to reach out to their members to support the pandemic control work.[82] In general, the NGO sector did not play any visible role during the pandemic, due both to the crackdown on NGOs in China since 2013 and the demand for social distancing,

78. Zhang Xiaosong, '习近平：干部重心下移，支援社区疫情防控', *Xinhua*, 10 February 2020, http://www.xinhuanet.com/politics/leaders/2020-02/10/c_1125556265.htm.

79. Cheng Rongxing Wang Chenglong, Li Yuan, Huang Lei, and Wu Chunxinxin, '武汉4.45万党员干部下沉防控一线', The People's Government of Hubei Province, 28 February 2020, http://www.hubei.gov.cn/hbfb/szsm/202002/t20200228_2161484.shtml.

80. He Bin, '西安疫情之下，社会组织都去哪里了？', 中国慈善家杂志, 5 January 2022, https://mp.weixin.qq.com/s/PnDMdX6flK6h99ynTDZ_Tw.

81. He Xin, '武汉1.7万余党员干部下沉社区大排查 确保应收尽收', *China Economic Net*, 11 February 2020, http://www.ce.cn/xwzx/gnsz/gdxw/202002/11/t20200211_34245935.shtml.

82. Yang Xiaoling, '陕西社会组织"合力抗疫"', The People's Government of Shaanxi Province, 31 December 2021, http://www.shaanxi.gov.cn/xw/ldx/bm/202112/t20211231_2206111_wap.html; 陕西省养生协会全媒体中心, '合力抗疫——陕西社会组织联合行动', 2 January 2022, https://www.sohu.com/a/513899176_255588.

although the spirit of volunteerism and charitable donations have continued and are highly visible in Chinese cities.[83] Through WeChat groups, volunteers in Guangzhou were assigned to RCs and, after some brief training, helped out at the many COVID-19 test centres.[84] Services that volunteers provided included looking after pets while their owners were placed under non-residential quarantine;[85] assisting with COVID-19 testing; providing online psychological therapy; or receiving calls from residents, registering their requests, and passing them on to *xiaoqu* leaders for further action.[86]

Making SaH Orders Work

The pandemic control work, particularly the enforcement of SaH orders at the micro-level in *shequ* and *xiaoqu*, requires a supporting macro environment to succeed. This includes a high degree of political trust, positive and consistent messaging, and effective legal enforcement. The disciplined participation of residents in and their support of SaH orders are often conditioned on the existence of a positive environment. Support would diminish or even evaporate if the larger environment changes when the government no longer has the trust of citizens.

Political trust

The relationship between social/political trust and levels of compliance with SaH orders and other SDMs is a contentious one. Some studies find positive correlations between trust and compliance. Thus, trust in decision-makers predicts higher levels of compliance with lockdown rules, with people in high-trust regions reducing their mobility significantly more than those in low-trust regions.[87] Others find a weak link. Mehari's study finds that people in traditionally high-trust countries behave more individualistically in defiance of SaH orders and, on the contrary, countries with low trust levels outperform their high-trust counterparts in following SaH orders—the fear of the virus and the mistrust of authorities may have forced people in low-trust countries to reach the conclusion that staying at home is the safest option.[88]

83. Ming Hu and Mark Sidel, 'Civil Society and COVID in China: Responses in an Authoritarian Society', *Nonprofit and Voluntary Sector Quarterly* 49, no. 6 (2020): 1173–1181.
84. '深度观察：广州社区防疫一线背后的志愿者力量', *Southern Metropolis Daily*, 4 June 2021, https://xw.qq.com/partner/vivoscreen/20210604A0B0XO00.
85. Yang, *Wuhan Lockdown*.
86. Some of the requests were urgent. One household reported that it has nothing left to eat except some sugar and another requested medicines for an elderly person who had recently gone through an operation. 张依依 (Zhang Yiyi), '封城七日：一位通化志愿者的迷与忙', *China Digital Times*, 25 January 2021, https://chinadigitaltimes.net/chinese/661993.html.
87. Olivier Bargain and Ulugbek Aminjonov, 'Trust and Compliance to Public Health Policies in Times of COVID-19', *Journal of Public Economics* 192 (2020), https://doi.org/10.1016/j.jpubeco.2020.104316.
88. Yeabsira Mehari, 'The Role of Social Trust in Citizen Mobility During COVID-19', SSRN 3607668, 20 May 2020, https://dx.doi.org/10.2139/ssrn.3607668.

Trust is an anomalous issue in China. While China is a low-trust society in terms of interpersonal relations due to the prevailing familism,[89] political trust is high, and the Chinese population, in general, has shown a high level of trust in institutions. However, the trust is hierarchical, and, in China's vertically fragmented state, people place their trust predominantly in the central government rather than local government.[90] As the pandemic control narrative and rules, like other rules, come down from the central to the grassroots level for enforcement, the level of trust in government diminishes. The Chinese pandemic control experiences both reflect and reinforce Chinese political trust, though the lockdown in Shanghai and sustained restrictions in the subsequent months when the rest of the world endeavoured to resume normalcy may have caused a fresh challenge to the long-held political trust in China, leading to nationwide protests against government policies.[91]

How is trust in government built and sustained? Facing a significant pandemic, the central government put its heart, head, and hands to work in designing the people's war and reiterated the priority of people's safety, health, and welfare.[92] This purposive mission, crystalised in a clear, positive, and confident tone, promoted solidarity and builds confidence.[93] At the city level, the people's war was multi-dimensional, combining paternalistic admonition with patient education, effective services, and punishment. There was close surveillance, but community surveillance was mostly embedded in and carried out through an interactive and dialogical process within the communities between sent-down officials, community leaders, volunteers, and residents. Residents under SaH orders were not mere recipients of a repressive system imprisoned in their homes just out of fear. They were active parties to a containment strategy that they shared and have confidence in. Despite the initial failures, dismal in some aspects, the Wuhan lockdown showcased the faith that people had in the Party and their resilience to carry SaH orders through regardless of their pains, sufferings, and grievances.[94]

---

89. Francis Fukuyama, *Trust: The Social Virtues and the Creation of Prosperity* (New York: Free Press, 1996), 87. For the development of the concept of amoral familism, see Michel Huysseune, 'Theory Travelling through Time and Space: The Reception of the Concept of Amoral Familism', *International Journal of Politics, Culture, and Society* 33 (2020): 365–388; and Robert D. Putnam, *Making Democracy Work: Civic Tradition in Modern Italy* (Princeton: Princeton University Press, 1993).

90. Gary Wu and Rima Wilkes, 'Local-National Political Trust Patterns: Why China Is an Exception', *International Political Science Review* 39, no. 4 (2018): 436–454; Lianjiang Li, 'Political Trust in Rural China', *Modern China* 230 (2004): 228–258. For a revised and more nuanced view, see Lianjiang Li, 'Reassessing Trust in the Central Government: Evidence from Five National Surveys', *The China Quarterly* 225 (2016): 100–121. For a study on the relationship between political trust and effective enforcement of pandemic control measures, see Chen Min, Fei Shen, Wenting Yu, and Yajie Chu, 'The Relationship between Government Trust and Preventive Behaviors during the COVID-19 Pandemic in China: Exploring the Roles of Knowledge and Negative Emotion', *Preventive Medicine* 141 (2020), https://doi.org/10.1016/j.ypmed.2020.106288.

91. Adam Minter, 'Lockdown Anger in Shanghai Won't Fade Anytime Soon', *Bloomberg*, 12 April 2022, https://www.bloomberg.com/opinion/articles/2022-04-12/shanghai-s-lockdown-anger-won-t-fade-anytime-soon.

92. Yu, 'An Analysis of China's Strategy'.

93. 'COVID-19 and China: Lessons and the Way Forward', editorial, *The Lancet* 396, no. 10246 (2020): 213.

94. Yang, *Wuhan Lockdown*, 79.

There were constant communications between the residents and community leaders through which concerns and anxieties were expressed, grievances aired, and suggestions made, all part of the semi-regulatory process of a close-knit community. Residents and the *shequ* leaders live together throughout the lockdown, sharing the same anxiety, fear, confidence and hope.[95] As the lockdown diaries have powerfully shown, residents followed and enforced all the pandemic control measures to protect their homes and their loved ones, and they cooperated 'out of a sense of civic responsibilities'.[96] Through the technologies-enhanced communicative process in crisis management, the communities became more transparent to the government, and their grievances, claims, and contentions became clear and better known. As a result, government controls and services became more tailor-made, subtle, and responsive. In an organic way, the grid system, which effectively embeds government control in service provisions and merges state surveillance of communities with residents' participation in neighbourhood affairs, offers a platform that has performed multiple and often conflicting functions in the grass-roots urban management. The grid is perhaps the most unique, effective, and significant instrument in the Party's toolkit of order maintenance.[97]

Standard and positive messaging

It requires more than adequate food and other daily necessities to maximise compliance and to make the lengthy and harsh SaH orders sustainable. Consistent with best practices in public health, the ability of a government to communicate with residents using clear and consistent messaging is indispensable to the effective enforcement of SDMs.[98] Indeed, a standardised and reassuring message was a Chinese strength unmatched by other countries, as the government was able to shape the tone of official and social media, with government officials, epidemiologists, reporters, and other stakeholders all speaking with one voice to the public.[99] President Xi himself reiterated the importance of strengthening Party propaganda to reinforce the guidance of public opinion in crisis management.[100] Clear messages about the infectious nature of the virus could create fear, which might then reduce risky behaviours, while guidance for citizens would reduce anxieties and build confidence at moments of panic, ensuring the smooth implementation of SDMs.[101] Local media, new and traditional, offered a psychological

---

95. Ibid.
96. Ibid., 220.
97. Tang, 'Grid Governance in China's Urban Middle-Class Neighborhoods'.
98. Arjen Boin, Allan McConnell, and Paul 't Hart, *Governing after Crisis: The Politics of Investigation, Accountability and Learning* (Cambridge: Cambridge University Press, 2008).
99. Schwartz, 'Compensating for the "Authoritarian Advantage"'.
100. Melanie Hart and Jordan Link, 'Chinese President Xi Jinping's Philosophy on Risk Management', Center for American Progress, 20 February 2020, https://www.americanprogress.org/article/chinese-president-xi-jinpings-philosophy-risk-management.
101. On how rumours caused panic in the society and reduced the effectiveness of the pandemic response in Taiwan in 2003, see Schwartz, 'Compensating for the "Authoritarian Advantage"'.

safe house for residents by providing guidance and health education of various kinds by experts and regular briefings on recent developments.[102] For the messages to be effective, they have to be convincing and credible in the eyes of their recipients.

Standardised messaging requires censorship, and the Chinese government has achieved this with rigour. It effectively silenced any alternative reporting, curbed public discussion and, in particular, punished rumour-mongering. Chinese law is well-equipped to subject anyone who spreads 'rumours' relating to the pandemic to police sanctions and criminal punishment, and police have been aggressive in placing those who spread rumours in police detention. In Beijing, for example, the police imposed the penalty of administrative detention, which could last for up to 15 days under Chinese law, on 610 individuals for violating pandemic control measures, and among them, 97 were for making or spreading pandemic-related rumours.[103]

In the meantime, government propaganda had been in full force to admonish residents not to generate, spread or believe in rumours, a message accompanied by regular clarification of facts and policies relating to the pandemic. This combination of proactive propaganda and education on the one hand, and rigorous censorship and police punishment on the other allowed the government to generate a single narrative, convincing people that whatever measures had been taken were absolutely necessary for public safety and beneficial to individual interests. Whether the official narrative could be effective and persuasive was largely contingent on the evolving threat that COVID-19 poses and China's relative international standing in pandemic control. The Shanghai lockdown seemed to have created a remarkable decline in the narrative power of the government as people demanded to follow the prevailing international practices to resume normal life in spite of pandemic risks.

Rigid enforcement

The rigidity in the enforcement of SaH orders was staggering, often leading to human tragedies commonly regarded as preventable by exercising discretion. The political goal to contain COVID-19 and the assignment of designated officials to specific *xiaoqu* generated tremendous pressure on local government and community leaders, in particular sent-down cadres, to enforce SaH orders with little concern for costs, consequences, or responsibilities. As it happened, officials who were held responsible for even a tiny COVID-19 breakout by international standards were punished harshly and swiftly, often with immediate removal from leadership positions if not criminal prosecution, sending a sharp message that the responsibility to contain the pandemic was absolute

---

102. Ni Zhang, Tianqin Shi, Heng Zhong, and Yijia Guo, 'COVID-19 Prevention and Control Public Health Strategies in Shanghai, China', *Journal of Public Health Management and Practice* 26, no. 4 (2020): 334–344, https://doi.org/10.1097/PHH.0000000000001202.

103. '2020年疫情防控以来查处扰乱正常防疫秩序类案件785起行政拘留513人', The People's Government of Beijing Municipality, 15 January 2021, http://www.beijing.gov.cn/ywdt/zwzt/yqfk/zxxx/202101/t20210115_2220826.html.

and that negligence would not be tolerated. The flip side was equally true that no major officials had been held liable for taking harsh and excessive measures to prevent the spread of the virus.

Given the zero-COVID-oriented incentives, it would not be surprising that there was a great deal of local variation with leaders racing to the bottom in competing to design and enforce the toughest measures to prevent a pandemic breakout or even a single positive case.[104] Thus, while rules made at the central or provincial levels may balance effectiveness, fairness, and humanity, when the same rules were enforced at lower levels, fairness and humanitarian concerns were watered down, and more restrictions and additional controls would be added. This may be repeated at every stage in the process, and when the rules were enforced at the grassroots level, excessiveness and distortion became abundant. Those manning the gates literally decided who was allowed to leave the compound, who was prohibited from entering, how one should behave in the community, and what infractions of rules warranted police intervention. Under the enabling Contagious Disease Control Law, often broadly interpreted and rigorously enforced, any lack of compliance with a SaH order or SDMs had the potential to be regarded as a violation of the law and thus subjected to police and criminal law sanctions.

New technologies, in particular the use of health codes, have enhanced China's capacity to monitor the travel and medical history of residents, track suspect cases for quarantine, and regulate social mobility in vulnerable times.[105] There is also the need to collect near-total information about citizens to make a sound assessment of public health risks and countries with different political systems have also used contact-tracing technologies to enforce pre-emptive and restrictive measures against the pandemic.[106] The Chinese government, working with tech giants, developed a monitoring design that can be easily and effectively used to determine whether a resident is entitled to leave their apartment and the degree of personal freedom that they can enjoy in public spaces. The deployment of the smartphone-based health code, coupled with the use of a massive surveillance system and AI-enhanced analytics, makes the Chinese *xiaoqu* the most closely monitored place in the world, 'rendering citizens to a state of permanent visibility'.[107]

There are few legal or political constraints on mass surveillance, and government surveillance and monitoring of individuals are taken for granted and commonly accepted if not welcomed. Personal data, in China's collective society, does not enjoy the same level of appreciation and protection as has been the case in liberal counterparts,

---

104. For an analysis of the distortion caused by target-oriented policy implementation, see Dali L. Yang, 'China's Illegal Regulatory State in Comparative Perspective', *Chinese Political Science Review* 2 (2017): 114–133.
105. Aditya Chaturvedi, 'The China Way: Use of Technology to Combat Covid-19', *Geospatial World*, 5 November 2020, https://www.geospatialworld.net/article/the-sino-approach-use-of-technology-to-combat-covid-19.
106. Fan Liang, 'COVID-19 and Health Code: How Digital Platforms Tackle the Pandemic in China', *Social Media + Society* 6, no. 3 (2020): 2.
107. Ibid., 3.

allowing the government to monitor citizens, gather their information, and develop a data-driven pandemic control strategy without giving much consideration to privacy.[108]

At the same time, the state has aggressively prosecuted and otherwise punished residents who may have violated social distancing rules. In 2020, there were 5,474 pandemic-related criminal trials in China,[109] and the number rose to 9,653 in 2021, a 76 per cent increase.[110] However, the number of prosecutions that were instituted by the procuratorate in pandemic-related cases witnessed a 63.7 per cent decline from 11,234 in 2020[111] to 4,078 in 2021,[112] indicating a likely decline in convictions in 2022.

The number of police punishments far exceeded that of criminal prosecutions. For example, the numbers of criminal detentions (which may lead to prosecution) and those of administrative detention were: 88 and 3,458 respectively in Heilongjiang between January and March 2020;[113] 74 and 1,910 in Inner Mongolia between January and February 2020;[114] 261 and 278 in Hunan between January and April 2020; 521 and 2,942 in Henan between January and March 2020.[115]

Conclusion

China's earlier success in containing COVID-19 relied on its ability to mobilise the entire society to participate in the people's war against the pandemic,[116] particularly in organising residents, through persuasion and discipline, into compliance. The social structure in place prior to the outbreak involves multiple government departments, commercial firms, and civil society organisations, combining state guidance and community volunteerism in developing co-governance at the grassroots urban level. That structure, energised by the strong will of the Party, has proved indispensable to China's containment strategies.[117] The same *shequ* system was used in the past to enforce the One Child Policy, root out 'evil cults' like Falun Gong, and keep suspicious outsiders at

---

108. Ibid.
109. '（两会受权发布）最高人民法院工作报告', *Xinhua*, 15 March 2021, http://www.xinhuanet.com/politics/2021lh/2021-03/15/c_1127212486.htm.
110. '最高人民法院工作报告', The Supreme People's Court of the People's Republic of China, 8 March 2022, https://www.court.gov.cn/zixun-xiangqing-349601.html.
111. '（两会受权发布）最高人民法院工作报告', *Xinhua*, 15 March 2021, http://www.xinhuanet.com/politics/2021lh/2021-03/15/c_1127212486.htm.
112. Ibid.
113. '黑龙江省公安机关办理4825起涉疫违法犯罪案件', *Baidu*, 15 March 2020, https://baijiahao.baidu.com/s?id=1661228712202321617&wfr=spider&for=pc.
114. '内蒙古快侦快破涉疫案件2078起', *Baidu*, 21 February 2020, https://baijiahao.baidu.com/s?id=1659127177068731591&wfr=spider&for=pc.
115. Li Guigang, '河南加强境外输入性疫情防控 查处6757宗涉疫犯罪案', *Eastday*, 12 March 2020, http://news.eastday.com/eastday/13news/auto/news/society/20200312/u7ai9153153.html.
116. '社区、社会工作、社会组织参与疫情防控专家谈（清华大学李强教授、南开大学关信平教授、上海交通大学徐家良教授）', 20 December 2021, https://www.163.com/dy/article/G39VSBKR0523N11P.html.
117. '社会力量在社区防疫中的作用和难题（中国社会科学院社会学研究所研究员、社会政策研究中心顾问杨团）', 1 April 2020, https://ishare.ifeng.com/c/s/v002PNvo9-_YcmquDjEqn9UmMDV49S0ulodYR-_ceabFN1dxw___.

a distance. City lockdowns and efficient hospitalisation are strategies that can be replicated in different societies, but the Chinese way of community organising and participation, based on the unique Chinese urban governance design and social ecosystem, as demonstrated in this chapter, is hard to transplant.[118]

Politics is also local in China, and it is at the basic level of SOs and RCs that millions of Chinese residents participate in national politics. Through socialised governance within their own gated communities, they interact with government departments, air their grievances, and settle their daily disputes. Life in the gated communities is rich, thick, and largely autonomous, forming what Yang refers to as the 'moral communities', the constant gaze of the state notwithstanding.[119]

Be they elderly residents, retired cadres, or the newly recruited grid monitors, all are simultaneously agents of the government and representatives of the communities, continuing to serve as a transmission belt to connect the Party with society. For the Party, these local agents make the numerous gated communities that dot Chinese cities observable, comprehensible and manageable. For citizens, their representatives provide easier access to power to have their personal and community concerns heard and maybe even addressed. The government, with all its power and resources, is too important to hide from and definitely not to be pushed away. Through the platform of the parastate, now actively organised by grid monitors, local welfare is promoted, and local problems are addressed, but more importantly, promoted and addressed with the participation and input of the local communities themselves.

China's pandemic control measures and the SaH orders take place within neighbourhood structures. Community mobilisation forms the core of the Chinese pandemic containment strategy and has proven to be the most crucial aspect of China's strategy to date. Even the experiences in Shanghai's lockdown in 2022, when the *shequ* system was stretched to a breaking point, proved, in a negative way, that there was no alternative to the existing urban design, calling for further solidification, reinforcement, and legitimisation of the existing social and political system of the Chinese neighbourhood in the post-crisis era. In coming out of the crisis, *shequ* governance, with all its innovation and upgrading, will remain a public-private partnership under the renewed leadership of the Party at the grassroots level.

---

118. '社会力量在社区防疫中的作用和难题（中国社会科学院社会学研究所研究员、社会政策研究中心顾问杨团）', 1 April 2020, https://ishare.ifeng.com/c/s/7vJmslTYe1N.
119. Yang, *Wuhan Lockdown*, 221.

11

The Hong Kong and Greater China Response to COVID-19

Richard Cullen

This chapter examines how the Hong Kong Special Administrative Region (HKSAR) developed and managed its response to the COVID-19 pandemic starting in early 2020.[1] This review includes a comparative discussion of COVID-19 responses in other jurisdictions in Greater China and Singapore.[2]

In June 2020, the International Monetary Fund said that the COVID-19 pandemic had generated 'a crisis like no other'.[3] The investigative approach in this chapter relies on an event-based evaluation of how this crisis unfolded in the HKSAR. The aim is to form an understanding of certain key elements that shaped what happened and to use this to discuss serious ongoing challenges and future pandemic-related choices.

The concept of the social contract,[4] discussed more fully in Chapter 6, is used below to help inform how particular approaches to dealing with the COVID-19 pandemic have evolved, especially in East Asia. The US political sociologist Barrington Moore advanced a version of 'class analysis' that argues that certain societal structures influence the primary protocols of a given social contract. Briefly, this argument holds

---

1. On 11 February 2020, the World Health Organization (WHO) announced that 'COVID-19' was the new official name for the disease caused by the deadly, novel coronavirus first identified in China in late December 2019; see 'WHO Says *COVID-19* Official Name of Coronavirus', *RTHK*, 12 February 2020, https://news.rthk.hk/rthk/en/component/k2/1508015-20200212.htm.

2. Greater China comprises mainland China (referred to as the mainland in the text), the HKSAR, the Macao SAR, and Taiwan.

3. International Monetary Fund (IMF), 'World Economic Outlook Update: A Crisis Like No Other, an Uncertain Recovery', June 2020, https://www.imf.org/en/Publications/WEO/Issues/2020/06/24/WEOUpdateJune2020.

4. The term 'social contract' dates back to the work of the English philosopher Thomas Hobbes (1588–1679) and was made explicit by Jean-Jacques Rousseau (1712–1778), who describes 'the desirable and usually mutually accepted forms of interaction among individuals and groups in their social environment. Modern political philosophers give the term a particular meaning: an unwritten agreement regarding rights and responsibilities between a state and its citizens'; *Oxford Reference*, 'Social Contract', accessed 15 September 2022, https://www.oxfordreference.com/view/10.1093/oi/authority.20110803100515301#:~:text=A%20term%20dating%20to%20the,groups%20in%20their%20social%20environment.

that operational political regimes are shaped by the social class structure of a given jurisdiction.[5]

One feature that emerges from the following discussion is how decision-making during the pandemic in Hong Kong has been significantly shaped by the priority given to securing the health and well-being of the 'grassroots' or the working class in Hong Kong. Given that government in pre-1997 British Hong Kong was long seen to favour the needs of the professional and elite business class—a trend continued after the creation of the HKSAR—this prioritising of the needs of the very large, vulnerable, working class in Hong Kong is not, at first glance, what one might expect. Yet it has happened—and this pattern has significantly tracked the approach adopted in the mainland. This matter is discussed again in the conclusion.

The next part discusses certain initial challenges and how these were addressed before examining how the first four COVID-19 waves were tackled in Hong Kong prior to discussing Hong Kong's struggle to cope with the devastating fifth wave in early 2022. A comparative review of basic responses in certain other jurisdictions (with a focus on Greater China) follows. After this, there is a wider review of the 'zero-COVID' and 'living with COVID' approaches, including a discussion of relevant political, social, and economic aspects.[6] Finally, this chapter considers ongoing and future challenges faced by Hong Kong, and lessons learnt from the COVID-19 pandemic.

The Onset of COVID-19

Background

In late February 2003, a medical doctor from Guangdong Province in China checked in with his wife at the Metropole Hotel in Hong Kong. He became very ill and went to a nearby hospital. He knew he was extremely sick and told the staff attending him that this was so. He died soon after. This doctor had recently been treating patients with what came to be known as Severe Acute Respiratory Syndrome (SARS) in Guangdong.[7] Infected guests from the Metropole Hotel subsequently spread the SARS virus both within Hong Kong and elsewhere, including in Canada, Singapore, and Vietnam. Before SARS was contained in Hong Kong, it infected around 1,800 people, of whom almost 300 died.[8]

Mainland China failed to provide timely advice following the primary commencement of SARS infections. Subsequently, an effective response was initiated (see Chapter

---

5. Barrington Moore, *Social Origins of Dictatorship and Democracy: Lord and Peasant in the Making of the Modern World* (Boston, MA: Beacon Press, 1966).
6. Zero-COVID is also now called Dynamic Zero-COVID, which signifies an aim to reduce COVID-19 infections to as close to zero as possible. The term Zero-COVID as used in this chapter encompasses achieving zero COVID-19 cases or securing an outcome as close to zero as possible.
7. S. H. Lee, 'The SARS Epidemic in Hong Kong' *Journal of Epidemiology and Community Health* 57, no. 9 (2003): 653–654, https://jech.bmj.com/content/57/9/652.
8. Ibid.

9). Altogether, SARS spread to around 30 jurisdictions worldwide, most widely in East Asia and Southeast Asia. Hong Kong, like many jurisdictions in East Asia, learnt a number of critical lessons from the SARS pandemic about how to track, trace, and control infections (through quarantining where needed).

Enter COVID-19

In December 2019, Hong Kong was still experiencing the impact of the constant political rioting, dating back to June, which had grown out of very large peaceful protest marches. This violent political upheaval was massively disruptive. By the end of December 2019, a new concern took hold. There was credible news of a novel flu-like illness that had first been recognised in Wuhan. This immediately brought back sharp memories of the SARS epidemic in 2002–2003. What swiftly became apparent were the differences between SARS and this new virus. Although COVID-19 was less lethal, it was significantly more infectious. With SARS, the virus did not survive well in temperatures above 25 degrees Celsius, especially accompanied by high humidity. Thus, the onset of summer in Hong Kong in 2003 helped bring the epidemic under control.[9] The COVID-19 virus, it transpired, did not face this problem.

As the concerns over COVID-19 grew, the Hong Kong government moved to suspend teaching at all levels from kindergarten through to university as part of their institutional social distancing programme. These closures commenced in January 2020 and were first applied on a week-by-week basis. As the COVID-19 threat in Hong Kong increased and the number of cases grew globally the closures were extended, first beyond Chinese New Year into February 2020, and later right through until the end of teaching in that academic year.

One development, which arose from the months of intense social upheaval beginning in June 2019, was a major lift in applications to register new Trade Unions in Hong Kong, all of which appeared to be related to the broad anti-government, or opposition, movement. One such new union was focused on those who worked for the Hospital Authority (HA)—the Hospital Authority Employees Alliance (HAEA).[10] By late January, the HAEA claimed to have recruited over 15,000 HA members including doctors and nurses. This number represented about 10 per cent of the total staff of the HA.

Also, by late January 2020, eight COVID-19 cases had been confirmed in Hong Kong. The mainland, meanwhile, had recorded around 6,000 cases with a death toll of about 130. The Hong Kong government began to restrict cross-border travel in the

---

9.   K. H. Chan, Malik J. S. Peiris, S. Y. Lam, L. L. M. Poon, K. Y. Yuen, and W. H. Seto, 'The Effects of Temperature and Relative Humidity on the Viability of the SARS Coronavirus', *Advances in Virology* (2011), https://www.ncbi.nlm.nih.gov/pmc/articles/PMC3265313.

10. Tony Cheung, 'Medical Group Aligned with Opposition in Hong Kong Comes under Official Scrutiny for Range of Criticisms', *South China Morning Post*, 15 September 2021, https://www.scmp.com/news/hong-kong/politics/article/3148868/medical-group-aligned-opposition-hong-kong-comes-under?module=perpetual_scroll_0&pgtype=article&campaign=3148868.

second half of January. Given the high numbers of people who depended on cross-border transit (students, businesspeople, and employees, for example) the authorities adopted a staged approach to closing down movement. By this time, the mainland had imposed intense lockdowns in Wuhan and across major centres in Hubei Province (starting from 23 January 2020). That is, China itself had taken drastic steps to contain the spread of COVID-19 within days of confirming person-to-person transmission (see Chapter 9). A most important control measure, which incidentally helped to protect the wider world, was imposed on the mainland.[11]

Still, there were deep concerns in Hong Kong about whether more restrictions were needed, including a complete closure of all mainland entry points. The most insistent calls come from the opposition camp that had explicitly or tacitly supported the months of vehement protesting. The HAEA was strident in its criticism of the failure of the government to close all borders with the mainland completely. In a move never before seen in Hong Kong, some HAEA members walked away from their HA posts, including frontline medical posts, and went on strike on 3 February. The HAEA insisted that they would increase their strike action unless the government agreed to their demands for an urgent, total border closure with the mainland. The pressure on the government arising from the crisis was immense.[12] Popular reaction proved to be against this HAEA industrial action. The strike was not extended. Fairly soon after, border controls with the mainland were made tighter until, in due course, almost all non-essential cross-border traffic was stopped.

The First Four COVID-19 Waves

The first wave of infections was minimal. One factor that assisted Hong Kong from the outset was a very wide understanding, drawing on the SARS experience, of the benefits of wearing masks, social distancing, and maintaining high personal hygiene standards. Unlike in much of the Western world, for example, wearing masks at such times is recognised as manifestly logical across East Asia—good for both the individual and the community. Outside of one's home, masks were widely worn indoors and outdoors and on public transport. A small second wave commenced in March 2020, arising from returning residents. There was a larger third wave of infections underway by July 2020, driven by sea crew and air crew arriving in Hong Kong and foreign domestic helpers returning to work in Hong Kong. For several days, more than 100 cases each day were reported.[13] In November 2020, a fourth, locally driven wave commenced that included a cluster of cases related to commercially run dance groups. Close contact without

---

11. Lily Kuo and Lillian Yang, '"Liberation" as Wuhan's Coronavirus Lockdown Ends after 76 Days', *The Guardian*, 7 April 2020, https://www.theguardian.com/world/2020/apr/07/liberation-as-wuhans-coronavirus-lockdown-ends-after-76-days.

12. 'Hong Kong Medical Staff Strike for Third Day as Locally Transmitted Virus Cases Rise', *Reuters*, 5 February 2020, https://www.reuters.com/article/china-health-hongkong-idUSL4N2A510T.

13. Tong B. Tang, 'The COVID-19 Response in Hong Kong', *The Lancet* 399, no. 10322 (2022): 357, https://www.thelancet.com/journals/lancet/article/PIIS0140-6736(20)32217-0/fulltext.

masks helped amplify infection levels. A similar cluster outbreak associated with a fitness studio arose in March 2021.[14]

It is well recognised that coronaviruses can adapt repeatedly as they spread. By the end of 2020, one new notably infectious COVID-19 variant, Delta, was detected in India. It soon spread around the world. Another, even more infectious variant, Omicron, was detected in South Africa in November 2021. Its spread around the globe was astoundingly swift and comprehensive. By early 2022, as the global total of COVID-19 infections rapidly exceeded 300 million, the Omicron variant was said to be responsible for a major surge in infection rates across much of the world. Although it is exceptionally infectious, the illness it induces was said to be less threatening than other variants.[15] Up until this time, Hong Kong had demonstrated a notable capacity to retain strong control of COVID-19 outbreaks. At the same point in time, infection rates in the United Kingdom and the United States were 90 to 100 times higher per capita than in Hong Kong.

The Fifth COVID-19 Wave

Control measures were sorely tested in January 2022 by an increasing number of Omicron cases. By early February, it was clear these measures were failing. Within just a few weeks, COVID cases in Hong Kong had jumped by a factor of 30. They kept growing rapidly, as did the death toll. Before examining how this terrible setback developed, it is useful to consider some of the factors that enabled Hong Kong to do as well as it did for the first two years of the pandemic. It is this otherwise commendable framework that the devastating fifth wave tested to breaking point.

The understanding of personal responsibility for maintaining personal health is one part of what underpinned the initial durable, positive outcome. Other intervention factors were also important. As the COVID-19 pandemic unfolded, the authorities in Hong Kong learnt from experience, especially within Hong Kong but also from across Greater China. Hong Kong was also well served by both its frontline and research-focused medical sectors. They became increasingly skilled in COVID-19 investigation, detection, tracing, isolation, and treatment.

Hong Kong did not endure a single city-wide lockdown during the first two years of the COVID-19 pandemic. But the operation of risk-zone venues, including bars, restaurants, teaching institutions, health centres, and sports centres were subject to varied opening, closing, and operational rules aimed at reducing infection hazards, as new COVID-19 waves emerged. Overnight lockdowns of large and small residential

---

14. Elizabeth Cheung, Kathleen Magramo, and Lilian Cheng, 'Coronavirus: Hong Kong's Fourth Wave of COVID-19 Cases Has Ended but Don't Ease Rules Yet, Government Pandemic Adviser Says', *South China Morning Post*, 29 May 2021, https://www.scmp.com/news/hong-kong/health-environment/article/3135325/coronavirus-hong-kongs-fourth-wave-COVID-19-cases.

15. 'World Passes 300 million COVID Cases as Omicron Breaks Records', *France 24*, 7 January 2022, https://www.france24.com/en/live-news/20220107-world-passes-300-million-COVID-cases-as-omicron-breaks-records.

blocks to test all inhabitants based on case and contact locations became common-place. Sewage sampling to detect COVID-19 related to particular buildings was used. Mandatory individual testing orders arising from contact tracing were increasingly used. Sometimes wider, district-based mandatory testing was applied.[16]

The very strict controls applied at Hong Kong's borders were another vital factor. For anyone coming to Hong Kong including from the mainland, these became among the strictest in the world. For the vast majority coming to Hong Kong during the COVID-19 period, comprehensive testing on arrival, followed by compulsory quarantine (either in a designated hotel or the public quarantine facilities) of up to 21 days became the norm. Given that Hong Kong is the primary International Financial Centre (IFC) for China and one of the leading IFCs worldwide,[17] this long-running stern approach generated significant criticism from within and outside of Hong Kong. Critics argued that these obstructive travel rules could put Hong Kong's IFC standing at risk, given that competing IFCs in, for example, Singapore, London, and New York had moved to a much less restrictive 'living with COVID' approach.[18] This matter is discussed further below.

Rapidly established medical and quarantine facilities also helped to protect Hong Kong. The North Lantau Hospital Infection Control Centre with over 800 beds was built within five months and opened in late February 2021. An additional temporary Community Treatment Facility (with 500–1,000 beds), which could be opened as required was established by the HA within the large AsiaWorld-Expo complex, located adjacent to the Hong Kong Airport.[19] Meanwhile, a purpose-built Quarantine Centre was constructed on vacant land at Penny's Bay, on Lantau Island. This provided over 3,400 units which could accommodate several thousand persons. The government was also operating other hotel-based quarantine facilities adding over 1,000 further units. These public quarantine facilities housed around 70,000 'confinees' during the first two years of the pandemic.[20] In addition, the government organised a designated hotel quarantine list, which catered to persons returning to Hong Kong (mainly residents) who were shown to be not infected with COVID-19 on arrival. By late 2021, over 12,000 rooms were provided under this scheme.

Then came Omicron.

---

16. Government of the HKSAR, 'Compulsory Testing for Certain Persons', https://www.coronavirus.gov.hk/eng/compulsory-testing.html.

17. Alex Lo, 'The Status Quo Is the Best and Worst Scenario for Hong Kong', *South China Morning Post*, 27 January 2022, https://www.scmp.com/comment/opinion/article/3164928/status-quo-best-and-worst-scenario-hong-kong.

18. Dan Strump, 'Foreign Executives in Isolated Hong Kong Head for Exit, Sick of Zero-COVID Curbs', *Wall Street Journal*, 23 January 2022, https://www.wsj.com/articles/foreign-executives-in-isolated-hong-kong-head-for-exit-sick-of-zero-COVID-curbs-11642950280.

19. Hospital Authority, 'Public Hospitals Gear up for the Challenging Epidemic', 31 December 2021, https://www.ha.org.hk/haho/ho/pad/211231Eng.pdf.

20. Centre for Health Protection, 'Quarantine Facilities', 19 January 2022, https://www.chp.gov.hk/files/pdf/quarantine_centre_en.pdf.

Singapore began to see a surge in Omicron cases by early January 2022, soon after recovering from a serious surge in Delta cases which extended from September into December 2021. Its approach largely protected Hong Kong from the Delta variant. Omicron, however, broke through due, primarily, to cross-infection because of breaches of protocols for returning travellers and quarantine hotels by some returning airline staff. Initially, Hong Kong managed to retain a level of control as the Omicron variant spread very rapidly through a large housing estate in Kwai Chung. This, however, proved to be an immense struggle, which was soon after lost.

The rapid spread of infections was unprecedented. The prevailing control model, based on testing, tracing, and isolation (close contacts) or hospitalisation, had worked well but it relied on having no more than a few hundred cases to handle per day. Thousands and then tens of thousands of new cases per day overwhelmed this system. It placed an alarming burden on Hong Kong's very large public hospital system. New patients had to wait outdoors in tents. Mortuaries began to overflow. These were scenes Hong Kong residents had watched unfold elsewhere, for example in New York in 2020. Now they were happening with frightening intensity in Hong Kong.

Apart from the extreme infectiousness of the Omicron variant, two other factors amplified the very grim impact of the fifth wave. First, is the far too low vaccination rate of the elderly in Hong Kong (see below). Next, one element that made the original control scheme so effective was the fact that the great majority of Hong Kong's population lives in very high-density high-rise tower blocks. This social housing reality facilitated test-and-trace targeting using sewage sampling, before Omicron. Unfortunately, this condition amplified Omicron infection rates. Hong Kong's very compact housing profile also presented serious problems in organising effective home quarantine as the fifth wave spread. The average living space per person in Hong Kong (at 12.9 square metres) is less than half that provided in Singapore, for example.[21]

One especially alarming aspect of the fifth wave, discussed further below, was the rapid escalation in the daily COVID death rate to one of the highest levels in the developed world.[22] By early February 2022, the Hong Kong government had reached out to seek help from the mainland in managing this dismaying COVID-19 surge.[23] That help proved to be wide-ranging and generous. A series of (largely mainland-funded) rapid building projects were commenced to lift hospital and quarantine accommodation levels as soon as possible. These combined with other government measures to increase

21. 'Hong Kong & Singapore Housing', *Hong Kong—Singapore*, https://sites.google.com/site/hongkong singaporehousings3wl/comparison-between-hk-and-singapore-housing-environment.

22. 'Hong Kong's Covid Death Rate Is Now One of the World's Highest', *The Standard*, 1 March 2022, https:// www.thestandard.com.hk/breaking-news/section/4/187684/Hong-Kong's-COVID-death-rate-is-now-one-of-the-world's-highest.

23. Twinnie Siu and Marius Zaharia, 'Mainland China to Help Overwhelmed Hong Kong with COVID Fight', *Reuters*, 12 February 2022, https://www.reuters.com/world/china/hong-kong-report-record-1510-COVID-cases-saturday-tvb-2022-02-12/.

public isolation accommodation capacity to over 70,000.[24] Other support included teams of mainland workers to assist in running testing services, stressed Residential Care Homes (RCH), and certain other staff-depleted services. A major project to ensure the timely, ongoing supply of medical items together with food and necessities into Hong Kong, shipped by road, rail and sea from the mainland, was soon implemented. A range of distinguished mainland experts visited to provide experienced-based advice. A number of local Hong Kong business leaders stepped forward, too, offering support in various ways.[25] The Hong Kong government also investigated organising the first (mainland-assisted) Compulsory Universal Testing scheme for the entire population. Strong local medical expert advice urging caution and logistical challenges resulted in this measure being postponed and then dropped.

Once Omicron had broken through the containing framework of the prevailing control system, it was clear that any swift return to the position previously secured by that system was inconceivable.

Vaccination

This section considers certain policy and practical aspects of the rollout of Hong Kong's COVID-19 vaccination programme. For a full review of the remarkable COVID-19 vaccination story, see Chapter 4.

Although Hong Kong worked well collectively to manage the COVID-19 pandemic for over two years, one area where it failed to advance expeditiously was mass vaccination. This disturbing lapse gravely amplified the lethal consequences of the fifth wave.[26]

An increasing range of vaccines was soon approved for emergency use around the world. By the end of February 2021, the Hong Kong government had taken delivery of sufficient vaccine supplies to begin a free mass vaccination programme. The two vaccines ultimately approved for emergency use in Hong Kong were the Pfizer-BioNTech vaccine from Europe (it was manufactured in Europe and the United States initially) and the Sinovac-CoronaVac vaccine (commonly known as Sinovac) from mainland China. The latter is a traditional, inactivated-virus vaccine and the former uses a new vaccine-making approach based on messenger RNA (or mRNA) methodology. Legal threats to mass vaccine usage that were once common, especially with new vaccines,

---

24. 'Hong Kong's COVID Isolation Plan Crumbles as Infections Soar', *The Standard*,1 March 2022, https://www.thestandard.com.hk/breaking-news/section/4/187663/Hong-Kong%E2%80%99s-COVID-isolation-plan-crumbles-as-infections-soar.

25. John Lee Ka-chiu (HKSAR Chief Secretary), 'We Are Determined to Win This Uphill Battle against COVID', *China Daily*, 7 March 2022, https://www.chinadailyhk.com/article/262401.

26. For a detailed review (based on an extended medical-survey) of certain key issues discussed here, see Jingyi Xiao, Justin K. Cheung, Peng Wu, Michael Y. Ni, Benjamin J. Cowling, and Qiuyan Liao, 'Temporal Changes in Factors Associated with COVID-19 Vaccine Hesitancy and Uptake among Adults in Hong Kong: Serial Cross-Sectional Surveys', *The Lancet (Regional Health—Western Pacific)* 23, no. 100441 (2022), https://doi.org/10.1016/j.lanwpc.2022.100441.

in the United States and elsewhere have now largely been curtailed by shield laws.[27] In keeping with widespread international practice, the Hong Kong authorities provided a significant level of indemnity for the vaccine manufacturers in the relevant procurement contracts,[28] and a Vaccine Injury Compensation Scheme was established for individual recipients.[29]

By late January 2022, as the Omicron fifth wave gained irresistible traction, Hong Kong had vaccinated (with at least two doses) over 70 per cent of its total population. This, however, was below the rate achieved by that time in a range of other jurisdictions including, Australia, Chile, Japan, and Singapore.[30] The sort of aggressive, rights-based, *anti-vaxxer* activism seen across much of the developed world had not been such a critical problem in Hong Kong. But the vaccination issue had still been subject to a degree of localised politicisation, resulting chiefly from the divisive months of political insurgency that immediately preceded the onset of the COVID-19 pandemic. Alarmist criticism in the media (and more widely) was, initially, comprehensively directed at both approved vaccines. Every possible risk was highlighted and the Sinovac vaccine was regularly portrayed as being tainted by development within the mainland. Fervent viewpoints influenced adverse opinion-shaping as the mass vaccination drive commenced.

The Hong Kong government gradually moved to mandate vaccination for most persons directly on the public payroll. A range of other semi-public and private organisations, including many teaching institutions, followed suit. But the government was wary about applying more wide-ranging mandatory vaccination measures. It preferred to rely on inducements and indirect pressures to drive greater vaccine acceptance, likely bearing in mind the long-term political experience in Hong Kong, which has consistently stressed significant deference to judicially protected, individual rights for more than 30 years. The most serious drawback arising from this approach proved to be the low vaccination uptake by the elderly in Hong Kong. By late January 2022, as the fifth wave commenced, over 70 per cent of those over 80 were unvaccinated and over 40 per cent of those aged 70 to 79 remained unprotected.[31] Making this shortfall even more acute was the fact that Hong Kong has the longest life expectancy in the world, surpassing Japan—It had gone from 72 years in 1971 to 85 years by 2020.

27. Richard Cullen, 'COVID-19 Vaccines, Litigation-Shield Laws Go Hand in Hand', *China Daily*, 4 January 2021, https://www.chinadailyhk.com/article/153929.

28. HKSAR Government, 'Government Makes Prevention and Control of Disease (Use of Vaccines) Regulation', Press Release, 24 December 2020, https://www.info.gov.hk/gia/general/202012/24/P2020122300963. htm.

29. HKSAR Government, 'Indemnity Fund for Adverse Events Following Immunization with COVID-19 Vaccines', Press Release, 16 June 2021, https://www.info.gov.hk/gia/general/202106/16/P2021061600808. htm.

30. See Our World in Data, 'Coronavirus (COVID-19) Vaccinations', accessed 15 September 2022, https:// ourworldindata.org/COVID-vaccinations?country=CHL.

31. Fiona Sun, 'Coronavirus Hong Kong: Why Are Elderly Not Getting Vaccinated? Families, Doctors and Government Not Doing Enough to Tackle Irrational Fears and Practical Obstacles, Say Social Workers', *South China Morning Post*, 13 February 2022, https://www.scmp.com/news/hong-kong/health-environment/ article/3166840/coronavirus-hong-kong-alone-afraid-and.

One reason for this poor vaccine response appears to be the success of Hong Kong's management of the COVID-19 pandemic. As each of the first four waves was brought under control relatively swiftly, the elderly felt less concerned about the need to be protected, while continuing to fret about possible and imagined vaccine side effects.[32] It seems, too, that both the families of older Hong Kong residents and their family doctors regularly advised caution with respect to using new vaccines.[33] Comparisons between possible vaccine side effects or zero side effects, provided a vaccine was refused, were regularly advanced. This was simply wrong, as one expert noted. The comparison should always have emphasised the difference between possible side effects and serious illness or death.

Looking back, wide-ranging, ill-judged advice, sometimes politically tilted, combined with government hesitation and inaction with respect to mandating (and providing) RCH and home-visit vaccinations, left far too many vulnerable residents gravely exposed to serious and lethal COVID-19 infection consequences as the fifth wave struck.[34] Around 75,000 people live in RCH facilities in Hong Kong. The daily COVID-19 death toll far exceeded 100 once the fifth wave took hold. Around 90 per cent of those who died were 65 or over and unvaccinated or not double-vaccinated. The magnitude of this problem becomes clear when one considers Singapore. About 95 per cent were vaccinated there as the Omicron surge unfolded and the daily death toll was 10 per cent of the daily death rate in Hong Kong.[35] At an individual level, the fact that a number of babies and young children perished in the fifth wave after being infected with the Omicron variant was particularly disturbing.[36]

Comparative Observations[37]

Mainland China, Hong Kong, Macao, and Taiwan, along with a range of other jurisdictions, including Australia, New Zealand, South Korea, and Singapore, effectively adopted a zero-COVID-19 policy from the outset of the pandemic. Subsequently, all the jurisdictions within Greater China retained this approach well after most of the rest of the world moved to a 'living with COVID' approach.

---

32. 'Is Hong Kong about to Host a Natural Experiment on Omicron's Severity?', *The Economist*, 12 January 2022, https://www.economist.com/the-economist-explains/2022/01/12/is-hong-kong-about-to-host-a-natural-experiment-on-omicrons-severity.

33. Sun, 'Coronavirus Hong Kong'.

34. Peter Kammerer, 'Ultimately, Vaccine Refuseniks Are to Blame for Omicron's Deadly Chaos in Hong Kong', *South China Morning Post*, 8 March 2022, https://www.scmp.com/comment/opinion/hong-kong/article/3169393/ultimately-vaccine-refuseniks-are-blame-omicrons-deadly.

35. 'Hong Kong's COVID Death Rate', *The Standard*, 1 March 2022.

36. 'COVID-19 Deaths among Hong Kong's Young Children Alarm Parents', *Straits Times*, 4 March 2022, https://www.straitstimes.com/asia/east-asia/COVID-19-deaths-among-hong-kongs-young-children-alarm-parents.

37. The COVID statistics quoted in the part are based on the information recorded at the COVID-19 Data Repository by the Center for Systems Science and Engineering (CSSE) at Johns Hopkins University, available at https://github.com/CSSEGISandData/COVID-19.

Singapore is widely regarded as having managed the COVID-19 pandemic well. By mid-July 2022, it had officially recorded a total of around 1.6 million cases within a total population of 5.7 million (over 28,000 infections per 100,000 persons) and close to 1,500 deaths. There was a spike (especially among visiting construction workers) in cases between April and August 2020 after which daily cases were brought down to low double-digit increases for about 12 months. Another major COVID-19 wave came around September 2021, with daily case numbers regularly exceeding 1,000, and the move to the 'living with COVID' followed. In January 2022 a major Omicron surge gained traction.

Taiwan witnessed case patterns like those in Hong Kong (pre-fifth wave). There was a new COVID-19 wave from May to June 2021, but it was brought under control. Until early April 2022, total recorded case numbers were contained to around 24,000 with about 850 deaths in a population of 23.6 million—an infection rate of around 100 infections per 100,000 persons. Taiwan announced a formula for opening up in 2021, as a first step towards 'living with COVID', based significantly on achieving certain vaccination levels. That plan was later suspended in the light of the rapid global spread of the Omicron variant, and Taiwan moved back to a zero-COVID management model.[38] Initially, unlike in Hong Kong—but like the mainland and Macao—Taiwan continued to maintain tight and effective controls despite the arrival of some imported Omicron cases. However, by late April 2022, Omicron infections began to rise dramatically in Taiwan. Case numbers peaked at around 90,000 per day in late May and were still running at around 25,000 per day in mid-July, by which time officially recorded total figures stood at around 4.4 million infections and 8,500 deaths (a case rate of around 18,500 per 100,000 persons). By this time, approximately 85 per cent of the population had been fully vaccinated. Taiwan announced, in May 2022 that it planned to gradually ease travel and local COVID controls and move away from its zero-COVID policy, noting that the Omicron variant, though highly infectious, was milder than previous strains.[39]

Macao, with a population of less than 700,000, has been particularly successful in containing the COVID-19 pandemic. Like the mainland, Hong Kong, and Taiwan, it adopted a zero-COVID strategy. After more than two years, in mid-June 2022, recorded COVID-19 infections totalled over 100 with zero deaths equal to an overall infection rate of around 18 infections per 100,000 persons. However, Macao had to impose mass testing, quarantine, and lockdown of certain neighbourhoods in mid-July 2022 as Omicron cases surged.

Mainland China is by far the largest jurisdiction in Greater China, with a population of over 1.4 billion. Total recorded COVID-19 infections by mid-July 2022

---

38. Victor Vincej, 'Taiwan Keeps Its "Zero-COVID" Approach as of Dec. 21', *Travelling Lifestyle*, 31 December 2021, https://www.travelinglifestyle.net/taiwan-is-opening-borders/.

39. Phoebe Zhang, 'COVID Cases Bounce back in Taiwan after Week of Declines', *South China Morning Post*, 11 June 2022, https://www.scmp.com/news/china/politics/article/3181343/covid-cases-bounce-back-taiwan-after-week-declines.

exceeded 900,000 with over 5,000 deaths resulting in an overall infection rate of around 70 infections per 100,000 persons.

Until mid-January 2022, COVID-19 infections in Hong Kong totalled below 14,000, in a population of about 7.5 million, with less than 220 deaths (around 190 infections per 100,000 persons). Within a few months, following the onset of the fifth wave, these numbers had grown exponentially to a recorded figure of more than 1.3 million cases (*estimated* to be much higher) and over 9,400 deaths (over 17,000 infections per 100,000 persons).

These figures show that, across Greater China, the overall COVID-19 infection rate was kept remarkably low for over two years. The highest infection rate, in Hong Kong, was still very low compared to most jurisdictions worldwide until the devastating fifth wave struck. The lowest rates, in mainland China and Macao, were exceptionally low, while the rate in Taiwan (until the recent major Omicron surge) fitted between these two 'bookends'. Until September 2021, Singapore (whose population is approximately 76% Chinese) fitted within this low-rate group. However, rising infections evident in September 2021, signalled a need to change from following a zero-COVID strategy to a 'living with COVID' approach.

Before moving on from these broad comparisons, two other points should be made. First, Hong Kong, Macao, Taiwan, and Singapore run public finance systems that are, comparatively, particularly sound. Fiscal reserves are typically strong, government debt is low, and private savings are high. There has been no need for recourse to extended public borrowing triggered by the pandemic, unlike what was commonly seen across much of the Western world. These East Asian jurisdictions have all long been prepared for a serious 'rainy day'. They have so far coped without the need to build up colossal new debt that taxpayers will need to cover in the future. Mainland China, given its massive development programmes, does carry large debt. But as the leading global trading economy, it also has the world's highest foreign exchange reserves (over US$3 trillion)—and a high-saving population.[40] Hong Kong has seen its total fiscal reserves reduced from around US$150 billion to around US$130 billion by COVID-19-related deficit spending. However, the HKSAR has retained in excess of one year's total government expenditure in the fiscal reserves.[41]

Experts advised, correctly, that, as COVID-19 spread around the world, the original virus would mutate. The greater the number infected (around 570 million in July 2022) the greater the possibility that new variants will emerge. Two new variants (Delta and Omicron) have shown themselves to be highly infectious. Greater China—and especially mainland China—by making zero-COVID policies work so well for so long, has significantly reduced the potential global, COVID-19 variant, incubation

40. Elvis Picardo, '10 Countries with the Biggest Forex Reserves', *Investopedia*, 4 June 2021, https://www.investopedia.com/articles/investing/033115/10-countries-biggest-forex-reserves.asp.

41. HKSAR Government, 'Financial Results for the 10 Months Ended January 31, 2022', Press Release, 28 February 2022, https://www.info.gov.hk/gia/general/202202/28/P2022022800418.htm#:~:text=The%20fiscal%20reserves%20stood%20at,profits%20tax%20and%20stamp%20duties.

pool. Greater China, led by the mainland, has also, significantly lowered the risk of the relevant health systems being overwhelmed by serious 'long-COVID' burdens in the future. Experts consider that these burdens, arising out of continuing later illnesses particularly affecting a number of those infected with earlier versions of COVID-19,[42] pose a potential major health system operational hazard in certain other jurisdictions, including the United States.

Zero COVID and Living with COVID

Zero-COVID and 'living with COVID' strategies create (differing) social and economic costs and benefits. In both cases, greater attention needs to be paid to assessing these costs and benefits thoroughly.

The *Economist* argued in mid-October 2021 that 'China has decided it does not want to live with the virus'.[43] This was a curious claim as China's top respiratory disease expert, Dr Zhong Nanshan, had already explicitly discussed the opening of China's borders, stressing the need for very high vaccination rates to be fully achieved. He spoke about the process of 'living with COVID' in China once this was accomplished.[44] In fact, all the zero-COVID jurisdictions in Greater China knew that they would need, in due course, to establish effective ways to re-open their borders to the rest of the world. They knew, too, that the success of their zero-COVID policies had saved many lives; avoided placing major, additional stress on medical facilities; measurably protected their economies; and assisted global economic performance (and health protection). This approach has also given Hong Kong and the three other jurisdictions time to plan ahead with respect to when they should open and to whom. Nevertheless, the *Economist* stated that other jurisdictions with zero-COVID policies had 'moved to relax them', while 'China is holding out'. The clear tilt in such stories is that the likes of Hong Kong, Macao, Taiwan, and mainland China are behind the times. This move-with-the-times narrative implicitly advanced the idea that the cited jurisdictions that have significantly eased their COVID controls have astutely done so after completing international comparative due diligence. In fact, all the named jurisdictions that have moved to 'living with COVID' have done so primarily out of necessity. In Singapore, Australia, and New Zealand, for example, the authorities lost control over the spread of COVID-19, despite their best efforts, after the arrival of more infectious variants. The explicable necessity of 'living with COVID' has since been re-presented, in a number of cases, as a distinct virtue.

---

42. Benjamin Mazer, 'Long COVID Could Be a "Mass Deterioration Event"', *The Atlantic*, 16 June 2022, https://www.theatlantic.com/health/archive/2022/06/long-covid-chronic-illness-disability/661285.
43. 'How Long Can China's Zero-COVID Policy Last?', *The Economist*, 6 October 2021, https://www.economist.com/china/2021/10/16/how-long-can-chinas-zero-COVID-policy-last.
44. Wallis Wang, 'Mainland Headed towards 80pc Jab Rate and Fully Open Borders', *The Standard*, 4 October 2021, https://www.thestandard.com.hk/section-news/section/11/234727/Mainland-heading-toward-80pc-jab-rate-and-fully-open-borders.

Arguments in favour of 'living with COVID' were vigorously advanced well before this term entered common usage. In September 2020, former Australian Prime Minister Tony Abbott said that 'Health Dictatorships' were failing to consider the economic costs of the crisis and that some elderly COVID-19 patients should be allowed to die naturally. Abbott stressed how costly it was to maintain certain lives and he cast serious doubt on the wisdom of striving to achieve very low or zero transmission rates.[45] At about the same time, WHO Director-General Tedros Adhanom Ghebreyesus took a strong position objecting to the view that high COVID-19 death rates for the elderly were not a major concern.[46]

China was the first responder to the COVID-19 pandemic. It struggled, initially, to cope with a new infectious disease and to act with level-headed transparency. But it quickly settled on a comprehensive response. The solution's focus swiftly and radically moved to containing and controlling the spread of the virus and, above all, saving lives (see Chapter 9). This imposed stringent personal controls and, initially, as the *Times* reported, it 'effectively stopped economic activity'.[47] However, as the same *Times* report highlighted, these powerful disease control measures laid the foundations for an early normalisation of production with Chinese exports posting their strongest growth in 18 months in August 2020. This was a post-COVID-19 outcome unmatched by any other major jurisdiction. China thus confirmed that the initial best economic response to the epidemic was also the most life-saving and humanitarian. This outcome depended on scientifically informed decisiveness applied within the effective, centralised, mainland mode of governance.[48]

In February 2022, Professor Li Bingqin, from the University of New South Wales, summarised both why the Chinese approach has worked so well and why it was still needed. Li stressed that maintaining the fitness of China's domestic health system was crucial. China, she argued, with 3.6 critical care beds per 100,000 people, is in a far more vulnerable position than the United States or Germany, with 29.4 and 38.7 such beds per 100,000, respectively. Moreover, as she noted, even with a high vaccination rate, in such circumstances, the risk of an overwhelmed health system remains high (a risk acutely confirmed in comparatively wealthy Hong Kong). Li also observed how

45. Patrick Wintour, 'Tony Abbott: Some Elderly COVID Patients Could Be Left to Die Naturally', *The Guardian*, 1 September 2020, https://www.theguardian.com/australia-news/2020/sep/01/tony-abbott-some-elderly-COVID-patients-could-be-left-to-die-naturally.

46. World Health Organization, 'COVID-19: Virtual Press Conference', 31 August 2020, https://www.who.int/docs/default-source/coronaviruse/transcripts/COVID-19-virtual-press-conference---31-august.pdf?sfvrsn=391fc93a_0.

47. Philip Aldrick, 'China Scores Hat-Trick of Export Gains', *The Times*, 8 September 2020, https://www.the-times.co.uk/article/china-scores-hat-trick-of-export-gains-lw52jz7qx.

48. A cogent argument that what went wrong with the management of the COVID-19 pandemic in the UK pivoted, inter alia, on a fundamental lack of 'governmental capacity' is made in David Campbell and Kevin Dowd, 'Disregard of the Empirical; Optimism of the Will; the Abandonment of Good Government in the COVID-19 Crisis', Studies in Applied Economics Working Paper, Johns Hopkins Institute for Applied Economics, Global Health, and the Study of Business Enterprise, March 2022, https://sites.krieger.jhu.edu/iae/files/2022/03/Working-Paper-202-in-Studies-in-Applied-Economics.pdf.

China's long-established, fine-grained community governance systems have helped to provide an effective platform for applying massive and successful rapid zero-COVID test-and-trace exercises (Chapter 10). Li, further confirmed what was argued in the *Times*: that China's zero-COVID approach had strengthened rather than weakened China's post-COVID-19 economic performance.[49]

The unfolding of very serious Omicron outbreaks in various Chinese cities, including Shanghai in the spring of 2022 severely tested the mainland's zero-COVID strategy, however. By early May, over 600,000 infections had been detected in Shanghai, with around 540,000 being asymptomatic carriers.[50] This massive outbreak was eventually brought under control but at a serious cost, over several months, to the economy and to freedom of movement for millions.[51] Lessons learnt from this harrowing experience are discussed further below.

In Shanghai, it was reported that less than 5 per cent of the almost 600 who died during the recent Omicron outbreak were vaccinated.[52] These were typically older patients with co-morbidities, confirming how the COVID-19 pandemic has most severely affected older persons and the infirm. Statistics show that 75 per cent of COVID-19 deaths in the United States have occurred among adults aged 65 years and older.[53]

It is important, at this point, to note another factor which has shaped Hong Kong's COVID-19 management approach. The total population living in low-cost, public rental housing is over 2.2 million. Those worst off, around 220,000 people, live in over 100,000 tiny, subdivided units. More than 1.4 million people, about 20 per cent of the population, are said to live (before government welfare interventions) below the poverty line.[54] Yet, Hong Kong has the longest life expectancy in the world, which now stands at 85 years. Studies that have looked at why this is so almost always note that wide access to good public health care is a key factor.[55]

Public hospitals and clinics in Hong Kong handle millions of individual outpatient cases every year. More than 40 public hospitals provide around 30,000 beds, over 70 per cent of the total in Hong Kong. These services are always stretched and waiting

49. Bingqin Li, 'China Clings to COVID-19 Zero', *East Asia Forum*, 27 February 2022, https://www.eastasiaforum.org/2022/02/27/china-clings-to-COVID-19-zero.

50. Xinxin Zhang, Wenhong Zhang, and Saijuan Chen, 'Shanghai's Life-Saving Efforts against the Current Omicron Wave of the COVID-19 Pandemic', *The Lancet* 399 (2022), https://www.thelancet.com/action/showPdf?pii=S0140-6736%2822%2900838-8.

51. Peter Jackson and Zubaidah Abdul Jalil, 'Shanghai Lockdown: China Eases COVID Restrictions after Two Months', *BBC*, 1 June 2022, https://www.bbc.com/news/world-asia-china-61647687.

52. Zhang et al., 'Shanghai's Life-Saving Efforts'.

53. Julie Bosman, Amy Harmon, and Albert Sun, 'As U.S. Nears 800,000 Virus Deaths, 1 of Every 100 Older Americans Has Perished', *New York Times*, 13 December 2021, https://www.nytimes.com/2021/12/13/us/COVID-deaths-elderly-americans.html#:~:text=Seventy%2Dfive%20percent%20of%20people,closer%20to%201%20in%201%2C400.

54. Oxfam Hong Kong, 'Poverty in Hong Kong', accessed 15 September 2022, https://www.oxfam.org.hk/en/what-we-do/development-programmes/hong-kong/povertyinhongkongandoxfamsadvocacywork.

55. Chinese University of Hong Kong, 'Why Hong Kong Has the Longest Life Expectancy in the World', *CUHK eNews*, January 2021, https://www.oal.cuhk.edu.hk/cuhkenews_202101_life_expectancy.

times are long for significant, non-emergency treatment. The lack of funding and development of primary health care and community health facilities adds to the huge day-to-day burden placed on this hospital-based regime.[56] This is the system that is fundamentally charged with the vital responsibility of looking after the medical welfare of Hong Kong's huge low-income population. The work pressures on staff within these institutions are always very high. Nevertheless, prior to the fifth wave, they continued to do the same often-unsung, extraordinary work. Hong Kong's successful zero-COVID approach, which endured for two years, underwrote the ability of this system to continue looking after its oversize, vulnerable client base so well, until early 2022.

Next, there is the crucial matter of travel between the mainland and Hong Kong, which has been conspicuously restricted in both directions for over two years. Measured by transit numbers, this is the most important border Hong Kong shares. Hong Kong's zero-COVID policy (which emulates the policy applied on the mainland) has been notably shaped by the need to re-open this border. In 2018, before the violent political upheaval began, over 50 million mainland visitors made up almost 80 per cent of the total arrivals of 65 million in Hong Kong. This is also the border that the vast majority of Hong Kong residents wish to see re-opened as a priority. And for many professional expatriates residing in Hong Kong, this is also a crucial business border.

By early 2022, Hong Kong was drawing close to a staged re-opening of this border. The devastating Omicron fifth wave sank these plans. Hong Kong soon found itself in a position where the basic well-being of its own health infrastructure was put at risk. Moreover, Hong Kong became a new, major threat (because of this massive outbreak) to maintaining the successful zero-COVID policy on the mainland. [57]

Both Hong Kong and Singapore saw their visitor numbers drop, by 2021, to a tiny fraction of what they were, following the onset of the COVID-19 pandemic: to less than 2 per cent of pre-pandemic levels in Singapore and around 3 per cent of the normal number of visitors in Hong Kong.[58] Both jurisdictions also experienced small but measurable reductions in total population in 2021: in Hong Kong a 1.2 per cent drop in population and in Singapore, a 4.1 per cent drop over the same period (amplified by the departure of low-wage contract workers).[59] As the Omicron fifth wave gripped

---

56. David Dodwell, 'Omicron Crisis: How a Lack of a Community-Based Primary Health Care System Doomed Hong Kong', *South China Morning Post*, 21 March 2022, https://www.scmp.com/comment/opinion/hong-kong/article/3171111/omicron-crisis-how-lack-community-based-primary-health.

57. Lau Siu-kai, 'Han's Message on Hong Kong COVID Fight Must Be Heeded', *China Daily*, 8 March 2022, https://www.chinadailyhk.com/article/262575.

58. See 'Visitors to Singapore Fall to Record Low in 2021', *The Standard*, 25 January 2022, https://www.thestandard.com.hk/breaking-news/section/6/186416/Visitors-to-Singapore-fall-to-record-low-in-2021; and 'Hong Kong Welcomed 91,000 Visitors Last Year, 97pc Less Than 2020', *The Standard*, 17 January 2022, https://www.thestandard.com.hk/breaking-news/section/4/186057/Hong-Kong-welcomed-91,000-visitors-last-year,-97pc-less-than-2020.

59. See King Man Ho and Cheng Yut You, 'Hong Kong's Population Falls for Second Year Running Amid Exodus', *Radio Free Asia*, 16 August 2021, https://www.rfa.org/english/news/china/falls-08162021154904.html; and *The Standard*, 'Singapore Shrinks as COVID Takes Shine off Expatriate life', 25 January 2020, https://www.thestandard.com.hk/breaking-news/section/6/186498/Singapore-shrinks-as-COVID-takes-shine-off-expatriate-life.

Hong Kong, departure numbers rose conspicuously, strengthened by an inviting new pathway to permanent residence in the United Kingdom opened up to Hong Kong residents by the British government.[60]

The downside of semi-closed international borders is plain to see. Extended quarantine periods, for example, make all travel—and especially business travel—significantly more difficult. They also have a clear adverse effect on separated families, and they add additional stress and expense to daily life. Moreover, cogent arguments have been made that this policy risks endangering Hong Kong's standing as a leading IFC. Such restrictions hamper hiring fresh talent (especially from outside Greater China) equipped with the skills needed in a principal IFC.[61] These drawbacks are real, but they are also selectively stressed. The wider, sustained benefits of the zero-COVID approach, noted above, are conspicuous. This is especially so in the case of mainland China, as well as in Hong Kong and Taiwan for over two years, until the ruinous fifth wave struck. A number of zero-COVID critics have paid insufficient attention to this complete picture: crucial benefits arising from this policy are regularly overlooked—or taken for granted.

Conclusion

Debating COVID

Hong Kong managed the COVID-19 pandemic by sustaining an effective zero-COVID policy for over two years, thus maximising the health protection and protection of the right to life for its most vulnerable residents over that period. This was in keeping with the maintenance of similar policies across Greater China. Hong Kong, however, lost its capacity to sustain this policy within just a few weeks, once the fifth wave slipped alarmingly beyond its control by February 2022.

All through the pandemic period in Hong Kong, there have been contesting opinions about what policies are best. The debate over moving to 'living with COVID' provides some examples. Once the fifth wave hit, both the range and volume of contesting opinions became significantly amplified. The global reality is that countless governments have faltered (most sooner than Hong Kong) trying to cope, especially with the Delta and Omicron variants, during the most intense international health crisis seen in more than 100 years.

Singapore and New Zealand are widely and rightly regarded as each having done as good a job as possible in pandemic management. Yet, in each case, they lost control while pursuing a zero-COVID strategy: in Singapore, with the arrival of the Delta variant and in New Zealand, as the Omicron variant rapidly spread, with cases rising

---

60. 'One-Way Flights out of the City Surge 300pc amid COVID Outbreak', *The Standard*, 15 March 2022, https://www.thestandard.com.hk/breaking-news/section/4/188144/One-way-flights-out-of-the-city-surge-300pc-amid-COVID-outbreak%C2%A0.

61. Strump, 'Foreign Executives'.

from around 200 a day to over 20,000 a day within a month.[62] In the case of Singapore, it is clear that strong, experienced governance capacity has been of central importance in meeting the shifting pandemic challenges so well, especially measured by the way it has kept the death rate low after moving, by October 2021, to 'living with COVID'.[63] But coping with this change of policy (after the arrival of the Delta variant) still generated, 'tension, division and fear' within Singapore.[64]

It needs to be remembered, too, that Singapore maintains some of the tightest media controls in the developed world. According to the Reuters Institute, print and broadcast media outlets in Singapore are largely run by two major corporations that are associated with the governing party, each of which maintains a dominant online presence.[65] Also, in 2019, Singapore introduced a robust anti-fake news law to counter falsehoods (especially online) aimed at 'exploiting' the city's 'fault lines'. This law has been already used to curtail certain negative, COVID-messaging related to Singapore.[66] The scope for regular, skewed reports about the claimed medical and political hazards of COVID-19 vaccines, for example, is far lower in Singapore than in Hong Kong.[67] Meanwhile, this problem of antagonistic messaging (anti-vaccine and encouraging infected persons to spread the virus, for example) has persisted in Hong Kong during the fifth wave.[68] In a recent report, Transparency International ranked Singapore within the top 2 per cent of least corrupt jurisdictions. At about the same time, the US-based, World Justice Report ranked Singapore within the top 11 per cent (globally) for rule of law compliance. Reporters Without Borders (RWOB), however, placed Singapore in the lowest 16 per cent of jurisdictions for press freedom.[69] Despite this RWOB ranking, the Reuters Institute ranked Singapore second highest in terms of media trust in the Asia-Pacific in 2021 (ahead of Australia, Japan, Hong Kong, and Taiwan).[70]

---

62. These COVID statistics are based on the information drawn from the Coronavirus Resource Center at Johns Hopkins University, 9 March 2022, https://coronavirus.jhu.edu/region.

63. Michelle Fay Cortez, Faris Mokhtar, and Low De Wei, 'Singapore Confronts the Division and Fear that Come from Living with COVID', *Bloomberg*, 15 October 2021, https://www.bloomberg.com/news/articles/2021-10-14/singapore-confronts-division-and-fear-bred-by-living-with-covid.

64. Ibid.

65. Edson C. Tandoc Jr., 'Singapore: 2019 Report', Reuters Institute Oxford, https://www.digitalnewsreport.org/survey/2019/singapore-2019/.

66. Edson C. Tandoc Jr., 'Singapore: 2021 Report', Reuters Institute Oxford, https://reutersinstitute.politics.ox.ac.uk/digital-news-report/2021/singapore.

67. Tony Kwok, 'Beware of Political Saboteurs When Combating COVID-19 Fifth Wave', *China Daily*, 11 March 2022, https://www.chinadailyhk.com/article/263049.

68. Selina Cheng, 'COVID-19: Hong Kong National Security Police Arrest Two for Sedition over Anti-vaxx Posts', Hong Kong Free Press, 25 February 2022, https://hongkongfp.com/2022/02/25/COVID-19-hong-kong-national-security-police-arrest-2-for-sedition-over-anti-vaxx-posts/.

69. Richard Cullen, *Hong Kong Constitutionalism: The British Legacy and the Chinese Future* (Abingdon: Routledge, 2020), 47.

70. Nic Newman, 'Executive Summary and Key Findings of the 2021 Report', Reuters Institute, https://reutersinstitute.politics.ox.ac.uk/digital-news-report/2021/dnr-executive-summary.

Social contracts

The social contracts across Greater China visibly differ. The mainland remains a singular party-state; Taiwan is home to a thriving democracy; and both Hong Kong and Macao have each been deeply shaped by their respective colonial legacies. Yet there has been a visible commonality in their responses to the COVID-19 pandemic. Professor Daniel Bell of Shandong University observed in May 2021 that '[t]he Confucian value of filial piety, or reverence for the elderly, helps [in part] to explain why East Asian countries took such strong measures to protect people from a disease that is particularly dangerous for the elderly'. It was increasingly evident, he argued (at that time), that East Asian societies had done notably better than most other jurisdictions in containing the spread of COVID-19 infections. Bell contrasted this focus with the prioritising of individual autonomy which, more than ever, lies at the core of social comprehension across most advanced Western nations.[71] One British writer captured this actuality with the observation that many today, in such societies, consider themselves to be the 'Sun King of their own soul'.[72]

As noted in Chapter 9, the paramount leadership in Beijing stressed in January 2020 that in tackling the pandemic, all governance levels throughout China 'should put people's lives and health first'.[73] In late December 2021, Professor Chan Changchuan from the National Taiwan University College of Public Health observed that 'the whole society in Taiwan has a zero-COVID mentality—the tolerance rate is so low and we cannot bear one case, not to mention ten or 100 cases'.[74] In essence, the right to life is regarded as preeminent across these jurisdictions. There is an emphasis on this right that is not evident, to the same degree, in the Western world. This viewpoint has shaped policy-making in response to the COVID-19 pandemic. First-rate public fiscal health has helped provide the resources to stress protecting the right to life in this way. The success of these zero-COVID policies has delivered fundamental health, human rights, and economic benefits. However, primary policy-makers across Greater China recognise that this approach cannot continue indefinitely. For Hong Kong, its leading IFC role is being hampered by this approach—and now the fifth wave has critically undermined the operation of its zero-COVID policy.

---

71. 'Pro-people Policies, Dutiful Citizens Effective in China's COVID-19 Fight: Daniel A. Bell', *Global Times*, 2 May 2020. See also Priscilla Leung Mei-fun, '"Dynamic Zero Infection" Model Much Closer to True Humanism', *China Daily*, 15 March 2022, https://www.chinadailyhk.com/article/263561.

72. Theodore Dalrymple, *How Other People's Rubbish Shapes Our Lives* (London: Gibson Square, 2011), 98.

73. See also 'Xi Jinping Honors China's Coronavirus Fighters, Says Saving Lives Was Foremost', *The Standard*, 8 September 2020, https://www.thestandard.com.hk/breaking-news/section/3/154959/Xi-Jinping-honors-China's-coronavirus-fighters.

74. Nicola Smith, 'Taiwan's "Zero-COVID" Strategy: How Much Longer Can It Keep Out Variants', *The Telegraph*, 20 December 2021, https://www.telegraph.co.uk/global-health/science-and-disease/taiwans-zero-COVID-strategy-much-longer-can-keep-variants.

Looking forward

Professor Chan, in Taiwan, is a firm advocate of clear-headed planning to begin the task of 'weaning the public off a zero-COVID mindset'. To achieve this sort of transition, he has stressed the need for:

- Maximum levels of vaccination
- Still wider testing, tracing, and controlling
- Maintaining a highly robust public health system

He notes that '[o]ur hygiene standards are high. The people are the heroes of our successful story of pandemic control until now.'[75] This observation about Taiwan (made before the recent massive rise in Omicron cases) can also be said of the rest of Greater China, including Hong Kong. It reflects a key, similar aspect embodied within the varied social contracts which apply. The arrival of new variants is placing these zero-COVID jurisdictions under far greater pressure, however, as we have seen in Hong Kong, Taiwan, and the mainland. But their success in managing the pandemic so well, especially over the first two years, means significant benefits have already been 'banked'. And this approach gave these jurisdictions time to plan how they can best manage their re-engagement with the rest of the world. Moreover, they have a wide range of real-life, 'living with COVID' experiments from around the world to study and learn from. Finally, it has given more time, too, for the potential development of improved COVID-19 vaccines and medical treatments.

Regrettably, Hong Kong and the mainland did not vaccinate enough of their elderly. One veteran Hong Kong commentator argued that 'vaccine refuseniks' were ultimately most to blame for laying the foundations for Omicron's alarmingly deadly impact in Hong Kong.[76] This does not, however, absolve the government of significant responsibility for the exceptionally high Omicron death rate in Hong Kong. Most critically, Hong Kong helped foster the creation of this acute hazard, by being so watchful about individual rights that it failed to think unflinchingly about how best to protect that most primary of all rights—the right to life.

Looking beyond Hong Kong, potentially even more important is the way that maintaining a zero-COVID policy may allow other jurisdictions across Greater China to open up *after* the COVID pandemic has largely peaked across the rest of the world. WHO Europe Director Hans Kluge observed in late January 2022 that the European region may be 'moving towards a kind of pandemic endgame'. The argument is that increasing vaccination and the boost to herd immunity arising from the highly contagious but less severe Omicron variant could, in combination, presage a steady move away from the COVID-19 pandemic towards it becoming an endemic illness more like

---

75. Ibid.
76. Kammerer, 'Ultimately, Vaccine Refuseniks Are to Blame'.

the seasonal flu.[77] Still, this development is uncertain—and new, more harmful variants could yet emerge.[78] Even when an illness does become endemic, this, in itself, does not mean it will no longer be highly dangerous to health and life: Malaria is a life-threatening endemic disease, for example (see Chapter 1).

Opening up comprehensively would pose significantly lower risks across Greater China if very high vaccination rates have been secured, including across most of the world, and the international travelling public is markedly less liable to carry a dangerous version of the COVID-19 virus. In fact, overall vaccination rates are now quite high in mainland China, but its huge population amplifies potential risks greatly. Almost 90 per cent of the entire population is double-vaccinated. However, it was reported in mid-May of 2022 that close to 50 million people aged over 60 (more than the total population of Spain) remain particularly vulnerable as they were still not fully vaccinated.[79]

This problem of the vulnerability of those of advanced age is confirmed by the Hong Kong experience. Hong Kong struggled badly to secure vaccination protection across its older population. Advice from the mainland and from within Hong Kong since the fifth wave struck has emphatically confirmed that fixing this shortfall is a fundamental priority both to emphasise saving lives and to build proper foundations for managing the transition to eventual opening up with the lowest risk. But why were so many older people left unvaccinated in China? One factor, it seems, was that a number of doctors counselled against vaccination for older patients with co-morbidities, especially as the zero-COVID strategy had contained the spread of COVID-19 so effectively. Professor Wang Feng, from the University of California Irvine, declared that 'China really missed an opportunity in the last two years'.[80] He observed that, unlike in so many other jurisdictions, vaccination of the elderly was not prioritised in China. It seems that the mainland reluctance to mandate—or at least drive—vaccinations for the elderly presents significant resonances with the HKSAR experience. While the mainland has so far managed to avoid the huge relative spike in elderly deaths seen in Hong Kong, this has been achieved at a substantial social and economic cost, especially in Shanghai. Recent acute experience in Hong Kong and the mainland, thus, highlights how the deep tension between (a) major economic and freedom of movement costs and (b) basic health and survival costs are amplified when there is a decisive shortfall in vaccination coverage.

In mid-2022, the matter of the full opening of the HKSAR borders remained both unresolved and subject to significant debate. The new chief executive of the HKSAR expressed the view, shortly before taking office in July 2022, that the primary Hong

77. 'Europe Could Be Headed for Pandemic "Endgame": WHO', *The Straits Times*, 24 January 2022, https://www.straitstimes.com/world/europe/europe-could-be-headed-for-pandemic-endgame-who.

78. 'Facing Uncertainties, Sticking to Zero-COVID Policy Remains China's Best Strategy: Epidemiologists', *Global Times*, 24 January 2022, https://www.globaltimes.cn/page/202201/1246794.shtml.

79. 'China's Unvaccinated Elderly Driving Force behind Unrelenting "Covid-Zero" Policy', *The Standard*, 17 May 2022, https://www.thestandard.com.hk/breaking-news/section/3/190220/China%E2%80%99s-unvaccinated-elderly-driving-force-behind-unrelenting-%22Covid-zero%E2%80%9D-policy.

80. Ibid.

Kong border opening to be resolved was that with the mainland.[81] How this complex process was set to be managed was linked to the manner and timing of Hong Kong's wider opening up to regular international travel. Later in 2022, however, the new HKSAR government prioritised opening the international border and Hong Kong refocussed on 'living with COVID'. The mainland government began radically moving in the same adapting to COVID direction, after some significant protests, at about the same time.

Lessons learnt

The experience with SARS in 2003 was effectively called upon as the COVID-19 pandemic began, 17 years later. Masking, social distancing, and enhanced personal hygiene were swiftly and widely adopted. Most residents understood that all these measures played a role in augmenting personal protection and public well-being.

It is highly likely that the world will see further virus-based pandemics. There is a large pool of different illness-causing viruses circulating within the animal and bird populations. In very particular (but unpredictable) circumstances, these viruses can transition across species so that they are eventually able to infect humans. In the most dangerous cases, such as with COVID-19, they can trigger very serious illness and establish a propensity for highly infectious, human-to-human transmission.

The Spanish Flu, as it is generally known, resulted in what is still widely regarded as one of the deadliest disease outbreaks in human history, killing, it is said, between 50 million and 100 million people after it began to spread in 1918. Research by the Australian virologist and Nobel Laureate Macfarlane Burnet concluded that the evidence was 'strongly suggestive' that the disease started (notwithstanding its common name) in the United States and spread to France with 'the arrival of American troops' to fight in World War I.[82] This hugely amplified the way it spread: it was taken around the world by personnel returning home from that terrible conflict. Persistent, official public lying across the United States, virtually mandated by the new Sedition Act, comprehensively covered up the terrible crisis, further aggravating the harmful outcome worldwide.[83]

Today, the scope for mass, international travel has vastly increased since 1918, which, in turn, has greatly amplified the potential for global pandemics to run ahead of standard control measures. One primary lesson learnt from this latest pandemic is how crucial it is to establish, as accurately as possible and as soon as possible; the morbidity, mortality, and infectiousness levels of any new virus. Where these are all deeply

---

81. "Reopening Borders with Mainland Is Top Priority, Says CE-Hopeful John Lee", *The Standard*, 5 May 2022, https://www.thestandard.com.hk/breaking-news/section/4/189865/Reopening-borders-with-mainland-is-top-priority.

82. John M. Barry, 'How the Horrific 1918 Flu Spread across America', *Smithsonian Magazine*, November 2017, https://www.smithsonianmag.com/history/journal-plague-year-180965222.

83. Ibid.

concerning, as with COVID-19, radical test, trace, and control responses (including mass quarantining in dedicated facilities) will be needed, wherever resources allow. Living, from the outset, with such a virus, either deliberately or as a consequence of poor management (when resources are ample) very likely will result in prominently increased hospitalisation demands, very widespread illness, and significantly elevated death rates. Rapidly applying very strong control measures, including robust, efficient vetting of all visitors, can strikingly reduce these adverse impacts. There is no question that such restrictions will have an unfavourable impact on normal economic activity. But accelerating mass morbidity and high death rates can be even more damaging to economic activity. Moreover, strong control measures have proved to be the best way to protect the right to life (and good health) across a given population, especially among the elderly and infirm.

An important, positive message delivered by the response to the COVID-19 pandemic is that developing virus-impeding vaccines can now be fast-tracked in ways not previously conceivable. Hong Kong worked commendably fast to take up the new vaccines created to fight the COVID-19 pandemic. These were distributed widely and at no cost—an excellent initiative. But the government failed to prevent a major short-fall in securing comprehensive vaccination of substantial, vulnerable segments of the population.

Hong Kong also did far worse than it might have in using the time gained by its durable first-rate control of COVID-19 infection rates to research intensively and project how it might best meet future challenges which could arise. The specific, exceptional potency of the Omicron variant was not foreseeable in detail, but Hong Kong should have used the time it had to be notably better prepared for infection challenges which would *not* fit within the prevailing control framework, which relied on managing case numbers typically well below 1,000 per day. It lacked the best sort of policy research infrastructure to conduct, relevant, ongoing advanced risk analysis.[84]

Although Hong Kong officials were steadfastly good at communicating statistics and certain details reliably and accurately, the government, as a whole, was distinctly less adept at maintaining a lucid and consistent, broader narrative about how the pandemic was being managed—and what the future options were.[85] This left still more space for harm to be done by the constant feed of negative, regularly misleading commentary, especially from the largely unchecked media—and social media—both local and international.

The challenges presented to governments by the onset of an exceptional, globalised public health emergency are extraordinary. The lessons outlined above do not provide any sort of magic bullet pandemic solution. They do emphasise the need for rapidly setting crucial initial and ongoing priorities so that extraordinarily grave harm

84. Lau Siu-kai, 'Enhancing SAR Government's Capability to Cope with Crises', *China Daily*, 22 March 2022, https://www.chinadailyhk.com/article/a/264579.
85. Ibid.

is minimised; the right to life is visibly respected; and the operation of normal life and the broad economy are both secured as far as is reasonably possible. All these plans and measures must, moreover, be effectively communicated to the people.

Finally, the way in which the COVID-19 pandemic has been managed in Hong Kong signals that certain, deep changes to the operating political framework in Hong Kong may have evolved since 1997. In a series of three significant books, Leo Goodstadt explained the extraordinary influence of business and professional elites on the governance of British Hong Kong and then the HKSAR.[86] He argued how 'business leaders in Hong Kong have always had a major influence on government policies and they have successfully thwarted many policies detrimental to their interests.'[87] That power of influential persuasion, dating back to the nineteenth century, remains significant today, but the experience with the COVID-19 pandemic signals that the dominance of these groups is no longer as distinct as it was.

The merits of Hong Kong's primary COVID-19 management policy have been intensely debated, but for well over two years the perceived rights of the huge number of low-income residents in Hong Kong have been prioritised by persisting with a zero-COVID influenced strategy over a strongly argued case by certain business and professional leaders and qualified commentators to move decisively away from that strategy. This approach has closely followed aspects of COVID-19 policy-making in the mainland. Further research is warranted on the complex factors which have shaped the choice of this prevailing management mode in the HKSAR. One interesting question which arises from a review of the established research on the elevated level of business and professional influence on government in Hong Kong is whether the COVID-19 pandemic may have been managed in a measurably different way had it struck while Hong Kong was still under British rule or during the early years of the HKSAR? What we can say, at this point, is that the handling of the COVID-19 pandemic has arguably provided evidence of an appreciable shift, since 1997, in certain operational precepts governing the social contract in Hong Kong. In this sense, too, it is possible that Hong Kong will no longer be entirely the same once closure on managing the pandemic is ultimately achieved.

---

86. Leo F. Goodstadt, *Profits, Politics and Panics: Hong Kong's Banks and the Making of a Miracle Economy, 1935–1985* (Hong Kong: Hong Kong University Press, 2007); *Poverty in the Midst of Affluence: How Hong Kong Mismanaged Its Prosperity* (Hong Kong: Hong Kong University Press, 2013); and *A City Mismanaged: Hong Kong's Struggle for Survival* (Hong Kong: Hong Kong University Press, 2018).

87. See Bart Wissink, Sin Yee Koh, and Ray Forrest, 'Tycoon City: Political Economy, Real Estate and the Super-Rich in Hong Kong', in *Cities and the Super-Rich: Real Estate, Elite Practices and Urban Political Economies*, ed. Ray Forrest, Sin Yee Koh, and Bart Wissick (New York: Palgrave Macmillan, 2017), 229–252.

12

A Comparative Perspective on the COVID-19 Response in Europe

Renu Singh

Chapter 6 introduces a central tenet to any society, describing the social contract as an agreement between individuals and their governments about their rights and duties to each other and the government's role in public service provision. This framework of the social contract helps us understand what happened in Europe during the COVID-19 pandemic—why we saw the controversies that we did, why certain countries adopted the public health measures that they did, and why they look different from the rest of the world.

This chapter aims to share the European pandemic experience to provide a comparative lens to varied COVID-19 responses. After the initial outbreak in China spread, this was the region first hit with the coronavirus and the region experienced high cumulative cases and deaths, only surpassed by the Americas.[1] Further, as we hope to learn how to better coordinate and respond to the next public health crisis as a global community, Europe provides an important case in regional crisis management and public health harmonisation that could provide lessons to other transnational efforts in the future.

The European COVID-19 Response

After the initial outbreak in China, Europe became the epicentre of the COVID-19 pandemic. Many European countries were ranked highly in their emergency preparedness and health security capabilities prior to the outbreak, but these did not prove to mean much in reality. Fifteen of the top 35 countries in the Global Health Security Index (GHSI) 2019 were from Europe, and yet they also had relatively higher reported cases per 100,000 people.[2] With some of the more comprehensive and established

---

1. World Health Organization (WHO), 'WHO Coronavirus (COVID-19) Dashboard', accessed 15 September 2022, https://covid19.who.int/table.
2. Matthew M. Kavanagh and Renu Singh, 'Democracy, Capacity, and Coercion in Pandemic Response: COVID-19 in Comparative Political Perspective', *Journal of Health Politics, Policy and Law* 45, no. 6 (1 December 2020): 997–1012, https://doi.org/10.1215/03616878-8641530.

welfare state systems, European countries may have been considered better prepared for a public health emergency, but in a globalised world, they were still incredibly vulnerable. Relatively strict lockdowns were put in place, although by the summer of 2020 most European countries had adopted a system of imposing and removing public health measures as the pandemic waxed and waned, especially once vaccines were available and successfully administered to majorities of their populations. The Omicron variant brought another surge in cases towards the end of 2021,[3] but the largely vaccinated populations seemed to have kept the death rates lower and facilitated the move towards 'living with COVID' and treating the disease as endemic. By the end of July 2022, there have been a total of over 241 million COVID-19 cases and 2 million deaths, with the top five countries for the total number of cases being France, Germany, the United Kingdom, Russia, and Turkey.[4]

Interestingly, even with the similarities in COVID-19 responses and the overarching role of the European Union, there were quite varied approaches established around the public health crisis, across the continent. Sweden chose to not follow most of the rest of the world in implementing lockdowns, closing schools, contact tracing, and other common public health measures as part of its national strategy. Swedes were even intentionally discouraged by their government from—and at times reprimanded for—wearing masks in an effort to avoid panic. It maintained fewer COVID-19 deaths per capita than the European average for long enough that it gained a reputation for having an alternative, laissez-faire, even 'holistic' response to COVID-19 focused on herd immunity. Unfortunately, this natural herd immunity was never reached and at the cost of numerous lives, especially among the most vulnerable populations, but the political leadership has steadfastly held to their strategy.[5] Meanwhile, the UK tried applying a similar strategy, only to go back and forth with the implementation of lockdowns and more stringent measures that have led its response to be considered 'too little, too late, [and] too flawed'.[6]

---

3. Monir Ghaedi, 'EU Countries Record COVID-19 Records as Omicron Spreads | DW | 30.12.2021', Deutsche Welle, 30 December 2021, https://www.dw.com/en/eu-countries-record-covid-19-records-as-omicron-spreads/a-60288621.

4. WHO, 'COVID-19 Situation in the WHO European Region', accessed 15 September 2022, https://www.arcgis.com/apps/dashboards/ead3c6475654481ca51c248d52ab9c61.

5. Johan Ahlander and Niklas Pollard, 'Sweden's COVID Response Was Flawed but Allowed Freedoms—Commission', *Reuters*, 25 February 2022, https://www.reuters.com/world/europe/sweden-pandemic-strategy-correct-early-response-flawed-commission-2022-02-25; N. Brusselaers, D. Steadson, K. Bjorklund, Sofia Breland, Jens Stilhoff Sörensen, Andrew Ewing, et al., 'Evaluation of Science Advice during the COVID-19 Pandemic in Sweden', *Humanities and Social Sciences Communications* 91, no. 9 (2022), https://doi.org/10.1057/s41599-022-01097-5; Gretchen Vogel, 'Sweden's Gamble: The Country's Pandemic Policies Came at a High Price—and Created Painful Rifts in Its Scientific Community', *Science*, 6 October 2020, https://www.science.org/content/article/it-s-been-so-so-surreal-critics-sweden-s-lax-pandemic-policies-face-fierce-backlash.

6. *BMJ*, 'UK's Response to Covid-19 "Too Little, Too Late, Too Flawed"', 15 May 2020, https://www.bmj.com/company/newsroom/uks-response-to-covid-19-too-little-too-late-too-flawed.

In contrast, Italy was the first country to be severely hit by the pandemic and the first to implement some of the strictest COVID-19 lockdown measures.[7] It was also not the last one to do so. For example, during Spain's first COVID-19 wave in March 2020, the government implemented a strict stay-at-home lockdown under its state of emergency that ordered all citizens to stay home with exceptions only for short shopping trips and essential business. This applied to all ages, including children, and did not include any exceptions even for exercising. Such draconian measures ultimately took a toll on the country's economy and led to a backlash among the public and political opposition, a sentiment reflected in the Spanish Constitutional Court's decision to deem the lockdown unconstitutional.[8] There has also been variation in the resistance of the public to such policies, as seen by the pushback from citizens protesting in the Netherlands, Germany, Belgium, and France, among others.[9]

As the pandemic progressed, the main issues of prevention and immediate crisis containment and response gave way to those concerning access to, administration of, and uptake of vaccines; socio-economic stimulus; and a debate over how viable a policy of 'living with COVID' would be. The European story of similar overall approaches to COVID-19 by the continent but varied strategies within domestic politics and policy has also continued beyond the initial responses to the public health crisis. By 2021, social contracts in the context of COVID-19 were not only being questioned by the public, as was already the case with the start of COVID-19 measures; the relationship and responsibilities of the public and the government to each other started to adapt and change in the context of the coronavirus.

By early 2021, multiple vaccines were starting to become accessible, and by the end of the year, 66 percent of people were fully vaccinated on the continent.[10] As vaccines became available and the pandemic raged on, public and political discourse made it clear that Europe was shifting towards a 'living with COVID' strategy. The Netherlands took a very literal interpretation of living with COVID-19 with the 'Dansen met Janssen' or 'Dancing with Janssen' initiative, where citizens were encouraged to get their vaccinations and then join in public celebrations immediately after. This strategy appears to have backfired and failed within two weeks, with coronavirus infections rising by 500

7. Iris Bosa, Adriana Castelli, Michele Castelli, Oriana Ciani, Amelia Compagni, Matteo M. Galizzi, et al., 'Response to COVID-19: Was Italy (Un)Prepared?', *Health Economics, Policy and Law* 17, no. 1 (January 2022): 1–13, https://doi.org/10.1017/S1744133121000141.

8. Joseph Wilson, 'Spain's Top Court Rules Pandemic Lockdown Unconstitutional', *AP News*, 14 July 2021, https://apnews.com/article/europe-business-health-government-and-politics-courts-a0a36ebadb24600e-122e2f1fb035011c.

9. 'French "Freedom Convoy" Gets under Way in Protest at Covid-19 Restrictions', *France 24*, 9 February 2022, https://www.france24.com/en/france/20220209-french-freedom-convoy-gets-under-way-in-protest-at-covid-19-restrictions; BBC News, 'Covid: Huge Protests across Europe over New Restrictions', 21 November 2021, sec. Europe, https://www.bbc.com/news/world-europe-59363256.

10. Our World in Data, 'Coronavirus (COVID-19) Vaccinations', accessed 15 September 2022, https://ourworldindata.org/covid-vaccinations.

percent after the immediate relaxing of restrictions were lifted on nightclubs on 26 June 2021.[11]

In order to encourage vaccine uptake, a number of European countries began to require proof of COVID-19 vaccination or of recent recovery from COVID-19 to enter public places including bars and restaurants. By mid-2021, many began to require a 'green pass', European COVID Digital Certificate, or other forms of digital or paper documentation. Such documentation increasingly became necessary for adults to attend large gatherings, nursing homes, bars, restaurants, hotels, theatres, sports facilities, and other public spaces.[12] While many countries had their own policies and documentation requirements, they generally converged—with some notable exceptions—on the need to have a version of a green pass to help contain the spread of the virus and allow for safer gatherings.

What they did not agree on was how much of a requirement protection from COVID-19 in some form (i.e., vaccination, recent illness, or regular testing) was required by the workforce, especially as people started to go back to in-person settings. This policy development and debate around green passes in Europe reflects how social contracts changed as a direct result of the pandemic—with the public being required or strongly encouraged in most countries to consider the collective concerns of spreading illness among each other and the resulting costs to the economy and the government, in turn, in a new light. However, there was much disagreement and a lack of coordination among the public and the governments within countries themselves, as well as in the overall European context, regarding all COVID-19 measures as vaccine mandates emerged and public health restrictions ebbed and flowed in parallel with rising and falling COVID-19 cases. And overall, protests, riots, and other expressions of pandemic fatigue were not uncommon across the continent, especially by the end of 2021 and into early 2022.[13]

A parallel development as vaccines were being produced and then rolled out across Europe was the global effort to share vaccines worldwide in order to reduce inequities and help end the pandemic. Europe as a bloc of mostly developed countries, several of whom were even vaccine producers and manufacturers and most of whom are high-income countries, had a particular role to play. It was clear from the beginning of the pandemic that equitable vaccine distribution was key to containing COVID-19, and yet this failed to happen at the scale needed. Countries in the EU and the UK ordered

---

11. Chloe Lovatt, '"Dancing with Janssen" Day after Jab Says Dutch Health Minister', *Dutch Review*, 1 July 2021, https://dutchreview.com/news/vaccination-certificate-the-day-after-janssen; Leo Cendrowicz, 'After the Party Ends: Coronavirus Infections in Netherlands Jump by 500% after Country Relaxes Restrictions', *The Independent*, 14 July 2021, https://www.independent.co.uk/news/world/europe/netherlands-pandemic-nightclubs-rules-coronavirus-b1883474.html.

12. Shannon McDonagh and Tim Gallagher, 'Green Pass: Which Countries in Europe Require a COVID Vaccine Pass to Get Around?' *Euronews*, 17 November 2021, https://www.euronews.com/travel/2021/10/12/green-pass-which-countries-in-europe-do-you-need-one-for.

13. *BBC News*, 'Covid: Huge Protests across Europe over New Restrictions', editorial, 21 November 2021, https://www.bbc.com/news/world-europe-59363256.

a surplus of vaccines for their populations, while other countries will have to wait years for full vaccination coverage. The EU ordered about 525 million extra full doses, while the UK ordered enough to vaccinate its population several times over. This stark global inequity is further compounded by the fact that countries in Europe have significant engagement with the World Health Organization, international development, and civil society groups interested in global health, and yet they have not pushed hard enough for the attainment of global vaccine equity.[14] The EU and UK also have access to greater production technologies and knowledge that they have not been willing to share with the rest of the world to increase the number of vaccines available. As such, Europe has failed to uphold the social contract shared among people and governments of other countries and humanity at large even as it has provided for its own as a bloc and as individual countries.

The Social Contract and the European Union

In order to fully understand the response to COVID-19 in Europe, we have to look to the role of the EU. As a regulatory superpower with 27 member states, it imposes several trade, monetary policy, consumer protection, environmental, single market, and even public health standards. As the only supranational entity with such legislative and regulatory power, it has the most unique social contract of them all with member states and their citizens in conjunction with the national social contracts that have preceded its existence.[15]

The initial COVID-19 response came through the European Commission's Directorate-General for Health and Food Safety and the Directorate-General for Research and Innovation, with their work already focusing on promoting public health and coordinating funding for issues including pandemic preparedness, respectively. As such, together with EU agencies such as the European Centre for Disease Control, the EU Civil Protection Mechanism, and the European Medicines Agency, the EU has the institutional and legal ability to respond to the crisis in some form.[16]

While the EU has been engaged in many global and public health efforts over the years, its member states are still predominantly responsible for healthcare and public health policy and services in their jurisdictions. The Maastricht Treaty (1992) and Amsterdam Treaty (1997) set the foundation for public health policy development in the EU by emphasising the facilitating and funding of cooperation among member

---

14. Robin Cohen, 'COVID Vaccines: Rich Countries Have Bought More Than They Need—Here's How They Could Be Redistributed', *The Conversation*, 9 February 2021, https://theconversation.com/covid-vaccines-rich-countries-have-bought-more-than-they-need-heres-how-they-could-be-redistributed-153732.
15. Renu Singh, 'How the Coronavirus Is Plaguing Autocracies and Democracies', *The Duck of Minerva*, 10 March 2020, https://www.duckofminerva.com/2020/03/how-the-coronavirus-is-plaguing-autocracies-and-democracies.html.
16. Rebecca Forman and Elias Mossialos, 'The EU Response to COVID-19: From Reactive Policies to Strategic Decision-Making', *Journal of Common Market Studies* 59, no. S1 (2021): 56–68, https://doi.org/10.1111/jcms.13259.

states to promote public health, but the legal harmonisation of public health measures across all countries involved have always faced strong restrictions.[17] Thus, the states ultimately maintain their central role in this arena. However, there is a clear contradiction for EU health policy since the EU also provides for the freedom of movement of people, goods, and services—including those involved in health services—across its member states' borders, and additionally, it has law and policy that applies to national health policy.

As such, the relationship between individuals within the EU and the governing institution itself is incredibly complex and intertwined with any social contract in place with their own national governments. The same was true during the response to COVID-19, where most policies arose at the national level and were risk mitigation responses implemented by the member states as they were exposed to SARS-CoV-2 at varying levels of intensity. While responses were administered by each country, they did converge (with the notable exceptions of the UK and Sweden) in their choices to implement stringent COVID-19 measures to suppress the virus as opposed to merely mitigating it.[18] Given the precedent of the SARS and H1N1 outbreaks, better EU coordination was a reasonable expectation, but the disconnect between EU and member state health policies made that virtually impossible. However, the EU did play a larger role once countries started to lift their public health measures. An exit strategy was coordinated by member states, the EU Commission, and the European Council in the form of the Joint European Roadmap for lifting COVID-19 measures. It provided criteria to use in assessing whether or not to begin relaxing the restrictive COVID-19 policies initially put in place to reduce the risk of spreading the virus.

Nevertheless, the COVID-19 pandemic has also questioned some of the most fundamental tenets of the EU social contract. Freedom of movement of people and goods within the Schengen zone is one of the defining characteristics of the Eurozone. And yet, the public health crisis has empowered populist political actors to question the borderless Schengen area of Europe that allows for the freedom of movement within the EU. EU member states did choose to adopt a council recommendation in October 2020, representing the EU head of state and government, that they then updated three times through January 2022 on a coordinated approach for restricting movement in the Schengen zone for safety concerns. However, it also provided the perfect excuse for the far right to question the very need for free movement and the 1985 Schengen Agreement altogether.[19] The right-wing Marine Le Pen called for a closure of the French

17. Singh, 'How the Coronavirus Is Plaguing Autocracies and Democracies'.

18. Alberto Alemanno, 'The European Response to COVID-19: From Regulatory Emulation to Regulatory Coordination?' *European Journal of Risk Regulation* 11, no. 2 (June 2020): 307–316, https://doi.org/10.1017/err.2020.44.

19. European Council, 'Council Recommendation (EU) 2020/1475 of 13 October 2020 on a Coordinated Approach to the Restriction of Free Movement in Response to the COVID-19 Pandemic (Text with EEA Relevance)', *Official Journal of the European Union*, 13 October 2020, http://data.europa.eu/eli/reco/2020/1475/oj/eng; European Commission, 'Council Agreement to Strengthen Coordination of Safe Travel', 25 January 2022, https://ec.europa.eu/commission/presscorner/detail/en/statement_22_544.

borders with Italy in early 2020, and Swiss populist Lorenzo Quadri stated his alarm at the EU's prioritisation of its open borders.[20] In addition, governments themselves became myopic in their attempts to protect their own citizens, as exhibited by Germany and France withholding medical supplies from their fellow member states.[21]

Italy's Response to COVID-19

As the first country in Europe to record COVID-19 cases and the one to bring the epicentre of the pandemic to Europe itself, Italy had a unique and particularly prominent role in the response to COVID-19 in Europe very early on in 2020.

On 31 January 2020, the day of the first government response, the Italian government declared a six-month national emergency when the first two COVID-19 cases were found in Rome. By 22 March 2020, the country had implemented a complete lockdown. As such, Italy was also the first country in Europe to employ very stringent public health measures in response to what was considered its most difficult crisis since World War II. Lockdowns started in specific hotspots or towns, and then expanded to regions before the country was completely locked in and shut down (i.e., schools were closed and all factories and non-essential production were closed). At the time, this was considered an immense economic and social sacrifice.[22] Italy had one of the worst death rates in the world and needed to come together.

These sorts of measures were unprecedented, but in general the public complied and accepted the government's role. During this time, Prime Minster Giuseppe Conte even attempted to reassure his citizens by stating, 'The state is here.'[23] This statement and the public's response reflects the social contract that Italy has between its people and government. This is also reflected in how the government generally approaches its healthcare system, providing a regionally based national health service that offers universal coverage free of charge at the point of service. This Servizio Sanitario Nazionale was established in 1978, based on the principles of universal access and free healthcare, mostly paid for by taxes. As such, there is an understanding in this society of the government playing a central role in ensuring healthcare, even if austerity measures have reduced some of its capacity over time.

At the same time, some Italians have been very vocal about their opposition to what they perceive to be infringements of their liberties.[24] This reflects the tension

---

20. Singh, 'How the Coronavirus Is Plaguing Autocracies and Democracies'.

21. Amie Tsang, 'E.U. Seeks Solidarity as Nations Restrict Medical Exports', New York Times, 7 March 2020, https://www.nytimes.com/2020/03/07/business/eu-exports-medical-equipment.html.

22. Jason Horowitz, Emma Bubola, and Elisabetta Povoledo, 'Italy, Pandemic's New Epicenter, Has Lessons for the World', New York Times, 21 March 2020, https://www.nytimes.com/2020/03/21/world/europe/italy-coronavirus-center-lessons.html.

23. Ibid.

24. Valentina Di Donato and Angela Dewan, 'Italy Protests Turn Violent as Anger Mounts over Covid-19 Measures', CNN, accessed 6 April 2022, https://www.cnn.com/2020/10/27/europe/italy-coronavirus-protests-intl/index.html.

that is more broadly visible in European countries: on the one hand expecting that the government will play a central role in one's health, but on the other that people will be allowed to do what they want. The Italian healthcare system is a robust one, and in terms of public health, it also has a mix of regulations on healthy behaviours.[25] Italians had been concerned about the unprecedented measures from the initial lockdowns in Italy to the regulations in October 2021 mandating green passes for all public and private sector workers and everyone over 50 starting in January 2022.[26] There was significant resistance and protesting to such measures for being overly draconian, with citizens claiming that the government exhibited too much regulatory power over their daily lives. The state had been relatively heavy-handed during the pandemic, and not all Italians approved of how their government chose to respond to the COVID-19 crisis.

Germany's Response to COVID-19

Home to the oldest welfare state, Germany has had a unique relationship with public health institutions and policy, and a strong historical precedent. This is evident in much of its public health infrastructure today and in its response to COVID-19 since the beginning of the pandemic.

Within days of the first case of COVID-19 in Bavaria being reported on 27 January 2020, Germany's government swiftly set up a system of reporting cases within its healthcare system, an inter-ministerial crisis management group at the federal level, contact tracing among travellers, and a system of regular updates through the country's public health institution (the Robert Koch Institute). Germany has been touted as a success in its initial response to COVID-19 and in its healthcare system's and government's preparedness for such a crisis.[27] It has also had a system of local and state-level public health institutions in place for decades, which was able to contribute to the monitoring of the situation, and a strong connection between government and scientific experts to advise policy.[28] However, rates of COVID-19 infections and deaths rose during the second wave at the end of 2020.

The vaccine rollout starting in December 2020 brought its own set of problems, with supply shortages, logistical challenges in inoculating the elderly first, and delays in

25. Nanny State Index, 'The Best and Worst Countries to Eat, Drink, Smoke & Vape in the EU'.
26. Angelo Amante, Giuseppe Fonte, and Gavin Jones, 'Italy Extends COVID Vaccine Mandate to Everyone over 50', *Reuters*, 6 January 2022, https://www.reuters.com/world/europe/italy-make-covid-jab-mandatory-over-50s-tighten-curbs-draft-2022-01-05.
27. Lothar Wieler, Ute Rexroth, and René Gottschalk, 'Emerging COVID-19 Success Story: Germany's Strong Enabling Environment', Our World in Data, 30 June 2020, https://ourworldindata.org/covid-exemplar-germany-2020.
28. Claudia Hanson, Susanne Luedtke, Neil Spicer, Jens Stilhoff Sörensen, Susannah Mayhew, and Sandra Mounier-Jack, 'National Health Governance, Science and the Media: Drivers of COVID-19 Responses in Germany, Sweden and the UK In 2020', *BMJ Global Health* 6, no. 12 (2021), https://dx.doi.org/10.1136/bmjgh-2021-006691.

getting vaccine appointments being three of the most predominant.[29] By March 2021, the UK had administered nearly six times as many single doses, and headlines were made of Germany's lagging position. An additional constraint was created by Chancellor Angela Merkel's insistence on ordering vaccines as an EU bloc, which backfired when other countries decided to create bilateral agreements with pharmaceuticals well before Germany jumped on the bandwagon. A further decision by Germany's Standing Committee on Vaccination to set an age cap on the use of AstraZeneca vaccines until further research was done also increased vaccine hesitancy among the public.[30]

Overall, the German public has had a mixed response to the country's pandemic response and changing social contract. Public health policy also has a complicated history in Germany given the strong Nazi influence on health during the Third Reich. As such, Germans are often more sceptical of public health interventions, despite their strongly established healthcare system, on issues ranging from obesity to tobacco policy as well.[31] In other words, their relationship with the social contract around public health is very sensitive to state influence given the historical context. In part for this reason, the domain of public health in Germany is predominantly delegated down to the 16 states or Länder, which has allowed for more accountability and tailoring of policy to local circumstances during the pandemic. While this involved greater coordination of the Länder among themselves and with the federal government during the first two COVID-19 waves, there were still differences of opinion and contentions over specific regulations and policies. For example, insufficient supplies of personal protective equipment brought about a competitive race for supplies among them early on. In addition, as cases continued to rise and the pandemic continued into its second year, decisions to re-open borders to the EU/Schengen countries and the UK and decisions to re-impose lockdowns, among others, were not coordinated across the Länder.[32]

The United Kingdom's Response to COVID-19

The UK also illustrated how the tension between the government's role as a guarantor of health and the protection of civil liberties created friction in the COVID-19 response of European countries. On the one hand, all legal residents of the UK are entitled to

29. Holly Ellyatt, 'Germany's Vaccine Rollout Is Not Going to Plan, Frustrating Officials and Experts', *CNBC*, 20 January 2021, https://www.cnbc.com/2021/01/19/germanys-vaccine-rollout-challenges-and-problems-in-vaccine-strategy.html; Sarah Dean, Fred Pleitgen, Nadine Schmidt, and Claudia Otto, 'Germany Should Have Led the World at Handling the Pandemic. But Experts Slam Merkel's Vaccine Response as a Disaster', 8 March 2021, https://www.cnn.com/2021/03/07/europe/germany-vaccine-disaster-grm-intl/index.html.
30. Sarah Dean, Fred Pleitgen, Nadine Schmidt, and Claudia Otto, 'Germany Should Have Led the World at Handling the Pandemic. But Experts Slam Merkel's Vaccine Response as a Disaster', *CNN*.
31. Renu Singh, 'Policy Change and the Politics of Obesity in Germany and the United States of America', Georgetown University Graduate School of Arts & Sciences, 2020.
32. Sabine Kropp and Johanna Schnabel, 'Germany's Response to COVID-19: Federal Coordination and Executive Politics', in *Federalism and the Response to COVID-19: A Comparative Analysis*, ed. Rupak Chattopadhyay, Felix Knüpling, Diana Chebenova, Liam Whittington, and Phillip Gonzalez (Abingdon: Routledge, 2022), 84–94.

healthcare through the National Health Service, paid for by taxes. The system emerged out of the post-war era, and the Minister of Health at the time, Aneurin Bevan, asserted the basic principles of the social contract being built by stating: 'The essence of a satisfactory health service is that the rich and poor are treated alike, that poverty is not a disability, and wealth is not advantaged.'[33] And the country's vaccine programme was effectively planned and implemented starting in December 2021. As such, the health of its citizens is an important responsibility of the UK government, reflected in its healthcare system and in part of its COVID-19 response.

And yet, the UK's response to the coronavirus pandemic has been described as one of the country's 'worst ever public health failures'.[34] The focus on achieving herd immunity via COVID-19 infections delayed the first national lockdown until late March 2020 and led to a much higher death toll than there would have been with a more efficient decision process. Basing the public health strategy on a fatalistic view of not being able to suppress the virus ended up leading to an overwhelmed National Health Service and thousands of preventable, COVID-19-related deaths. An inquiry led by two parliamentary committees led to the release of a 150-page report in late 2021 which found that: 'Decisions on lockdowns and social distancing during the early weeks of the pandemic—and the advice that led to them—rank as one of the most important public health failures the United Kingdom has ever experienced.'[35]

In understanding the overall context for the UK, it is also important to note that all of this was happening during Brexit. As such, much political capital was focused on another national crisis. Concurrently, the response to COVID-19 further deepened divisions created by Brexit among Scotland, England, Wales, and Northern Ireland, as major decisions on public health measures were often devolved to each region to decide for itself.[36] In addition, there was widespread distrust in the government's ability to address the public health crisis, given a number of mishaps, and especially the very public breaching of lockdown rules by the then Prime Minister's main adviser, Dominic Cummings.[37]

Overall, the UK has had the worst per capita COVID-19 mortality in Europe. Much of this has been attributed to the fact that it was relatively faster in relaxing public

33. The Nuffield Trust, 'NHS Reform Timeline', 8 July 2019, https://www.nuffieldtrust.org.uk/health-and-social-care-explained/nhs-reform-timeline.
34. Ian Sample and Peter Walker, 'Covid Response "One of UK's Worst Ever Public Health Failures"', The Guardian, 11 October 2021, https://www.theguardian.com/politics/2021/oct/12/covid-response-one-of-uks-worst-ever-public-health-failures.
35. Holly Ellyatt, 'Lawmakers Slam UK's Covid Response, Say "Herd Immunity" Strategy a Public Health Failure', CNBC, 12 October 2021, https://www.cnbc.com/2021/10/12/uks-herd-immunity-covid-strategy-a-public-health-failure-inquiry.html.
36. Clive Grace, 'Perfect Storm: The Pandemic, Brexit, and Devolved Government in the UK', in Federalism and the Response to COVID-19: A Comparative Analysis, ed. Rupak Chattopadhyay, Felix Knüpling, Diana Chebenova, Liam Whittington, and Phillip Gonzalez (Abingdon: Routledge, 2022), 229–238.
37. Ben Davies, Fanny Lalot, Linus Peitz, Maria S. Heering, Hilal Ozkececi, Jacinta Babaian, et al., 'Changes in Political Trust in Britain during the COVID-19 Pandemic in 2020: Integrated Public Opinion Evidence and Implications', Humanities & Social Sciences Communications 8, no. 166 (2021), https://www.nature.com/articles/s41599-021-00850-6.

health restrictions and re-opening compared to other European countries and that it lagged on vaccine rollout to adolescents and children.[38] As mentioned earlier, Sweden and the UK fall on one side of the spectrum of living with COVID to zero-COVID, and they very intentionally chose to prioritise certain individual liberties and freedoms over collective restrictions in an effort to abate the spread of the pandemic.

The story of the UK shows how having a strong social contract and precedent for the government's role in prioritising the health of its citizens is never enough to guarantee it stays that way going forward. The social contract is a fluid concept and relationship that needs to be consistently reassessed and adjusted for the time and the context.

Conclusion

Europe was one of the regions most visibly affected by the COVID-19 pandemic. Understanding how states responded and how the public reacted can be facilitated by thinking through the relationship between individuals and society put forward by the social contract. In the EU, there was little history of the regulatory body directly involving itself in matters of healthcare and public health. As such, it was not as much of a surprise when pandemic policies were driven by national governments. However, the EU does have the institutional and legal ability to respond to such a global health crisis, and there are many more lessons to be learnt if the future of public health harmonisation is to be strengthened in order to better serve the citizens of the bloc. The response of governments has also been varied due to the existing social contracts in place, often reflected in precedents in public health and health services provision, and due to emerging and changing public opinion on the role of government in public health, crises in general, and health policy. This chapter also highlights how many European countries struggled with inherent tension baked into their social contracts between guaranteeing health for their citizens and protecting personal liberties. This tension often complicated the pandemic response and will remain a challenge for addressing public health challenges in the future. Going forward, balancing the benefits of strict public health measures with the necessity of maintaining the public's trust should play a central role in determining responses to public health crises.

---

38. Yueqi Yang, 'Why Are U.K. Covid Cases So High Compared to the Rest of Europe?' *Bloomberg*, 18 October 2021, https://www.bloomberg.com/news/articles/2021-10-18/u-k-falls-behind-europe-on-covid-19-as-mutation-draws-focus-kuwlrzjo.

13

Observations and Conclusion

Christine Loh with contributions from other authors

COVID-19 has been a humbling experience. Many experts from around the world have written about the large number of lessons that could be drawn from the pandemic. The most obvious overarching lesson is that authorities around the world need to do the right things and do them right very quickly whenever there is an infectious disease outbreak. Speed is important because of the mathematics of exponential spread.

COVID-19 was a shock to the world, but a pandemic should not have been a surprise. Many countries had pandemic plans on the shelf—the risk of a pandemic is a 'known known'—but having plans is one thing, rolling them out successfully is another matter altogether.

A new coronavirus, named SARS-CoV-2, was first identified in China at the very end of 2019 and by 20 January 2020, China was going all-out to fight this highly transmissible disease. A number of countries and jurisdictions took early effective action by closing borders and imposing testing, tracing, and various social distancing restrictions to cut the spread of the virus. Many others did not. Once the World Health Organization (WHO) declared COVID-19 a pandemic in mid-March 2020, communities around the world went into lockdowns with enormous social and economic consequences. The speed and magnitude of the 'big pause' were disconcerting—there was nothing like it in living memory.

COVID-19 became more than a public health threat—it was an economic threat, as most people became homebound; and a social threat, as family life and many work and social activities had to adapt, in-person events were cancelled, and social gatherings discouraged or even disallowed. Schools were closed for an extended period and children all around the world lost many months of education. Tensions increased, particularly in places where the population was divided between those who stressed protecting the society from the pandemic (by lockdowns and other stringent public health measures), and those stressing individual freedom. COVID-19 was a political threat too. The emergence of a new disease accompanied by high fatalities and deaths, the scale and speed of its impact, and the myriad terrifying unfolding outcomes in real time tested every leader and health system—many failed in controlling transmission when the opportunity was there in the early days. Cases and fatalities continued to mount. Governments had to step in with massive subsidies to help people through tough times as economies collapsed. COVID-19 went into a second year and new variants emerged, creating renewed havoc. Vaccines became available at the start of the second year in richer economies and were crucial to bringing about a certain level of immunity and reducing mortality rates as public health measures were progressively relaxed. The pandemic recovery was interrupted by subvariants of Omicron in the third year of the pandemic in 2022 that continued to disrupt lives, business, travel, and global supply chains.

This concluding chapter provides insights from the authors of this book. While some of the chapters contain specific recommendations relevant to the topic under discussion, the purpose of this chapter is to pull key general insights together. COVID-19 was and remains a deeply personal experience. We all know people whose lives were disrupted by the pandemic. Indeed, our own lives had been disrupted.

Choices Are Political

The COVID-19 pandemic provided examples from around the world of what to do and what not to do. Chapters 9 to 12 show the diversity of the responses to the pandemic in Greater China (Mainland China, Hong Kong, Macao, and Taiwan), the United States, Europe, and the United Kingdom. Those chapters seek to explain through the lens of good governance why various countries reacted so differently. Chapter 7 looks at the socio-economic consequences of COVID-19—the pandemic was extremely expensive for the world.

A number of factors were at play: firstly, the concept of the 'social contract' had a role in the governance practices of a jurisdiction. An element of good governance is that governments are supposed to be at least somewhat prepared for known risks ahead of time. People will often accept constraints and inconveniences for the greater good, especially in emergencies. Chapter 6 provides a discussion about the concept of the social contract and its relevance in good governance and political decision-making (although it is unclear that this stage what contribution the pandemic may make to the concept of the social contract), while Chapters 9 to 12 discuss how it manifested itself in various jurisdictions in light of COVID-19.

Second, political trust was important too (see Chapter 1). Those societies where the people trusted the government's performance and/or trusted each other to act in the public interest were more willing to abide by restrictions in crises. Research showed the level of political trust was a useful indicator of a successful response to COVID-19. On the whole, the Greater China and Asia-Pacific jurisdictions had higher political trust in governments and/or within society. In Europe, some countries had higher political trust than others and those with higher trust tended to do better in their pandemic response, as government and citizens were better aligned. Societies with low political trust were more polarised and less accepting of pandemic restrictions. The lesson here is political and socio-cultural systems that encourage the reduction of division would help in emergencies, such as dealing with a pandemic.

Third, leaders and governments have to make political choices when facing several waves of outbreaks with respect to COVID-19. The quality of leadership affected the response. Chapter 5 shows transmission of a disease needs to be contained quickly; otherwise, exponential growth can become unstoppable. Reducing the rate of spread at an earlier point in an epidemic cut the incidence of the disease dramatically. Those who acted early reaped the benefits in both public health and socio-economic terms. Staying vigilant for over three years tested every jurisdiction and its leaders. Chapter 7 notes rich economies threw money at the problem to provide massive subsidies that often did not reach those most in need. Poor economies had few options.

Preparedness vs. Leadership

The quality of leadership and governance practices at the time of crisis made the difference. COVID-19 showed a new infectious disease outbreak requires the immediate application of very tough actions from governments. Acting decisively and mobilising available resources, even in lower-income economies and irrespective of the type of political system, made a measurable difference in terms of infections and deaths.

The Global Health Security Index 2019 (GHSI 2019), published on the eve of the COVID-19 outbreak, noted that the world as a whole was poorly prepared (see Chapter 1). According to its ranking method, the United States and the United Kingdom came out as the top two countries with respect to the potential they had to deal with a pandemic. That potential may have been there, but preparedness simulations carried out by those two countries in recent years showed how unprepared they were. The United Kingdom's *Exercise Cygnus* in 2016, and America's *Crimson Contagion* in 2019, identified serious failures in many areas of pandemic preparedness. The United States and the United Kingdom turned out to be among the worst performers in the first two years of the pandemic. The GHSI continued to use the same assessment method after COVID-19 had already emerged for its 2021 report (GHSI 2021). The United States remained in first place, while the United Kingdom dropped to seventh place, still ranking ahead of others who did very much better. The countries that did well were in the Greater China and Asia-Pacific regions of diverse political systems and cultures, encompassing rich and middle- and lower-income countries. The designers of the GHSI acknowledged in GHSI 2019 and GHSI 2021 that their ranking systems could not assess the quality of leadership needed in times of emergency, which is understandable for such an index— but going forward, it may be better if the GHSI did not rank countries against each other and focused instead on how a country progresses without reference to others. High scores may give leaders an unrealistic sense of confidence.

Case for a Strong Initial Reaction

During the SARS outbreak in 2003, Dr Henk Bekedam, then the director of Health Sector Development, WHO, Western Pacific Regional Office, made it clear that to fight an infectious disease outbreak, one cannot be just 100 per cent ready, one needs to be 300 per cent ready. COVID-19 reminded us that with every outbreak, it is challenging to have a fully accurate risk assessment at the start of the outbreak. It is, therefore, prudent to act quickly and be ready for the worst—that is, the disease could be a highly transmissible and virulent disease. However, governments may not want people to panic and there can be resistance to applying tough restrictions in the early stages of a new outbreak, as the disease may not turn out to be of great concern. Stringent actions may turn out to be an overreaction. This is a universal phenomenon albeit with different cultural manifestations. The problem is no one knows at the start of an outbreak what the disease would be like. If COVID-19 taught us anything, it is that we do need to be prepared to react strongly.

Therefore, preparedness should surely mean having the governance capacity and capability to react aggressively at the beginning of an outbreak. Closing borders or reducing travel intensity initially can buy time for a more complete risk assessment. Other preparedness measures that would be important in the early days of the next pandemic—if not before—include building capacity in advance of an outbreak for testing and tracing, having sufficient personal protective equipment (PPE) for frontline health workers, and providing consistent messaging that gives information that helps people to stay calm because they are informed about what to expect and do rather than to tell people they don't need to worry—'it's just the flu'. The COVID-19 experience showed many examples at the start of the outbreak of what to do and what to avoid in diverse political systems and richer and poorer economies. Leaders in Greater China, Singapore, South Korea, Thailand, Vietnam, Australia, and New Zealand provided good examples of acting quickly and messaging clearly, while leaders in the United States and the United Kingdom took considerable time to acknowledge the seriousness of the outbreak and acted late.

Perhaps something similar to extreme weather warning systems could be developed for infectious diseases, where people become familiar with what to do as signals are issued. Hong Kong's typhoon warning system is an example of a successful, long-standing system where residents understand what to do as higher signals are posted alongside well-practised explanations about the likely trajectory of the typhoon, and what people should be aware of and be ready for. The Hong Kong signalling system is designed by meteorological experts and signals are raised in accordance with set conditions and not by politicians. Once a signal is posted, institutions and the public know what they need to do. Obviously, an infectious disease outbreak communication system would have to be designed differently, but once there is a system, people can get used to it and a standardised governance system can be developed. The advantage of such a system is that it is managed by subject experts.

Bringing the COVID-19 Pandemic to an End

As noted in Chapter 4, investing in COVID-19 vaccines and antiviral drugs was worthwhile. Having effective vaccines and drugs that became available in the second year of the pandemic meant that public health measures could be used more sparingly. Many higher-income countries achieved high levels of vaccination uptake in adults by early 2022, with third and even fourth and fifth doses being offered to maintain those high levels of protection. When breakthrough infections do occur in vaccinated individuals, they tend to be mild, and the high levels of population immunity conferred by vaccinations and also natural infections in most parts of the world meant that COVID-19 posed much less of a threat from 2022 onwards than it did earlier in the pandemic. However, when the Omicron variant emerged in late 2021, although it was seen as a milder variant, its increased rate of transmission and ability to evade prior immunity led to many infections occurring in a very short space of time. Even though each of those infections was—on average—milder, there were so many infections that the number of serious cases requiring hospital care at the epidemic peak still reached or exceeded levels in previous epidemics in some locations.

As time goes by, ensuring that vaccine coverage remains high will be a priority. One of the challenges for governments is to get the most vulnerable groups vaccinated early—this was far from easy in the light of the vaccine hesitancy experienced in many jurisdictions. In economies where vaccines are available, instead of monitoring the proportion of the population with two doses, three doses, or four doses, attention might instead switch to monitoring the proportion of older adults who have had a vaccination dose within say the last six months and encouraging regular booster doses to keep immunity at higher levels. It is likely that COVID-19 will continue to circulate; what is less clear is how frequently new variants or subvariants will emerge. We cannot rule out the possibility that some public health measures will have to be re-instituted to deal with resurgences in COVID-19 transmission perhaps in upcoming winters in temperate locations. In other words, in fighting infectious diseases, vaccines are not necessarily the silver bullet—they become part of a package of political, social, and economic measures that are needed in the arsenal.

Mathematics for Policy-makers

Chapter 5 provides a thorough discussion of the mathematics of infectious diseases, including the use of mathematical epidemiological models to predict the effects of alternative policies to contain the spread of the disease. In the early stage of an outbreak, reducing the rate of spread cuts the number of cases, which lowers the pressure on hospitals and reduces fatalities—and also reduces adverse economic impacts. In the later stages of the epidemic, especially if a vaccine or a medication is developed that reduces infectiousness, the models forecast a slowdown in growth and eventually dwindling numbers of cases. In this phase, the same models help to decide which segment of the population should be vaccinated first, where hospital facilities, healthcare workers, and medical equipment need to be increased (or can be decreased) and other actions.

Even more important than deploying mathematical models during an epidemic should be deploying them before the next epidemic. Running mathematical models without the stress of having to keep up with a concurrent pandemic and benefiting from the robust data sets obtained from the last pandemic and those before it, should enable the models to be more accurate than they could be while a pandemic is raging. Alternative public policy scenarios can be tested, including branching decision processes constructed in a kind of a flow chart, in which a public policy is tried early when disease parameters are not well known yet, and responses both from the disease and the public can be gauged—and alternative paths of the branching process taken depending on the response of the disease and the public. Giving as much attention to this process in advance of the next pandemic as was paid to it during the last one should enable the world to be much better prepared for the next one.

Managing PPE Supplies and Emergency Products

Chapter 8 emphasises the vital importance of having adequate PPE supplies for health workers during a pandemic as a matter of good governance. If health workers are not adequately protected, it can lead to the breakdown of the healthcare system at a time of massive demand. The authors used the United States, the world's richest economy, for their investigation, which holds a lesson for many other economies, especially those that do not produce PPE domestically or have little production capacity to do so. While the chapter focuses on PPE, the same could be said for other products vital in health emergencies.

Good governance in public health security must include policies that identify the range of goods that are required for a pandemic because that is when there is massive global demand for the same goods at the same time. Therefore, having some capacity for domestic production that could be ramped up quickly represents good governance. Hence, policies are needed for governments to work with reliable domestic producers even if they are of higher cost than imports. This approach involves elements of an industrial policy, as developing manufacturing capacity requires enabling an 'ecosystem' of designers, R&D centres, engineers, production engineers, and technicians that can be deployed to scale up production in times of need.

In the United States and others in similar situations, where domestic brands produce PPE overseas, governments could also consider policies to encourage companies to create hybrid supply chain structures to support domestic firms to sustain their global supply chains that serve the healthcare markets around the globe. Policies could also consider encouraging companies to bring back at least some of their offshore manufacturing capacity. It would not be practical to massively reshore manufacturing operations, as reshoring requires companies to develop many capabilities at scale, but they would benefit from hybrid supply chains with the flexibility to operate their supply chain in a cost-effective or time-efficient manner. Even if capacity is created domestically, raw materials and/or intermediate products may still have to depend on imports. A possible solution is for policies to provide R&D support to develop new materials and innovative production processes to ensure a shorter domestic supply chain. In addition, most economies have some sort of PPE stockpiling arrangement to determine the amount of inventory needed in case of a future pandemic. The procurement process should consider the value of the product (e.g., quality, whole lifecycle cost, and environmental cost). Doing so can create incentives for domestic companies to develop and produce innovative PPE products.

A lesson from COVID-19 is that governments must consider how citizens can help curb the spread of future viruses. The availability of affordable at-home rapid test kits can make individual responsibility easier to bear, as people could test themselves at home and take steps to avoid spreading the virus. Hence, easy-to-use home-testing kits could be another essential pandemic product. Policies should also include a communication strategy with online platforms to enable a coordinated response to quickly identify and match supply sources and demand locations on the one hand, and allow individual citizens and citizen groups to coordinate on the other hand.

Importance of Global Health Governance

A vital part of global health security and governance is provided by the WHO. As the author of Chapter 2 asks: If not the WHO, then who? Chapter 2 provides an extensive discussion of recommendations that have been made before and during the COVID-19 pandemic—as many ideas relating to improving the WHO are not new. Reforms will not come immediately, but if the discussion is delayed, then the danger is that the momentum and urgency might wane, as it has in the past.

There is a strong case to be made for strengthening the existing WHO, which operates by consensus of its member states who come together at regular meetings to review matters. One measure is to agree on a new pandemic treaty under the WHO. Issues that are on the table include:

More open governance: The governance of the WHO could be reformed to include more voices as non-voting non-state actors in the WHO's governing body, such as from non-government and philanthropic institutions.

Widen expertise: The WHO could maintain its technical focus but could broaden its expertise to include more input from political scientists, urban designers, lawyers, logisticians, philosophers, economists, and information technology specialists.

Reporting system: There are many practical suggestions regarding future pandemic outbreaks, such as defining a pandemic more precisely, and using a gradient of warnings to encourage countries to share information.

Financial resources: Funding the WHO represents value for money—for every US$1 invested in it, the WHO provides a return of US$35 in societal value. Member states are in principle agreeable to improving the WHO financing model and giving it more flexibility to deliver on its mandate.

The next step in creating a new pandemic treaty involves more negotiations and consultation hearings with a progress report to be delivered to the WHO's 2023 World Health Assembly, and an outcome document for the assembly in 2024.

Protect Public Health Policy from Harmful Industries

Beyond infectious diseases and pandemics, non-communicable diseases (NCD) are growing in relevance, currently causing 60 per cent of global deaths. Some voices have called for the role of the WHO to be cut back to focus on infectious diseases, which would limit global governance on NCDs and other threats to wellbeing. It became clear during the COVID-19 pandemic that harmful industries, most notably tobacco, took advantage of the situation to promote their businesses that related to NCDs. Chapter 3 provides an in-depth discussion of that exploitation and hence its relevance in a book about the experience of COVID-19. The key message is that governments should have a whole-of-government approach to protect public health policy against tobacco and other harmful industries, especially during epidemics and pandemics.

Chapter 3 provides specific recommendations that include governments being aware that they must stop interactions with those negative industries and reject their corporate social responsibility activities, as those are a form of promotion and/or method to gain influence in a crisis. Needless to say, governments must reject any form of agreement to collaborate, and there should not be any incentives or preferential treatment given to those industries. State-owned tobacco enterprises should be treated like any other tobacco company, and governments should divest from the tobacco industry. It would be helpful for governments to implement a code of conduct with clear guidance on interactions with the tobacco industry. Indeed, there is no reason why the tobacco industry should not be compelled to provide information about its business, marketing, lobbying, and philanthropic activities in order to enhance transparency for greater accountability. Non-government organisations must continue to be encouraged to research and expose industry interference with public health policy. While they can research and expose the industry, it is the governments that are ultimately responsible for curtailing unhealthy industries and their influence on public health policy.

Finger Pointing Is Unhelpful

There has been too much unhelpful politicising and moralising. COVID-19 tested every leader and government. Humility and cooperation are needed to deal with the various Omicron subvariants, which are continuing to spread. Hence, the post-pandemic picture was murky as this book went to print at the end of 2022. The Russia-Ukraine war that started on 24 February 2022 has created many more disruptions and uncertainties, and it has also heightened geopolitical tensions that are affecting relations between the major powers in the world. The temptation to use COVID-19 to finger-point at opponents should be resisted, as it would be unhelpful. We need to call upon our better angels to enhance the potential for cooperation.

US-China Cooperation Is Better Than Conflict

Chapter 9 asked what level of cooperation may still be possible at a time of intensifying conflict between China and the United States. The very poor state of relations between them has a major spill-over effect on the world, as they are the two major powers with enormous capabilities in many areas of technology and production. They have a combined share of about 45 per cent of the world's GDP.

The two countries have a history of collaboration that has fallen by the wayside in the light of deteriorating relations. Notably, the experience of SARS in 2003 led to expanded health cooperation between China and United States, and between China and the wider international community. China and the United States forged a multi-year partnership through the Chinese Ministry of Health, renamed the National Health Commission in 2018, and the US Department of Health and Human Services (HHS). The United States established a health attaché at its embassy in Beijing in 2003, which was the main point of contact for health diplomacy.

The year 2005 was particularly noteworthy: China and the United States established a Joint Initiative on Avian Influenza, they inaugurated the Collaborative Program on Emerging and Re-emerging Infectious Diseases, and they also established the US–China Health Care Forum to address bilateral commercial, trade, and policy issues relating to health. In 2006, the then Ministry of Health and HHS further expanded their collaboration on biomedical research with a memorandum of understanding on research, technology, training, and personnel exchange, as well as cooperation on HIV/AIDS. Cooperation between the two countries also moved beyond bilateral governmental cooperation to the participation of non-governmental philanthropic organisations that funded health projects. With respect to the H1N1 pandemic in 2009, China and the United States shared information and technology to facilitate national monitoring of influenza spread and vaccine development, and China became the first country to roll out an H1N1 vaccine. In 2009, the two countries pledged to 'deepen cooperation on global public health issues, including human and avian influenza prevention, surveillance, reporting and control, and on HIV/AIDS, tuberculosis, and malaria'. The outbreak of the Ebola virus in West Africa in 2014 posed a new global health challenge for the world community. The cooperation between China and the United States was helpful beyond their own borders, including their expert teams collaborating on the ground in Africa, and it led to further mutual pledges to 'leverage our respective strength and work with the rest of the international community to help affected countries to strengthen capacity-building on health and epidemic prevention so as to place the epidemic under control as soon as possible'.

The current concern is that while much can be done through cooperation, COVID-19 could be further politicised, and this will stand in the way of cooperation. Some obvious steps in a positive direction include reviving the US-China Health Care Forum and the Collaborative Program on Emerging and Re-emerging Infectious Diseases to help with identifying the origin of COVID-19, collaborating on biosecurity laboratory standards, and the mass production and distribution of COVID-19 vaccines in low-income economies, just to name a few.

Further Reading

Chapter 2

Chaumont, C. 'Opinion: 5 Ways to Reform the World Health Organization'. *Devex*, 5 August 2020. https://www.devex.com/news/opinion-5-ways-to-reform-the-world-health-organization-97843.

Gavi. 'COVAX'. Accessed 9 September 2022. https://www.gavi.org/covax-facility.

Gostin, Lawrence O., Harold Hongju Koh, Michelle Williams, Margaret A. Hamburg, Georges Benjamin, William H Foege, et al. 'US Withdrawal from WHO Is Unlawful and Threatens Global and US Health and Security'. *Lancet* 396, no. 10247 (1 August 2020): 293–295. https://www.thelancet.com/journals/lancet/article/PIIS0140-6736(20)31527-0/fulltext.

McKee, Martin. 'Coronavirus Has Killed 30,000 Americans, and All Trump Can Do Is Blame the WHO'. *Guardian*, 16 April 2020. https://www.theguardian.com/world/commentisfree/2020/apr/16/coronavirus-30000-americans-trump-blame-who.

Maxmen, Amy. 'Why Did the World's Pandemic Warning System Fail When COVID-19 Hit?'. *Nature*, 23 January 2021. https://www.nature.com/articles/d41586-021-00162-4.

Ravelo, Jenny Lei. 'On His First Day in Office, Biden Retracts US Withdrawal from WHO'. *Devex*, 21 January 2021. https://www.devex.com/news/on-his-first-day-in-office-biden-retracts-us-withdrawal-from-who-98961.

STOP. 'Trading "Philanthropy" for Favors: Tobacco Industry CSR During COVID-19'. 17 August 2020. https://exposetobacco.org/news/ban-ti-csr/?utm_source=Stopping+Tobacco+Organizations+and+Products+%28STOP%29&utm_campaign=891101c19c-Stop_Newsletter_8.25.20&utm_medium=email&utm_term=0_a7474fe40f-891101c19c-354163305#utm_source=mailchimp&utm_medium=email&utm_campaign=COVID-19-accountability.

United Nations. 'United Nations Comprehensive Response to COVID-19'. June 2020. https://www.un.org/sites/un2.un.org/files/un_comprehensive_response_to_COVID-19-19_june_2020.pdf.

United Nations Development Programme. 'COVID-19 Pandemic'. Accessed 9 September 2022. https://www.undp.org/coronavirus.

World Bank. 'World Bank Group's Operational Response to COVID-19 (Coronavirus)—Projects List'. 24 September 2021. https://www.worldbank.org/en/about/what-we-do/brief/world-bank-group-operational-response-COVID-19-coronavirus-projects-list.

World Health Organization. 'Coronavirus Disease (COVID-19) Pandemic'. Accessed 9 September 2022. https://www.who.int/emergencies/diseases/novel-coronavirus-2019.

World Health Organization. 'COVAX: Working for Global Equitable Access to COVID-19 Vaccines'. Accessed 9 September 2022. https://www.who.int/initiatives/act-accelerator/covax.

World Health Organization. 'How WHO Is Funded'. Accessed 9 September 2022. https://www.who.int/about/funding.

Chapter 3

Assunta, Mary. 'Global Tobacco Industry Interference Index 2021'. Global Center for Good Governance in Tobacco Control. Bangkok, Thailand. November 2021. https://exposetobacco.org/global-index/.

Campaign for Tobacco Free Kids. 'Big Tobacco Is Exploiting COVID-19 to Market Its Harmful Products'. Accessed 9 September 2022. https://www.tobaccofreekids.org/media/2020/2020_05_COVID-marketing.

Collin, Jeff, Rob Ralston, Sarah Hill, and Lucinda Westerman. 'Signalling Virtue, Promoting Harm: Unhealthy Commodity Industries and COVID-19'. NCD Alliance, SPECTRUM. 2020. https://ncdalliance.org/sites/default/files/resource_files/Signalling%20Virtue%2C%20Promoting%20Harm_Sept2020_FINALv.pdf.

STOP (Stopping Tobacco Organizations and Products). 'Tobacco Industry Involvement in COVID-19 Science'. Tobacco Tactics. Accessed 9 September 2022. https://tobaccotactics.org/wiki/COVID-19/#database.

World Health Organization. 'Article 5.3'. Framework Convention on Tobacco Control. Accessed 9 September 2022. https://fctc.who.int/who-fctc/overview.

World Health Organization. 'Commercial Determinants of Health'. 5 November 2021. https://www.who.int/news-room/fact-sheets/detail/commercial-determinants-of-health.

Chapter 5

Acevedo, Miguel A., P. Forrest, P. Dillemuth, Andrew J. Flick, Matthew J. Faldyn, and Bret D. Elderd. 'Virulence-Driven Trade-Offs in Disease Transmission: A Meta-analysis'. *Evolution* 73, no. 4 (2019): 636–647.

Adam, David. 'The Effort to Count the Pandemic's Global Death Toll'. *Nature* 601 (2022): 312–315.

Alizon, Samuel, Amy Hurford, Nicole Mideo, and Minus Van Baalen. 'Virulence Evolution and the Trade-Off Hypothesis: History, Current State of Affairs and the Future'. *Journal of Evolutionary Biology* 22, no. 2 (2009): 245–259.

Alizon, Samuel, and Yannis Michalakis. 'Adaptive Virulence Evolution: The Good Old Fitness-Based Approach'. *Trends in Ecology & Evolution* 30, no. 5 (2015): 248–254.

Anastassopoulou, Cleo, Lucia Russo, Athanasios Tsakris, and Constantinos Siettos. 'Data-Based Analysis, Modelling and Forecasting of the COVID-19 Outbreak'. *PloS ONE* 15, no. 3 (2020): e0230405.

Anderson, Roy M., and Robert M. May. 'Coevolution of Hosts and Parasites'. *Parasitology* 85, no. 2 (1982): 411–426.

Brauer, Fred. 'Compartmental Models in Epidemiology.' In *Mathematical Epidemiology*, edited by Fred Brauer, Pauline van den Driessche, and Jianhong Wu, 19–79. Heidelberg: Springer Berlin, 2008.

Burki, Talha. 'China's Successful Control of COVID-19.' *The Lancet Infectious Diseases* 20, no. 11 (2020): 1240–1241.

Cowling, Benjamin J., Sheikh Taslim Ali, Tiffany W. Y. Ng, Tim K. Tsang, Julian C. M. Li, Min Whui Fong, et al. 'Impact Assessment of Non-Pharmaceutical Interventions against Coronavirus Disease 2019 and Influenza in Hong Kong: An Observational Study.' *The Lancet Public Health* 5, no. 5 (2020): e279–e288.

Cressler, Clayton E., David V. McLeod, Carly Rozins, Josée Van Den Hoogen, and Troy Day. 'The Adaptive Evolution of Virulence: A Review of Theoretical Predictions and Empirical Tests.' *Parasitology* 143, no. 7 (2016): 915–930.

Doumayrou, Juliette, Astrid Avellan, Rémy Froissart, and Yannis Michalakis. 'An Experimental Test of the Transmission-Virulence Trade-Off Hypothesis in a Plant Virus.' *Evolution: International Journal of Organic Evolution* 67, no. 2 (2013): 477–486.

Endo, Akira. 'Implication of Backward Contact Tracing in the Presence of Overdispersed Transmission in COVID-19 Outbreaks.' *Wellcome Open Research* 5 (2020): 239. https://doi.org/10.12688/wellcomeopenres.16344.3.

Endo, A., S. Abbott, A. J. Kucharski, and S. Funk. 'Estimating the Overdispersion in COVID-19 Transmission Using Outbreak Sizes outside China.' *Wellcome Open Res.* 5 (2020): 67. https://doi.org/10.12688/wellcomeopenres.15842.3.

Ewald, Paul W. 'Host-Parasite Relations, Vectors, and the Evolution of Disease Severity.' *Annual Review of Ecology and Systematics* 14, no. 1 (1983): 465–485.

Ferguson, Neil M., Daniel Laydon, Gemma Nedjati-Gilani, Natsuko Imai, Kylie Ainslie, Marc Baguelin, et al. 'Impact of Non-pharmaceutical Interventions (NPIs) to Reduce COVID-19 Mortality and Healthcare Demand.' Imperial College London, 16 March 2020. https://www.imperial.ac.uk/mrc-global-infectious-disease-analysis/covid-19/report-9-impact-of-npis-on-covid-19.

Ferguson, Neil M., Derek A. T. Cummings, Christophe Fraser, James C. Cajka, Philip C. Cooley, and Donald S. Burke. 'Strategies for Mitigating an Influenza Pandemic.' *Nature* 442, no. 7101 (2006): 448–452.

Germann, Timothy C., Kai Kadau, Ira M. Longini, and Catherine A. Macken. 'Mitigation Strategies for Pandemic Influenza in the United States.' *Proceedings of the National Academy of Sciences* 103, no. 15 (2006): 5935–5940.

Ghani, Azra C., Christl A. Donnelly, David R. Cox, J. T. Griffin, C. Fraser, T. H. Lam, et al. 'Methods for Estimating the Case Fatality Ratio for a Novel, Emerging Infectious Disease.' *American Journal of Epidemiology* 162, no. 5 (2005): 479–486.

Goldman, Emanuel. 'How the Unvaccinated Threaten the Vaccinated for COVID-19: A Darwinian Perspective.' *Proceedings of the National Academy of Sciences of the United States of America* 118, no. 39 (2021): e2114279118. https://doi.org/10.1073/pnas.2114279118.

Guan, Wei-jie, Zheng-yi Ni, Yu Hu, Wen-hua Liang, Chun-quan Ou, Jian-xing He, et al. 'Clinical Characteristics of Coronavirus Disease 2019 in China.' *New England Journal of Medicine* 382, no. 18 (2020): 1708–1720.

Hethcote, Herbert W. 'The Mathematics of Infectious Diseases.' *SIAM Review* 42, no. 4 (2000): 599–653.

Huang, Chaolin, Yeming Wang, Xingwang Li, Lili Ren, Jianping Zhao, Yi Hu, et al. 'Clinical Features of Patients Infected with 2019 Novel Coronavirus in Wuhan, China'. *The Lancet* 395, no. 10223 (2020): 497–506.

IHME COVID-19 Health Service Utilization Forecasting Team and Christopher J. L. Murray. 'Forecasting COVID-19 Impact on Hospital Bed-Days, ICU-Days, Ventilator-Days and Deaths by US State in the Next 4 Months'. *medRxiv* (2020). https://doi.org/10.1101/202 0.03.27.20043752.

Kucharski, Adam. *The Rules of Contagion: Why Things Spread—And Why They Stop*. New York: Basic Books, 2020.

Leung, Kathy, Joseph T. Wu, and Gabriel M. Leung. 'Real-Time Tracking and Prediction of COVID-19 Infection Using Digital Proxies of Population Mobility and Mixing'. *Nature Communications* 12, no. 1 (2021): 1–8.

Li, Qun, Xuhua Guan, Peng Wu, Xiaoye Wang, Lei Zhou, Yeqing Tong, et al. 'Early Transmission Dynamics in Wuhan, China, of Novel Coronavirus–Infected Pneumonia'. *New England Journal of Medicine* 382 (2020): 1199–1207. https://doi.org/10.1056/NEJMoa2001316.

Liu, Ying, Albert A. Gayle, Annelies Wilder-Smith, and Joacim Rocklöv. 'The Reproductive Number of COVID-19 Is Higher Compared to SARS Coronavirus'. *Journal of Travel Medicine* 27, no. 2 (2020). https://doi.org/10.1093/jtm/taaa021.

Lloyd-Smith, James O., Sebastian J. Schreiber, P. Ekkehard Kopp, and Wayne M. Getz. 'Superspreading and the Effect of Individual Variation on Disease Emergence'. *Nature* 438, no. 7066 (2005): 355–359.

Master, Ryan K., Laudan Y. Aron, and Steven H. Woolf. 'Changes in Life Expectancy between 2019 and 2021: United States And 19 Peer Countries'. *medRxiv* (2022). https://doi.org/1 0.1101/2022.04.05.22273393.

Méthot, Pierre-Olivier. 'Why Do Parasites Harm Their Host? On the Origin and Legacy of Theobald Smith's "Law of Declining Virulence"—1900–1980'. *History and Philosophy of the Life Sciences* (2012): 561–601.

Mossong, Joël, Niel Hens, Mark Jit, Philippe Beutels, Kari Auranen, Rafael Mikolajczyk, et al. 'Social Contacts and Mixing Patterns Relevant to the Spread of Infectious Diseases'. *PLoS medicine* 5, no. 3 (2008): e74. https://doi.org/10.1371/journal.pmed.0050074.

Park, Minah, Alex R. Cook, Jue Tao Lim, Yinxiaohe Sun, and Borame L. Dickens. 'A Systematic Review of COVID-19 Epidemiology Based on Current Evidence'. *Journal of Clinical Medicine* 9, no. 4 (2020): 967. https://doi.org/10.3390/jcm9040967.

Tolles, Juliana, and ThaiBinh Luong. 'Modeling Epidemics with Compartmental Models'. *Jama* 323, no. 24 (2020): 2515–2516.

Tufekci, Zeynep. 'This Overlooked Variable Is the Key to the Pandemic'. *The Atlantic* 30 (2020). https://www.theatlantic.com/health/archive/2020/09/k-overlooked-variable-driving-pandemic/616548/.

Tuite, Ashleigh R., and David N. Fisman. 'Reporting, Epidemic Growth, and Reproduction Numbers for the 2019 Novel Coronavirus (2019-nCoV) Epidemic'. *Annals of Internal Medicine* 172, no. 8 (2020): 567–568.

Walker, Patrick G. T., Charles Whittaker, Oliver J. Watson, Marc Baguelin, Peter Winskill, Arran Hamlet, et al. 'The Impact of COVID-19 and Strategies for Mitigation and Suppression in Low- and Middle-Income Countries'. *Science* 369, no. 6502 (2020): 413–422.

Wu, Joseph T., Kathy Leung, and Gabriel M. Leung. 'Nowcasting and Forecasting the Potential Domestic and International Spread of the 2019-nCoV Outbreak Originating in Wuhan, China: A Modelling Study'. *The Lancet* 395, no. 10225 (2020): 689–697.

Wu, Joseph T., Kathy Leung, Mary Bushman, Nishant Kishore, Rene Niehus, Pablo M. de Salazar, Benjamin J. Cowling, et al. 'Estimating Clinical Severity of COVID-19 from the Transmission Dynamics in Wuhan, China'. *Nature Medicine* 26, no. 4 (2020): 506–510.

Zhou, Yibiao, Honglin Jiang, Quanyi Wang, Meixia Yang, Yue Chen, and Qingwu Jiang. 'Use of Contact Tracing, Isolation, and Mass Testing to Control Transmission of Covid-19 in China'. *bmj* 375 (2021): n2330. https://doi.org/10.1136/bmj.n2330.

Chapter 7

Gates, Bill. *How to Prevent the Next Pandemic*. New York: Knopf, 2022.

Smil, Vaclav. *How the World Really Works: The Science Behind How We Got Here and Where We're Going*. New York: Viking, 2022.

Tooze, Adam. *Shutdown: How Covid Shook the World's Economy*. New York: Viking, 2021.

Chapter 8

Bender, M., and R. Ballhaus. 'How Trump Sowed Covid Supply Chaos'. *Wall Street Journal*, 31 August 2020.

Chandler, K. 'Oregon Gets Old, Faulty Masks; Other States Get Faulty Equipment from National Stockpile'. Katu.com, 14 April 2020. https://katu.com/news/coronavirus/oregon-gets-old-faulty-masks-other-states-get-flawed-equipment-from-national-stockpile.

Choi, T., D. Rogers, and B. Vakil. 'Coronavirus Is a Wake-Up Call for Supply Chain Management'. *Harvard Business Review*, 27 March 2020. https://hbr.org/2020/03/coronavirus-is-a-wake-up-call-for-supply-chain-management.

Cohen, D. 'Why a PPE Shortage Still Plagues America and What We Need to Do about it'. CNBC News. 22 August 2020. https://www.cnbc.com/2020/08/22/coronavirus-why-a-ppe-shortage-still-plagues-the-us.html.

Dai, T. L., and C. S. Tang. 'Needed: A PPE Industrial Commons'. EE Times. 27 May 2020. https://www.eetimes.com/needed-a-ppe-industrial-commons/#.

Dai, T. L., and C. S. Tang. 'The U.S. Medical Supply Chain Isn't Ready for a Second Wave'. *Barron's*, 28 June 2020. https://www.barrons.com/articles/the-u-s-medical-supply-chain-isnt-ready-for-a-second-wave-51592953230.

Dwyer, C., and A. Aubrey. 'CDC Now Recommends Americans Consider Wearing Cloth Face Coverings in Public'. NPR News, 3 April 2020. https://www.npr.org/sections/coronavirus-live-updates/2020/04/03/826219824/president-trump-says-cdc-now-recommends-americans-wear-cloth-masks-in-public.

Feuer, W. 'House Panel Opens Probe of White House Trade Advisor Navarro after Abrupt Cancellation of Ventilator Contract'. CNBC News, 31 August 2020. https://www.cnbc.com/2020/08/31/coronavirus-house-panel-opens-probe-of-white-house-trade-advisor-navarro-after-cancellation-of-ventilator-contract.html.

Gardner, G., and E. Garsten. 'Trump Orders General Motors to Make Ventilators—After the Automaker Reiterated Plans Do So with Ventec'. *Forbes*, 27 March 2020. https://

www.forbes.com/sites/greggardner/2020/03/27/gm-ventec-press-forward-to-expand-ventilator-output-despite-trump-tweets/#1a62eb5429ab.

Hufford, A., M. Maremont, and L. Lin. 'Over 1,300 Chinese Medical Suppliers to U.S.—Including Mask Providers—Use Bogus Registration Data'. *Wall Street Journal*, 12 June 2020. https://www.wsj.com/articles/over-1-300-chinese-medical-suppliers-to-u-s-including-mask-providersuse-bogus-registration-data-11591991270?adobe_mc=MCMID%3D139 50680188438669153529629032510089933%7CMCORGID%3DCB68E4BA55144CA A0A4C98A5%2540AdobeOrg%7CTS%3D1599010920.

IFC Report. 'Covid-19—PPE Demand & Supply Perspectives'. March 2021. https://www.ifc.org/wps/wcm/connect/1d32e536-76cc-4023-9430-1333d6b92cc6/210402_FCDO_GlobalPPE_Final+report_v14updated_gja.pdf?MOD=AJPERES&CVID=nyiUnTU.

International Monetary Fund. 'A Crisis Like No Other, An Uncertain Recovery'. World Economic Outlook Update, June 2020. https://www.imf.org/en/Publications/WEO/Issues/2020/06/24/WEOUpdateJune2020.

Karlinsky, A., and D. Kobak. 'The World Mortality Dataset: Tracking Excess Mortality across Countries during the COVID-19 Pandemic, Version 3'. *medRxiv*. Preprint. Revised 4 June 2021. https://doi.org/10.1101/2021.01.27.21250604.

Lee, Ho-Jeong. 'Key Face Mask Material Can Now Be Exported'. *Korea JoongAng Daily*. 5 August 2020. https://koreajoongangdaily.joins.com/2020/08/05/business/economy/mask-mask-export-covid19/20200805160800954.html.

Loh, C., and C. S. Tang. 'HK versus Los Angeles: A Tale of Two Cities amid COVID-19'. 24 July 2020. https://www.chinadailyhk.com/article/137837#HK-versus-Los-Angeles:-A-tale-of-two-cities-amid-COVID-19.

Loh, C., and C. S. Tang. 'It's Time to Plan for a Messy U.S.-China Divorce'. *Barron's*, 10 June 2020. https://www.barrons.com/articles/the-u-s-is-headed-for-a-messy-china-divorce-without-a-plan-51591807403.

Loh, C., and C. S. Tang. 'Rather than Decouple, China and the US Must Find Ways to Coexist'. *South China Morning Post*, 21 June 2020. https://www.scmp.com/comment/opinion/article/3089651/rather-decouple-china-and-us-must-find-ways-coexist.

Ma, J. 'Coronavirus: China's First Confirmed Covid-19 Case Traced back to November 17'. *South China Morning Post*, 13 March 2020. https://www.scmp.com/news/china/society/article/3074991/coronavirus-chinas-first-confirmed-covid-19-case-traced-back.

Nickelsburg, M. 'Ventec and GM, 2 Months Later: How a Startup Took on the Ventilator Shortage, and Where It Stands Now'. GeekWire, 2 June 2020. https://www.geekwire.com/2020/ventec-gm-2-months-later-startup-took-ventilator-shortage-stands-now.

O'Kane, S. 'How GM and Ford Switched out Pickup Trucks for Breathing Machines'. The Verge, 15 April 2020. https://www.theverge.com/2020/4/15/21222219/general-motors-ventec-ventilators-ford-tesla-coronavirus-covid-19.

Pisano, G. P., and W. Shih. 'Restoring American Competitiveness'. *Harvard Business Review*. July–August 2009.

Reich, R. 'Why the U.S. Needs an Industrial Policy'. *Harvard Business Review*. January 1982.

Sanger, D., Z. Kanno-Youngs, and N. Kulish. 'A Ventilator Stockpile, with One Hitch: Thousands Do Not Work'. *New York Times*, 1 April 2020.

Schmidt, C., and Undark. 'Coronavirus Researchers Tried to Warn Us'. *The Atlantic*, 13 June 2020. https://www.theatlantic.com/health/archive/2020/06/scientists-predicted-coronavirus-pandemic/613003.

Siddiqui, F. 'The U.S. Forced Major Manufacturers to Build Ventilators. Now They're Piling Up Unused in a Strategic Reserve'. *Washington Post*, 18 August 2020. https://www.washingtonpost.com/business/2020/08/18/ventilators-coronavirus-stockpile.

Sodhi, M. S., and C. S. Tang. 'Build Capability, Not Just Stockpiles, to Fight Future Pandemics'. Working Paper, UCLA Anderson School of Management, 2020.

Sodhi, M. S., and C. S. Tang. *Managing Supply Chain Risks*. New York: Springer, 2012.

Sodhi, M.S., and C. S. Tang. 'Rethinking Industry's Role in a National Emergency'. *MIT Sloan Management Review*, 27 May 2021. https://sloanreview.mit.edu/article/rethinking-industrys-role-in-a-national-emergency.

Stone, W., and C. Feibel. 'COVID-19 Has Killed Close to 300 U.S. Health Care Workers, New Data from CDC Shows'. NPR News, 28 May 2020. https://www.npr.org/sections/health-shots/2020/05/28/863526524/covid-19-has-killed-close-to-300-u-s-health-care-workers-new-data-from-cdc-shows.

Tang, C. S. 'Domestic Manufacturing Is Critical to Maintaining Emergency Supplies'. *Barron's*, 10 April 2020. https://www.barrons.com/articles/domestic-manufacturing-coronavirus-supply-chain-emergency-supplies-masks-51586549335.

Tang, C. S. 'The Key to Investing in the Everything Shortage'. *Barron's*, 3 November 2021. https://www.barrons.com/articles/the-key-to-investing-in-the-everything-shortage-51635951797.

Wells, C., M. Fitzpatrick, P. Sah, A. Shoukat, A. Pandey, and A. El-Sayed. 'Projecting the Demand for Ventilators at the Peak of the COVID-19 Outbreak in the USA'. *Lancet*, 20 April 2020. https://doi.org/10.1016/S1473-3099(20)30315-7.

World Health Organization. 'Preferred Product Characteristics for Personal Protective Equipment for the Health Worker on the Frontline Responding to Viral Hemorrhagic Fevers in Tropical Climates'. 2018. https://apps.who.int/iris/handle/10665/272691.

Chapter 9

Arbuthnott, George, and Jonathan Calvert. *Failure of State: The Inside Story of Britain's Battle with Coronavirus*. London: HarperCollins, 2022.

Ashton, John. *Blinded by Corona: How the Pandemic Ruined Britain's Health and Wealth and What to Do about It*. London: Gibson Square, 2020.

Baldwin, Peter. Fighting *The First Wave: Why the Coronavirus Was Tackled So Differently across the Globe*. Cambridge: Cambridge University Press, 2021.

Farrar, Jeremy, and Anjana Ahuja. *Spike: The Virus vs. The People—the Inside Story*. London: Profile Books, 2021.

Gottlieb, Scott. *Uncontrolled Spread: Why Covid-19 Crushed Us and How We Can Defeat the Next Pandemic*. New York: HarperCollins, 2021.

Gupta, Sanjay. *World War C: Lessons from the Covid-19 Pandemic and How to Prepare for the Next One*. New York: Simon & Schuster, 2021.

Horton, Richard. *The Covid-19 Catastrophe: What's Gone Wrong and How to Stop It Happening Again*. Cambridge: Polity Press, 2020.

Kahl, Colin, and Thomas Wright. *Aftershocks: Pandemic Politics and the End of the Old International Order* New York: St Martin's Press, 2021.

Lewis, Michael. *The Premonition: A Pandemic Story*. New York: W. W. Norton & Company, 2021.

Li, Linda Chelan, ed. *Facts and Analysis: Canvassing Covid-19 Responses*. Hong Kong: City University of Hong Kong Press, 2021.

Loh, Christine, ed. *At the Epicentre: Hong Kong and the SARS Outbreak*. Hong Kong: Hong Kong University Press, 2004.

Mackenzie, Debora. *Covid-19: The Pandemic that Never Should Have Happened and How to Stop the Next One*. New York: Hachette Books, 2020.

Markson, Sharri. *What Really Happened in Wuhan: A Virus Like No Other, Countless Infections, Millions of Deaths*. Sydney: HarperCollins, 2021.

Micklethwait, John, and Adrian Wooldridge. *The Wake-Up Call: Why the Pandemic Has Exposed the Weakness of the West, and How to Fix It*. New York: HarperCollins, 2020.

Monroe, Megan. *Notes in Wuhan: Life During Covid-19 Lockdown*. Hong Kong: The Hong Kong Literary Press, 2021.

Slavitt, Andy. *Preventable: The Inside Story of How Leadership Failures, Politics, and Selfishness Doomed the U.S. Coronavirus Response*. New York: St Martin's Press, 2021.

State Council Information Office. 'Fighting -19: China in Action'. 7 June 2020.

Witt, John Fabian. *American Contagions: Epidemic and the Law, from Smallpox to COVID-19*. New Haven, CT: Yale University Press, 2020.

Woodward, Bob. *Rage*. New York: Simon & Schuster, 2020.

Woodward, Bob, and Robert Costa. *Peril*. New York: Simon & Schuster, 2021.

World Health Organization. *Report of the WHO-China Joint Mission on Coronavirus Disease 2019 (Covid-19)*. 16–24 February 2020.

Yang, Guobin. *The Wuhan Lockdown*. New York: Columbia University Press, 2022.

Zhang, Li. *The Origins of COVID-19: China and Global Capitalism*. Stanford, CA: Stanford University Press, 2021.

Zhou, Wang. *The Coronavirus Prevention Handbook: 101 Science-Based Tips That Could Save Your Life*. New York: Skyhorse Publishing, 2020.